Children and Exercis

Children and Exercise XXVII presents the latest scientific research into paediatric sport and exercise science and medicine including contributions from a wide range of leading international experts and early career researchers. The book begins with chapters devoted to the 5 invited keynote lectures followed by 43 of the peer-reviewed presentations which are arranged into 6 thematic sections addressing:

- exercise physiology
- physical activity and health
- exercise and medicine
- testing and performance
- young athlete and sports participation
- methodology in longitudinal research.

The 48 chapters offer a review of current topics and ongoing research in paediatric sport and exercise science and medicine. The book is therefore a key text for all researchers, lecturers, paediatricians, health professionals and students with an interest in the exercising child in health and disease.

Craig Williams is Associate Professor of Paediatric Exercise Physiology and Co-Director of the Children's Health and Exercise Research Centre at the University of Exeter.

Neil Armstrong is Professor of Paediatric Physiology and Director of the Children's Health and Exercise Research Centre at the University of Exeter. He is also Vice-President and Senior Deputy Vice-Chancellor of the University of Exeter.

Children and Exercise XXVII

The Proceedings of the XXVIIth International Symposium of the European Group of Pediatric Work Physiology, September, 2011.

Edited by

Craig A. Williams and Neil Armstrong

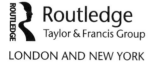

Routledge
Taylor & Francis Group

LONDON AND NEW YORK

First published 2012
by Routledge
2 Park Square, Milton Park, Abingdon, Oxon OX14 4RN

Simultaneously published in the USA and Canada
by Routledge
711 Third Avenue, New York, NY 10017

Routledge is an imprint of the Taylor & Francis Group, an informa business

British Library Cataloguing in Publication Data
A catalogue record for this book is available from the British Library

Library of Congress Cataloging in Publication Data
Pediatric Work Physiology Meeting (27th : 2007 : University of Exeter)
Children and exercise XXVII : the proceedings of the XXVIIth International Symposium of the European Group of Pediatric Work Physiology, September, 2011 / edited by Craig Williams and Neil Armstrong.
p. cm.
1. Exercise for children--Congresses. 2. Children--Physiology--Congresses. 3. Paediatric sports medicine--Congresses. I. Williams, Craig. II. Armstrong, Neil. III. Title. IV. Title: Children and exercise 27. V. Title: Children and exercise twenty-seven.
RJ133.P422 2012
617.1027083--dc23
2011020639

ISBN: 978-0-415-57859-2 (hbk)
ISBN: 970-0-203-85202-6 (ebk)
Typeset in Times New Roman by Craig A. Williams and Neil Armstrong

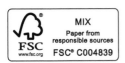

Printed and bound in Great Britain by
CPI Antony Rowe, Chippenham, Wiltshire

Contents

PREFACE

Children and Exercise XXVII contains the Proceedings of the XXVIIth International 'Children and Exercise' Symposium of the European Group of Pediatric Work Physiology (PWP) held in Mawgan Porth, Cornwall, UK. The Symposium was hosted by the Children's Health and Exercise Research Centre, University of Exeter, UK which celebrated its 25th Anniversary during the meeting. Associate Professor Craig Williams chaired the Symposium.

The European Group of Pediatric Work Physiology has organised the following international symposia:

Symposium	Date	Place	Chair
I	1968	Dortmund, Germany	J. Rutenfranz
II	1969	Liblice, Czechoslovakia	V.S. Seliger
III	1970	Stockholm, Sweden	C. Thoren
IV	1972	Netanya, Israel	O. Bar-Or
V	1973	De Haan, Belgium	M. Hebblinck
VI	1974	Sec, Czechoslovakia	M. Macek
VII	1975	Trois Rivieres, Canada	R.J. Shephard
VIII	1976	Bisham Abbey, UK	C.T.M. Davies
IX	1978	Marstand, Sweden	B.O. Eriksson
X	1981	Jousta, Finland	J. Ilmarinen
XI	1983	Papendahl, Netherlands	R.A. Binkhorst
XII	1985	Hardenhausen, Germany	J. Rutenfranz

XIII	1987	Hurdal, Norway	S. Oseid
XIV	1989	Leuven, Belgium	G. Beunen
XV	1989	Seregelyes, Hungary	R. Frenkl
XVI	1991	St Sauves, France	J. Coudert/ E. Van Praagh
XVII	1993	Hamilton, Canada*	O. Bar-Or
XVIII	1995	Odense, Denmark	K. Froberg
XIX	1997	Exeter, UK	N. Armstrong
XX	1999	Rome, Italy	A. Calzolari
XXI	2001	Corsedonk, Belgium	D. Matthys
XXII	2003	Porto, Portugal	J. Maia
XXIII	2005	Gwatt, Switzerland	S. Kriemler/ N. Farpour-Lambert
XXIV	2007	Tallinn, Estonia	T. Jürimäe
XXV	2009	Le Touquet, France	G. Baquet/ S. Berthoin
XXVI	2010	Niagara, Canada*	B. Timmons
XXVII	2011	Mawgan Porth, UK	C.A. Williams

*joint meetings with the North American Society of Pediatric Exercise Medicine

The XXVIIth International Symposium followed PWP tradition with an emphasis on discussion of issues and new research relating to children and exercise. This volume reflects the formal programme and contains the 5 keynote presentations and 43 of the free communications. If it stimulates further interest in the exciting study of the exercising child in both disease and health it will have served its purpose.

ACKNOWLEDGEMENTS

International Scientific Committee

Assoc Prof C.A. Williams, University of Exeter, UK (Chair)
Prof N. Armstrong, University of Exeter, UK
Dr A.R. Barker, University of Exeter, UK
Dr A. Middlebrooke, University of Exeter, UK
Dr R. Winsley, University of Exeter, UK
Dr M. De Ste Croix, University of Gloucestershire, UK
Dr S. Ratel, University of Clermont-Ferrand, France
Prof W. van Mechelen, Free University of Amsterdam, Netherlands
Dr T. Takken, University Medical Center Utrecht, Netherlands
Dr N. Farpour-Lambert, Geneve University Hospital, Switzerland
Assoc Prof K. Froberg, University of Southern Denmark, Denmark
Prof M.J Coelho-e-Silva, University of Coimbra, Portugal
Prof T. Rowland, Baystate Medical Centre, USA
Prof B. Falk, Brock University, Canada

Local Organising Committee

Assoc Prof Craig Williams
Dr Alan Barker
Zoe Saynor
Dr Richard Winsley

Prof Neil Armstrong
Dr Andy Middlebrooke
Owen Tomlinson
Dr Caroline Wragg

Principal Sponsor

The Organising Committee gratefully acknowledges the support of the Healthy Heart Research Trust.

Part I

The Josef Rutenfranz Lecture

THE JOSEF RUTENFRANZ LECTURE

Professor Dr Josef Rutenfranz was the leader of the group of eight scientists who conceived PWP in a café in Berlin in 1967. He organised and chaired the first PWP Symposium in Dortmund in 1968 and remained the unofficial 'Chairman of the Board' until his untimely death, at the age of 60, on 28 February 1989. At PWP XV in Hungary later that year it was decided, in his honour, that each subsequent PWP Symposium should begin with the Josef Rutenfranz Lecture.

The following lists the lecturers and their presentations:

1991	**Per-Olaf Astrand:**	Children and Adolescents: Performance Measurements, Education
1993	**Dan M. Cooper:**	New Horizons in Paediatric Exercise Research
1995	**Oded Bar-Or:**	Safe Exercise for the Child with a Chronic Disease
1997	**Han C.G. Kemper:**	A Scientific Voyage through Research in Children's Health – From Heart via Muscle to Bone
1999	**Frank Galioto:**	The Challenges of the Future; Are We Ready?
2001	**Anna Farkas:**	What About Girls?
2003	**Gaston Beunen:**	Physical Growth, Maturation and Performance: Back to the Future

The 2011 Josef Rutenfranz Lecture

FROM PLAYGROUND TO PODIUM

N. Armstrong

Children's Health and Exercise Research Centre, University of Exeter, UK

1.1 INTRODUCTION

Participation in organized, competitive sport often begins as early as 6-7 years of age and by their teens some young people have experienced several years of intensive training and high-level competition. Initial selection for, and retention in, elite sport takes place within a matrix of biocultural characteristics, which include health status, family size, parental support, socio-economic status, and psychological readiness. However, performance in sport during childhood and adolescence is underpinned by a range of physical, biochemical and physiological factors which operate in a sport-specific manner and are dependent on individual biological clocks. Experimental techniques initially pioneered with adults and new non-invasive technologies have been successfully modified for use with children and adolescents. These developments have opened up new avenues of research into exercise performance during youth but data on elite young athletes are sparse. This paper will briefly reference what we do and don't know in key areas in order to inform and challenge paediatric exercise scientists involved in supporting elite young athletes.

1.2 GROWTH AND MATURATION

Body size, body shape, and body composition are key components of success in chronological age-group sport and most elite young athletes have physiques that favour their sport. There are, however, wide individual variations in the timing of the initiation and the rate of progress through puberty. Puberty is characterized by a growth spurt in stature followed by a spurt in body mass. In most sports elite young athletes have statures that equal or exceed population median values with gymnastics and figure skating the only sports where elite participants are consistently smaller than population median values. The increase in boys' body mass is primarily due to gains in muscle mass and skeletal tissue with fat mass declining from about 16 % to 12-14 % of body mass. Peak muscle growth follows peak mass velocity and over the age range 7-

5

17 years boys' relative muscle mass increases from 42-54 % of body mass. During the growth spurt girls experience a rise in fat mass from about 18-25 % but elite young female athletes are generally leaner than their peers with values as low as 14 % fat recorded for gymnasts. Girls' muscle mass increases from 40-45 % of body mass between 5-13 years but then, in relative terms, declines due to body fat accumulation during adolescence. Boys' muscle strength increases in an almost linear manner from early childhood until about 13-14 years when there is a marked acceleration through the late teenage period followed by a slower increase into their 20s. Girls experience a less marked but almost linear increase in strength with age with no clear evidence of an adolescent spurt. Superior strength often differentiates the elite young athlete from the less successful performer and provides a significant advantage to earlier-maturing boys in many sports. Sparse data suggest that boys have 8-15 % more type II muscle fibres than girls and during the transition from moderate-to-high intensity exercise younger and/or less mature individuals of both sexes appear to recruit fewer type II fibres than older and/or more mature individuals. This phenomenon probably contributes to the metabolic responses to exercise in relation to sex, age and maturation described later (Armstrong and McManus, 2011; McManus and Armstrong, 2011).

Sex differences in body shape and the effect on performance become marked during adolescence. For example, girls' greater hip breadth is one of the reasons why they tend to throw out their heels when they run, as their thighs have to create a greater angle to bring their knees together. Earlier-maturing boys are generally taller, heavier, have higher mass-to-stature ratios, and broader shoulders than later-maturing boys. In addition to greater body size, earlier-maturing boys enjoy changes in body composition and shape that are advantageous in most sports. Increases in muscle size are reflected by strength increases and even small differences in shoulder breadth can result in large increases in upper trunk muscle. When, for example, greater upper body muscle is combined with the greater leverage of longer arms the advantages in throwing, racquet sports and rowing become readily apparent. The physical and physiological characteristics of earlier-maturing boys at the same chronological age as later-maturing boys enhance performance in most sports, particularly during the age range 13-16 years when participation in elite youth sport is at its peak. Since selection for youth sport is generally based on chronological age, few later-maturing boys are successful during early adolescence, except in sports such as gymnastics. Earlier-maturing girls have advantages in sports that are reliant on body size and strength but their broader hips, relatively shorter legs and greater body fatness are characteristics which can be disadvantageous in some sports. Later-maturing girls present linear physiques, less body fat, relatively longer legs, and lower hip-to-shoulder ratios which are more suitable for success in many sports. Earlier-maturing girls are therefore less dominant than earlier-maturing boys in youth sport (Armstrong and McManus, 2011; McManus and Armstrong, 2011).

1.3 EXERCISE METABOLISM

Sport performances of varying intensities and durations are supported by different energy systems and the relative contribution of these systems is dependent on age and maturation. Direct knowledge of children's adenosine triphosphate (ATP), phosphocreatine (PCr), and glycogen stores is limited to a series of muscle biopsy studies of boys aged 11.6-15.5 years, carried out in the 1970s by Eriksson and colleagues. There are no comparable data on girls. Eriksson observed that resting ATP stores in the quadriceps femoris were invariant with age at around 5 mmol· kg^{-1} wet weight of muscle, and very similar to values others had recorded in adults. Eriksson commented that boys' PCr concentration at rest was similar to that of adults but closer scrutiny of the data reveals an age-dependency with PCr concentrations rising from 14.5 mmol· kg^{-1} wet weight of muscle at age 11 to near adult values of 23.6 mmol· kg^{-1} wet weight in the 15-year-olds. Muscle glycogen concentration at rest averaged 54 mmol·kg^{-1} wet weight of muscle at 11 progressively increasing to 87 mmol·kg^{-1} wet weight at 15 years, which is comparable to values recorded in adults (Eriksson, 1980).

More recent muscle biopsy studies have investigated enzyme activities and have allowed the exploration of the ratio of selected glycolytic/oxidative enzyme activities. Berg and Keul (1988) reported ratios of pyruvate kinase/fumarase to be 3.59, 3.20 and 2.26 for adults, adolescents and children respectively. Haralambie's (1982) data allow a comparison of the activity of the potential rate-limiting enzymes of glycolysis and the tricarboxylic acid cycle, namely phosphofructokinase and isocitrate dehydrogenase respectively. He reported the ratio to be 93 % (and significantly) higher in adults than in adolescents at 1.63 and 0.84 respectively.

Following heavy exercise, Eriksson (1980) observed a decrease in glycogen at all ages but the decrease was three times greater in the oldest compared to the youngest boys. In contrast, during exercise below the lactate threshold data from work using ^{13}C stable isotopes and respiratory exchange ratio values have consistently supported a higher free fatty acid substrate contribution in children than in adults (Boisseau and Delmarche, 2000; Timmons et al., 2003). It has been suggested that the development of an adult substrate utilization profile occurs sometime in the transition between mid- and late-puberty and is complete on reaching full maturity (Stephens et al., 2006).

The weight of evidence therefore indicates that in terms of substrate utilization, enzyme activity and high energy phosphate stores children are disadvantaged, compared to adolescents who are, in turn, disadvantaged compared to adults, in sports involving short-duration, high-intensity events. Young people, however, appear well-equipped for performance in long duration, low-to-moderate-intensity sporting activities.

1.4 SHORT-TERM MAXIMAL INTENSITY EXERCISE

The ability to perform short-term maximal intensity exercise is fundamental to virtually all sports but the difficulty of measuring physiological variables under these conditions has limited understanding of the mechanisms underpinning performance in relation to sex, age and maturation. Research has focused on the assessment of external power output and the Wingate anaerobic test (WAnT), which allows the determination of cycling peak power (CPP) usually over a 1 s, 3 s or 5 s interval and cycling mean power (CMP) over the 30 s test period, has emerged as the most popular test of young people's maximal intensity exercise. Cross-sectional data show that in both sexes, there is an almost linear increase in CPP from age 7 until about age 13 years when, in boys but not girls, a second and steeper linear increase in CPP through to young adulthood is observed (van Praagh, 2000). Longitudinal data have emphasized the sex difference in power output in relation to age and maturation by showing 12-year-old boys and girls, respectively, to generate 45 % and 60 % of the CPP and 47 % and 63 % of the CMP they achieved at 17 years. In the same longitudinal study, Armstrong *et al.* (2001) observed that, over the age range 12-17 years, CPP and CMP increased by 121 % and 113 % in boys and 66 % and 60 % in girls whereas increases in peak oxygen uptake (peak VO$_2$) were somewhat less at 70 % and 50 % for boys and girls respectively. These data indicate that there are age- and sex-related changes in predominantly anaerobic and predominantly aerobic performance which are not synchronous and suggest that during adolescence both sexes experience a more marked increase in the ability to perform anaerobically than aerobically. However, metabolic profiles founded on CPP and peak VO$_2$ tests are the sum of numerous factors and do not provide the granulation of data required to tease out the subtle age- and maturation-related changes in exercise metabolism which support sport performance.

1.5 INCREMENTAL EXERCISE TO EXHAUSTION

Magnetic resonance spectroscopy using the phosphorus nucleus (^{31}P MRS) is able to interrogate the muscle and monitor the molecules which play a central role in exercise metabolism, namely ATP, PCr, and inorganic phosphate (Pi), in real time. Exercise within a magnetic bore is challenging for young people but recent studies have provided new insights into developmental muscle metabolism. During exercise Pi increases with a corresponding decline in PCr and the expression of muscle Pi/PCr against power output provides an index of mitochondrial function. The chemical shift of the Pi spectral peak relative to the PCr peak reflects the acidification of the muscle and allows the determination of the intracellular pH which gives an indication of muscle glycolytic activity. Incremental exercise results in non-linear changes in the ratio Pi/PCr plotted against power output and in pH plotted against power output. In both cases as power output increases, an initial shallow slope is followed by a second steeper slope and the transition point is known as the intracellular threshold (IT). Exercise below the Pi/PCr or pH IT which, in children, occurs at ~ 60 % of peak power output, is termed moderate-intensity exercise and above the Pi/PCr or pH IT high-intensity exercise (Barker and Armstrong, 2010).

During incremental quadriceps exercise to exhaustion with 9-12-year-olds and adults, Barker *et al.* (2010) normalized power output to quadriceps muscle mass and observed that the power output and the energetic state at the ITs were independent of age. However, during exercise above the ITs age-related differences in the muscle phosphates and pH were apparent with adult men and women exhibiting a greater anaerobic contribution to exercise metabolism than boys and girls. Maturational effects on metabolism were not demonstrated in boys but the earlier-maturing girls were showed to display pH dynamics akin to those of adult women. More research, perhaps addressing incremental muscle fibre type recruitment, is required to substantiate these findings but they do indicate that the metabolism supporting exercise performance above the Pi/PCr and pH ITs is age and maturation dependent.

1.6 PEAK OXYGEN UPTAKE

Peak VO_2, the highest VO_2 elicited during an exercise test to exhaustion, is recognized as the best single criterion of young people's aerobic fitness. The peak VO_2 of children and adolescents has been well-documented, secure data are available on young people from 8-18 years and they are remarkably consistent. Cross-sectional data show a progressive increase in boys' peak VO_2 ($L \cdot min^{-1}$) with age, and girls demonstrate a similar but less consistent trend with a tendency to level-off from about 14 years of age. Longitudinal studies of aerobic fitness provide a more informative analysis of peak VO_2 but few studies have coupled rigorous determination of physiological variables with substantial sample sizes. Nevertheless, boys' data are consistent and show a >120 % increase in peak VO_2 from 8-16 years, with some studies showing the largest annual increases occurring between 13 and 15 years. It has been suggested that the greatest annual increase in boys' aerobic fitness accompanies the attainment of peak height velocity (PHV) but other studies have observed a consistent growth in peak VO_2 from 3 years before to 2 years after PHV. Girls' data are equivocal but, in general, peak VO_2 appears to rise from 8-13 years and then level-off from about 14 years.

The increase in peak VO_2 with age reflects the increase in body size during the transition from childhood into young adulthood. When peak VO_2 is expressed in ratio with body mass ($mL \cdot kg^{-1} \cdot min^{-1}$) a different picture emerges from that apparent when absolute values ($L \cdot min^{-1}$) are used. Boys' mass-related peak VO_2 remains essentially unchanged at $\sim$ 48-50 $mL \cdot kg^{-1}.min^{-1}$ from 8-18 years, whilst girls' values decline from $\sim$ 45-35 $mL \cdot kg^{-1} \cdot min^{-1}$ over the same time period. Boys demonstrate higher mass-related peak VO_2 than girls throughout childhood and adolescence with the sex difference being reinforced by girls' greater accumulation of body fat during puberty. Although mass-related peak VO_2 remains an important measure in relation to sports which require the movement of body mass, the use of this ratio standard has clouded physiological understanding of aerobic fitness during growth. Rather than removing the influence of body mass, ratio scaling 'overscales' thereby favoring light children and penalizing heavy children. When appropriately analysed the data show that, in conflict with the conventional interpretation (using ratio scaling), there is a progressive rise in peak VO_2 in both sexes independent of body size. With body size appropriately controlled boys' peak VO_2 is higher than that of girls, and sex differences increase during growth.

As young people grow they also mature and the physiological responses of adolescents must be considered in relation to biological as well as chronological age. Early studies using the ratio standard concluded that mass-related peak VO_2 was unrelated to stage of maturation, indicating no additional effect of maturation on aerobic fitness above that due to growth. However, more recent studies using appropriate statistical techniques have demonstrated that although fat-free mass appears to be the predominant influence in the increase of peak VO_2 through adolescence both chronological age and stage of maturation are additional explanatory variables, independent of body mass. This is in accord with observed sport performance. Boys' peak VO_2 values both in absolute terms and adjusted allometrically for differences in body size have been shown to be consistently higher than those of girls by late childhood and the sex difference becomes more pronounced as young people progress through adolescence, reaching $\sim$ 37 % at 16 years of age (Armstrong et al., 2008).

1.7 BLOOD LACTATE ACCUMULATION

Despite its origins in anaerobic metabolism, blood lactate accumulation is a valuable indicator of aerobic fitness and it can be used to monitor improvements in muscle oxidative capacity with training in the absence of changes in peak VO_2. However, although blood lactate accumulation is commonly used to reflect muscle lactate it cannot be assumed to have a consistent quantitative relationship with muscle lactate production. At the onset of moderate exercise, there are minimal changes in blood lactate accumulation but as exercise intensity increases blood lactate increases almost linearly until a point is reached where subsequent blood lactate values rise rapidly until exhaustion. The point at which blood lactate increases non-linearly is referred to as the lactate threshold. The maximal lactate steady state (MLSS) defines the highest exercise intensity which can be maintained without incurring a progressive accumulation of blood lactate and the MLSS represents the highest point where blood lactate diffusion and removal are in equilibrium. Exercise can continue for prolonged periods at, or just below, the MLSS and it provides a sensitive measure of sub-maximal aerobic fitness. Although data on children's blood lactate during exercise are equivocal, a consistent finding is that children accumulate less blood lactate than adults during both maximal and sub-maximal exercise. There is a negative correlation between lactate threshold as a percentage of peak VO_2 and age and, in most studies, the MLSS has been reported to occur at a lower absolute level of blood lactate but at a higher relative exercise intensity in young people than in adults. These findings indicate a higher glycolytic contribution to a similar exercise stress in adults. However, although studies examining specific relationships between maturation and blood lactate indices of aerobic performance are sparse, they have consistently failed to identify an independent maturation effect (Armstrong and Welsman, 2008).

1.8 OXYGEN UPTAKE AND PHOSPHOCREATINE KINETICS

Peak VO_2 underpins maximal aerobic performance but in sporting situations involving rapid changes of pace it is the VO_2 kinetics of the non-steady state [which, in children, and adolescents are unrelated to peak VO_2] which best assess the integrated responses of the oxygen delivery system and the metabolic requirements of the exercising muscle. During exercise below the lactate threshold the VO_2 kinetic response to a step change in exercise intensity is significantly faster in children compared with adults, resulting in a smaller absolute and relative oxygen deficit. Children's faster increase in VO_2 to a new steady state and therefore lower contribution to ATP re-synthesis from anaerobic sources during the non-steady state reflects a more efficient oxygen delivery system, enhanced oxygen utilization or both compared to adults. During heavy exercise [i.e. above the lactate threshold but below the MLSS] children have a shorter time constant than adults and boys have a faster response time than girls. This response suggests a developmental influence on the mitochondrial oxygen utilization potential that supports enhanced oxidative function during childhood (Fawkner and Armstrong, 2003, 2004).

Barker *et al.* (2008a) have demonstrated that children's PCr kinetics during prone quadriceps exercise and VO_2 kinetics during upright cycle ergometer exercise are similar, at least during moderate-intensity exercise. To date only two published ^{31}P MRS studies have examined age-related differences in PCr kinetics during exercise. During step changes at the onset of exercise both below and above the Pi/PCr IT no significant age- or sex-related differences in PCr kinetics were detected (Barker et al., 2008b, Willcocks et al., 2010). In conflict with data from VO_2 kinetic studies, these data suggest that skeletal muscle metabolism is not related to age. However, it is worth noting that during the transition to heavy exercise a 42 % difference in PCr time constants was reported between boys and men which while not statistically different infers possible biological significance. Furthermore, unpublished data from our laboratory indicate that boys have significantly faster PCr time constants than men in response to the onset of very high-intensity exercise (Willcocks et al., unpublished). More research using breath-by-breath respiratory gas analysis and ^{31}P MRS is required to gain further insights into developmental muscle metabolism (Armstrong and Barker, 2009; Barker and Armstrong, 2010).

1.9 ENDURANCE TRAINING

Cross-sectional studies have reported that trained young athletes of both sexes have higher peak VO_2 than their untrained peers and focused studies have observed higher peak VO_2 than untrained youth in cyclists, swimmers, runners, cross-country skiers and canoeists. Elite young male athletes tend to have higher peak VO_2 than their female peers and, although this is probably due to the sex differences described earlier, variations in training volume cannot be ruled out. The precise mechanisms are still to be elucidated but training-induced increases in peak VO_2 appear to be primarily a function of enhanced oxygen delivery to the muscles through an increased maximal stroke volume.

In adults, training results in a faster VO_2 response time but no prospective data are available on young people. Nevertheless, research comparing trained female swimmers with untrained girls and Premier League Academy footballers with untrained boys has demonstrated faster response times in the young athletes. The mechanism underpinning the improvement in VO_2 kinetics is likely to be enhanced oxygen utilization in the muscles.

Data consistently demonstrate that trained young athletes accumulate less lactate in the blood than untrained youth at the same relative sub-maximal exercise intensity [i.e. their lactate threshold occurs at a higher % of peak VO_2]. The primary mechanism underlying a reduction in blood lactate accumulation following training appears to be an increase in oxidative capacity.

Peak VO_2 is the only component of aerobic fitness on which there are sufficient rigorously determined data to estimate a dose-response relationship with endurance training. The balance of evidence indicates that with an appropriate training programme there are no age, maturation or sex differences in responses. There is a small but significant inverse relationship between baseline (pre-training) peak VO_2 and training-induced percentage changes in peak VO_2. Little is known about the influence of genetics on responsiveness to training in youth but it has been estimated that almost half the change in peak VO_2 with exercise training is related to heredity. All aspects of a training prescription are important but exercise intensity is crucial. Based on the evidence of rigorously designed and executed studies, an appropriate training programme to improve the peak VO_2 of children and adolescents by about 7-8 % should include a mixture of interval and continuous exercise using large muscle groups, for a minimum of 12 weeks, four times per week, with the intensity of the sessions in the range 85-90 % of maximal heart rate. With elite young swimmers an endurance training programme has been reported to increase peak VO_2 by 29 % over a 52 week period (Armstrong and Barker, 2011).

1.10 HIGH-INTENSITY AND RESISTANCE TRAINING

Resistance and high-intensity training are safe and effective methods of developing young people's muscle strength and power output provided that exercises are carried out under appropriate supervision. Despite early studies suggesting the contrary it is now well-established that with appropriate resistance training pre-pubertal children are capable of similar relative strength gains to adolescents and adults, although they usually present smaller absolute strength gains. Potential mechanisms underlying strength gains from resistance training include muscle hypertrophy, neural drive, and motor unit synchronization but the relative contribution of these factors varies with age, sex and maturation as well as the volume of training. The balance of evidence suggests that pre-pubertal children display less muscle hypertrophy but show greater neurological adaptations than adolescents following resistance training. Overall, muscle strength gains of 10-40 % are generally observed in children and adolescents following a relatively short-term (< 20 weeks) resistance training programme.

Data on the effects of high-intensity exercise training on power output are sparse and evidence-based, optimal training programmes for children and adolescents are not currently available. Nevertheless, sparse data indicate that high-intensity exercise programmes are effective in increasing the power output of both children and adolescents with gains ranging from 5-12 % reported (Ratel, 2011).

1.11 CONCLUSION

Performance in sport during childhood and adolescence is dependent on a range of physical and physiological variables which are age-, maturation- and sex-related. Earlier-maturing boys are generally taller, heavier, and more muscular than boys of the same chronological age who mature later. Earlier-maturing boys also benefit from changes in body shape which are advantageous in many sports. In some sports earlier-maturing girls benefit from enhanced size and muscle strength compared to similar aged later-maturing girls but in other sports the body shape and size of later-maturing girls is advantageous. Increases in muscle strength and power are expressed in both sexes during adolescence but the changes are much more marked in boys. The muscle enzyme profile needed to promote the anaerobic generation of energy is enhanced as boys and girls move through adolescence into young adulthood. Aerobic performance benefits from age- and maturation-related increases in peak VO_2 which are more marked in boys. Children and adolescents of both sexes improve performance with training and there is no evidence to suggest that endurance, high-intensity or resistance training adversely affect growth and maturation. Evidence-based, optimal training programmes for elite athletes during growth and maturation are not currently available.

Further research is necessary to tease out the physiological factors determining elite sport performance during youth. The development of techniques and technologies, such as ^{31}P MRS and breath-by-breath respiratory gas kinetics, has unleashed the potential to provide new insights into the mechanisms underlying performance but few studies have included elite young athletes.

Many young people achieve success in youth sport but other talented children are denied access to elite age-grouped sport through selection policies which are influenced by factors related to growth and maturation. Other youngsters drop-out prematurely through ill-advised early specialization in sports which turn out to be inappropriate for their late-adolescent physiology or physique. Coaches and scientists who work with young people should be aware of and alert to the effects of sex, age, growth, maturation and exercise training on sports performance. A successful journey from school playground to Olympic podium has many stops and starts and twists and turns but it is ultimately dependent on fostering participation in sport for all, indentifying talent, and nurturing it irrespective of the ticking of individual biological clocks.

1.12 REFERENCES

Armstrong, N. and Barker, A.R., 2009, Oxygen uptake kinetics in children and adolescents: A review. *Pediatric Exercise Science*, **21**, pp. 130-147.

Armstrong, N. and Barker, A.R., 2011, Endurance training and elite young athletes. *The Elite Young Athlete*, edited by Armstrong, N. and McManus, A.M. (Basel: Karger), pp. 59-83.

Armstrong N. and McManus A.M, 2011, The physiology of elite young male athletes. *The Elite Young Athlete*, edited by Armstrong, N. and McManus, A.M. (Basel: Karger), pp. 1-22.

Armstrong, N., McManus A.M. and Welsman, J.R., 2008, Aerobic fitness. *Paediatric Exercise Science and Medicine*, edited by Armstrong, N. and van Mechelen, W. (Oxford: Oxford University Press), pp. 269-282.

Armstrong, N. and Welsman, J.R., 2008, Aerobic fitness. In *Paediatric Exercise Science and Medicine*, edited by Armstrong, N. and Van Mechelen, W. (Oxford: Oxford University Press), pp. 97-108.

Armstrong, N., Welsman, J.R. and Chia, M., 2001, Short-term power output in relation to growth and maturation. *British Journal of Sports Medicine*, **35**, pp. 118-125.

Barker, A.R. and Armstrong, N., 2010, Insights into developmental muscle metabolism through the use of ^{31}P-magnetic resonance spectroscopy: A review. *Pediatric Exercise Science*, **22**, pp. 350-368.

Barker, A.R., Welsman, J.R., Fulford, J., Welford, D. and Armstrong, N., 2008a, Muscle phosphocreatine and pulmonary oxygen uptake kinetics in children and adults at the onset of moderate intensity exercise. *European Journal of Applied Physiology*, **102**, pp. 727-738.

Barker, A.R., Welsman, J.R., Fulford, J., Welford, D. and Armstrong, N., 2008b, Muscle phosphocreatine kinetics in children and adults at the onset and offset of moderate-intensity exercise. *Journal of Applied Physiology*, **105**, pp. 446-456.

Barker, A.R., Welsman, J.R., Fulford, J., Welford, D. and Armstrong, N., 2010, Quadriceps muscle energetics during incremental exercise in children and adults. *Medicine and Science in Sports and Exercise*, **42**, pp. 1303-1313.

Berg, A. and Keul, J., 1988, Biochemical changes during exercise in children. In *Young Athletes*, edited by Malina, R.M. (Champaign, IL: Human Kinetics), pp. 61-78.

Boisseau, N. and Delmarche, P., 2000, Metabolic and hormonal responses to exercise in children and adolescents. *Sports Medicine*, **30**, pp. 405-422.

Eriksson, B.O., 1980, Muscle metabolism in children. A review. *Acta Physiologica Scandinavica*, **283**, pp. 20-28.

Fawkner, S.G. and Armstrong, N., 2003, Oxygen uptake kinetic response to exercise in children, *Sports Medicine*, **33**, pp. 651-669.

Fawkner, S.G. and Armstrong, N., 2004, Longitudinal changes in the kinetic response to heavy intensity exercise, *Journal of Applied Physiology*, **97**, pp. 460-466.

Haralambie, G., 1982, Enzyme activities in skeletal muscle of 13-15-year-old adolescents. *Bulletin of European Physiopathology and Respiration*, **18**, pp. 65-74.

McManus, A.M. and Armstrong, N., 2011, The physiology of elite young female athletes. In *The Elite Young Athlete*, edited by Armstrong, N. and McManus, A.M. (Basel: Karger), pp. 23-46.

Ratel, S., 2011, High intensity and resistance training in elite young athletes. In *The Elite Young Athlete*, edited by Armstrong, N. and McManus, A.M. (Basel: Karger), pp. 84-96.

Stephens, B.R., Cole, A.S. and Mahon, A.D., 2006, The influence of biological maturation on fat and carbohydrate metabolism during exercise in males. *International Journal of Sports Medicine*, **16**, pp. 166-179.

Timmons, B.W., Bar-Or, O. and Riddell, M.C., 2003, Oxidation rate of exogenous carbohydrate during exercise is higher in boys than men. *Journal of Applied Physiology*, **94**, pp. 278-284.

van Praagh, E., 2000, Development of anaerobic function during childhood and adolescence. *Pediatric Exercise Science*, **12**, pp. 150-173.

Willcocks, R.J., Williams, C.A., Barker, A.R., Fulford, J. and Armstrong, N., 2010, Age-and sex-related differences in muscle phosphocreatine and oxygenation kinetics during high-intensity exercise in adolescents and adults. *Nuclear Magnetic Resonance in Biomedicine*, **23**, pp. 569-577.

Part II

Keynote Lectures

EVIDENCE-BASED PHYSICAL ACTIVITY INTERVENTIONS IN CHILDREN

A.S. Singh, E.A.L.M. Verhagen,
M.J.M. Chinapaw, and W. van Mechelen
VU University Medical Center, Amsterdam

2.1 INTRODUCTION

The current generation of children is more overweight and obese than any other generation before. For instance, according to US CDC, '*Childhood obesity has more than tripled in the past 30 years. The prevalence of obesity among children aged 6 to 11 years increased from 6.5 % in 1980 to 19.6 % in 2008. The prevalence of obesity among adolescents aged 12 to 19 years increased from 5.0 % to 18.1 %*' (http://www.cdc.gov/healthyyouth/obesity/). At a meeting in Washington DC (July 2009) Michelle Obama stated to the 'Weight of the Nation' meeting, '*The trend is alarming. For the first time our youngest generation is predicted to live a shorter life span than their parents because of the growth in childhood obesity and its related diseases.*' Was this news? No, in 2005 Olshansky *et al.* had stated in the NEJM, '*Unless effective population-level interventions to reduce obesity are developed, the steady rise in life expectancy observed in the modern era may soon come to an end and the youth of today may, on average, live less healthy and possibly even shorter lives than their parents.*' Also in Europe we are faced with high rates of childhood overweight and obesity. In 2003 Lobstein and Frelut published results from a pan-European study showing prevalence rates for overweight in 7-11 year olds to vary from 10-34 % depending on country, whereas for 14-17 year olds the prevalence varied from 9-22 % (Lobstein and Frelut, 2003). A recent 2010 OECD report showed that now 'Across most EU countries, one in seven 11-15 year old children are overweight or obese' (OECD, 2010). From our own research we know that the increase in overweight and obesity rates in adults is not linear, but exponential (Nooyens *et al.*, 2009). It is not farfetched that the same holds true for children.

The consequences of the exponential increase in overweight and obesity in children are enormous, both for the individual, as well as for society. Obese children will become obese adults (Singh *et al.*, 2008), who will have a higher prevalence of associated morbidity compared to non-obese, which also has great economic consequences for society. In the Netherlands for instance, for the adult population the direct, medical cost associated with obesity was calculated at Euro 500 million, whereas the indirect cost due to lost productivity was estimated to be 4-fold, i.e. 2 billion Euros (RVZ, 2002). From other studies we know that there is an inverse relationship between obesity and long spells (> 7 days) of sickness leave from work (van Duijvenbode *et al.*, 2009). Needless to say the stakes are high for effective prevention of overweight and obesity already starting at an early age.

The root cause of the overweight and obesity problem is related to energy balance, or rather energy imbalance: i.e. too much food intake, too much sitting, or too little daily physical activity (PA), or all three. Because this chapter relates to evidence-based PA interventions, the food intake issue will not be further addressed. Furthermore, there are some indications that over time total energy intake has dropped, suggesting the overweight and obesity epidemic to be primarily a lack-of-energy-expenditure problem, i.e. too much sitting and low levels of daily PA (GCTV, 2002). If it comes to levels of daily PA of European children, there is also reason for concern. The above mentioned OECD report stated on the basis of a 2005-2006 comparative survey that 'Only one in five children in EU countries undertake moderate-to-vigorous exercise regularly', where regular moderate-to-vigorous exercise was defined as 'exercising for a total of at least 60 minutes per day over the past week'. This means that the vast majority of European kids are not sufficiently active and that there is a need for effective PA interventions in children. Engaging in PA entails a certain injury risk. Therefore at the same time interventions should be developed to prevent PA and sports-related injuries in children.

Like for any other Public Health intervention such interventions should be evidence-based, meaning that they need to be developed systematically, i.e. by applying the Intervention Mapping (IM) method (see below). Evidence-based also means that interventions should be tested first for effectiveness, preferably in a randomised controlled trial, before they can be implemented at a broader scale.

The purpose of this paper is to give a narrative overview on evidence-based PA interventions for children. In a comparable manner attention will be paid to the flip side of the same coin; i.e. interventions aimed at preventing PA and sports-related injuries in children. Also, the IM method will be briefly explained. Finally, one should realise that PA is a behaviour. For policy making it is of importance to provide an answer to the question whether physical inactivity is abnormal behaviour in a normal environment? Or, if we are dealing with normal behaviour in an abnormal environment? This answer has an important bearing on how we address this Public Health problem of physical inactivity and associated overweight and obesity.

2.2 EVIDENCE-BASED PHYSICAL ACTIVITY INTERVENTIONS

Although PA is thought of as an important and modifiable factor that influences young people's health, many young people do not achieve public health guidelines (Cavill *et al.*, 2009). Three recent reviews have dealt with the evidence on the effectiveness of interventions promoting PA among young people.

Van Sluijs *et al.* (2007) reported on the effectiveness of interventions promoting PA in children and adolescents. In this review 57 studies, solely controlled trials of which 33 aimed at children and 24 at adolescents, were included. The majority of the studies described school-based interventions. Significant results of these interventions ranged from an increase of 2.6 minutes during PE-classes to a 42 % increase in participation in regular PA and an increase of 83 minutes per week of moderate-to-vigorous PA. They concluded that among children there is limited evidence for an effect of interventions targeting children with a low socio-economic background. It was also concluded that there is limited evidence for environmental PA interventions among children. Among adolescents, there is strong evidence that multi-component interventions and interventions that involve both school and family or community can increase PA levels.

De Meester *et al.* (2009) reviewed 20 studies on the evidence of PA interventions among European teenagers. Most studies were conducted in school. Although the majority of studies reported positive effects on PA, these effects could not be sustained over a longer period of time. They also concluded that the reported improvements were generally limited to school-related PA, while PA during leisure time was not significantly affected. This finding links to another important conclusion, namely that PA interventions including parental involvement might be better in improving leisure time PA levels among teenagers. They suggested that the promising results of two interventions that involved peers and included links with the wider community should be confirmed by further research.

Dobbins *et al.* (2009) included 26 studies on school-based PA programmes for promoting PA and fitness, focused on both children and adolescents. They concluded that there is good evidence that school-based PA interventions have a beneficial effect on time spent on PA in young people, particularly during school hours. They also concluded that there is no evidence that these interventions are also effective in increasing leisure time PA among young people.

Summarising the above, one can conclude that there is evidence that school-based interventions aimed at children and adolescents can be effective in increasing PA levels. These findings are however, mostly limited to improvements of PA levels in the school setting. Another limitation is that the majority of studies do not provide evidence on the sustainability of these effects. A clear message is that interventions in the school setting provide promising results and a good starting point. However, involvement of the social environment of children and adolescents is a promising component for future interventions aimed at increasing PA levels in young people.

2.3 EVIDENCE-BASED PHYSICAL ACTIVITY INJURY PREVENTION INTERVENTIONS

Although the health benefits of a physically active lifestyle outweigh the negative consequences in terms of injury, there is a flip side that should not be neglected. With the current focus on a physically active lifestyle, an increasing number of sports and PA related injuries can be expected (Parkkari *et al.*, 2001). Moreover, recent evidence suggests that inactive children are at increased risk for injury when they engage in PA and sports (Verhagen *et al.*, 2009; Collard *et al.*, 2010). As a consequence sports and PA related injuries are an issue when our efforts towards increasing PA levels in children succeed. This makes prevention of injuries a vital component of PA interventions. Successful prevention of injuries will minimise negative experiences with PA and sports (and thus reduce potential drop-out), will reduce the absolute number of injuries, and will prevent injury recurrence risk and prolonged periods of impairment.

The above statement may sound very dramatic, but a recent prospective study in 10-12 year old Dutch children showed that in a single school year 1 out of 10 children suffered an injury due to either sports, physical education (PE) or leisure time PA (Verhagen *et al.*, 2009). Although injury incidence density was lowest during leisure time activities (0.39/1,000 h; 95 % CI 0.28 - 0.50), due to the overall high exposure about half of all registered injuries occurred during such free play activities. In young children it may be those activities one wants to promote in order to increase their PA levels and health status. However, the injury risk entailed by participation in sports or PE should also not be neglected.

Preventive measures must be based upon proven risk factors and aetiological causes of injury. However, the information about the aetiology of sports and PA related injuries in children is very limited. Nevertheless a great number of measures to prevent injuries have been suggested. With respect to acute sports injuries Smith *et al.* (1993) suggested the application of warm-up, the enhancement of compliance with (safety) rules, the improvement of adult knowledge about game rules (adults oversee paediatric sports participation), equipment and healthy sports behaviour, and the qualification of coaches and trainers. In addition, modification of the rules according to the physique of athletes, avoidance of excessive pressure from parents on winning, use and maintenance of certified safety equipment, and the supervision of all competitive sports are advocated preventive measures. Regarding prevention of overuse injuries, a reduction of training intensity (especially during periods of rapid growth) has been suggested (Baxter-Jones *et al.*, 1993). Other suggested measures include the use of padded protective devices (Meyers 1993), matching children according to age, maturity, skill, weight, and height and supervision of all competitive sports (Smith *et al.*, 1993). Furthermore, the 10 % rule is advised, i.e. in consecutive weeks the increase in training time, distance covered or number of repetitions performed should not exceed 10 % (see Smith *et al.*, 1993).

Although the preventive measures mentioned above seem logical and plausible, the 'true' effects of many of these measures remain to be established in the paediatric sports setting. Nevertheless, despite this lack of aetiological information and lack of proven preventive measures, there is one crucial factor that has an important role in the prevention of sports and PA injuries in children. Behaviour plays a very important role in the aetiology of injury. However, risky behaviour concerns not only the active child, but also all persons involved in the child's activities (e.g. other children, parents, coaches, physical therapists etc.). A young child is growing, learning and developing his or her skills. During this process the youngest children (6-12 years) 'evolve' from participants in joyful play to participants in competitive sports. Everything these children learn in this phase about preventive measures, listening to their own body, safe play, and fair play, will reflect in sports and PA participation at later ages. Especially during childhood, copying the behaviour and techniques of professional role models (who are at the other side of the sports spectrum), may lead to risky situations in team sports where there are great differences between children in body size, skill level, strength, etc. Coaches and parents should remember that their 'pupils' are not miniature Olympic athletes and should emphasise joyful and safe play.

Although the behavioural role has only been recognised in the sports injury area fairly recently, there has long been recognition of the importance of the need to address behavioural factors by general injury researchers (see Trifiletti *et al.*, 2005). In an attempt to reduce the risks associated with physical activities and sports we should learn from expertise that is available from other injury prevention settings. After all, the same theoretical concepts and principles apply. Regarding the role of behaviour in the prevention of sports and PA related injuries in children only 2 randomised controlled trials in the area sports medicine are available.

Backx (1991) showed that a prevention programme that incorporated behavioural change strategies, improved knowledge about injury prevention in pupils of a secondary school (12-18 years). It also improved attitude regarding sport injury prevention, which was suggested to have a favourable effect on injury incidence. Collard *et al.* (2010) conducted a cluster randomised controlled trial in which they evaluated an injury prevention programme in 2,200 10-12 year old children from 40 primary schools. This intervention programme was developed according to the IM protocol (see section 2.4). The 8-month intervention programme focused on both children and parents and aimed to improve motor fitness, as well as knowledge, attitude, and self-efficacy toward the prevention of PA injuries. A substantial and relevant reduction in injuries was found. The effect was strongest for the children with low levels of PA, which also happened to be the children with the highest injury risk.

Therefore, from a public health perspective this simple behavioural intervention may have serious impact.

2.4   INTERVENTION   MAPPING: THE   DUTCH   OBESITY INTERVENTION IN TEENAGERS – AN EXAMPLE

As has been illustrated above, interventions in the school setting provide promising results and a good starting point. However, the underlying mechanisms of successful PA and sports injury prevention interventions are not yet fully understood since only a few studies have provided sufficient details on the intervention contents and theoretical models they were based on to achieve the behavioural change. Often, more energy is devoted to the evaluation of poorly defined interventions of limited general applicability, than to the appropriate development of these interventions (MRC, 1997). Unless the development of the interventions and the theoretical models on which they are based are sufficiently identified and described more accurately, it will be difficult to conclude which interventions are effective and whether or not they have a solid theoretical basis (Hardeman et al., 2000). It is suggested that carefully tailored, theoretically well-supported interventions are essential for successful behavioural changes.

IM describes a stepwise process, mapping the path from recognition of a health problem to the identification of a solution, e.g. the evaluation of a PA intervention aimed at children. Intervention Mapping (IM) should be regarded as a tool for the planning and development of health promotion interventions in general. The DOiT (Dutch Obesity Intervention in Teenagers) study was developed using the IM protocol (Singh, 2008). Following the IM protocol it was decided to develop a school-based intervention, aimed at the prevention of overweight among adolescents from low SES background. The DOiT-intervention focussed on: 1. reduction of the consumption of sugar-sweetened beverages; 2. reduction of energy intake from snacks; 3. decreasing the levels of sedentary behaviour, and; 4. increasing the levels of PA (i.e. active transport behaviour and sports participation). The DOiT-intervention consisted of an individual classroom-based component (i.e. an educational programme, covering 11 lessons of both biology and PE classes), and an environmental component (i.e. encouraging and supporting changes at the school canteens, as well as offering additional PE classes). The DOiT-intervention lasted one year.

The effectiveness of the DOiT-intervention was evaluated among 1,100 Dutch adolescents, using a RCT design. Eighteen schools were randomly assigned to the intervention condition (DOiT) or the control condition (regular curriculum). Immediately after the end of the school year (8-month follow-up) and 1 year later (20-month follow-up) the girls in the intervention schools showed a significantly smaller increase in sum of skin folds. In boys, increases in waist circumference (8-month follow-up) and triceps, biceps, and subscapular skin fold thickness (at 20-month follow-up) were significantly smaller in the intervention group. Boys and girls in the intervention group consumed 250 mL. less sugar-containing beverages than the control group (8- and 12-month follow-up). At the 20-month follow-up boys in the intervention group reported 25 min. less screen-viewing behaviour (i.e. television viewing and computer use) than the control group. No significant intervention effect was found on consumption of snacks or active transport. It was concluded that the DOiT-intervention showed beneficial effects on measures of body composition and energy balance-related behaviours related to preventing excessive weight gain both in the short and long term (Singh, 2008).

The process evaluation of the DOiT-intervention programme indicated immense difficulties in the recruitment of schools, but the reach among adolescents of participating schools was high. Furthermore, it was found that the classroom intervention was implemented successfully in the trial setting and that a large proportion of the teachers and adolescents rated the DOiT-intervention as positive. Possibly most important, the majority of the teachers planned to implement the DOiT-intervention as they perceived DOiT feasible for prevocational education students. Besides this postive feedback, the process evaluation showed that: 1. teachers preferred the intervention to be spread over 2 school years (instead of 1); 2. that the materials could be better adapted to the specific needs of the target population, i.e. more structure within and across the lessons and; 3. that parents should be more involved in the intervention.

2.5 PROMOTING PHYSICAL ACTIVITY: SELF-REGULATION AND SELF-RESPONSIBILITY OR A NANNY STATE?

When promoting healthy behaviour, including a physically active lifestyle, there are basically two approaches one can take. One approach is to identify those with unfavourable behaviours and to subsequently expose them to a targeted intervention, aimed at the individual. The other approach is to shift the health behaviour of the entire population into the desired direction. This can also be done by interventions targeted at the individual. However, the alternative approach is to intervene at a systems level, in which generic measures are taken affecting the entire population. Such systems measures refer to the physical and socio-economic environment, but also to normative thinking about a healthy lifestyle at a population level.

So far many interventions to get children more active have been targeted mainly at the individual. In principle individualised interventions assume that physical inactivity is 'abnormal behaviour in a normal environment'. If this statement holds true for physical inactivity then surely individuals, including children and their parents, should be able to self-regulate their 'abnormal' physical inactivity behaviour. The alternative line of reasoning is that one is dealing in the case of physical inactivity with 'normal behaviour in an abnormal environment'. If this holds true, then interventions aimed at the individual are bound to fail in the long term and instead the environment needs to be changed.

When looking at the global exponential increase of overweight and obesity one wonders if PA interventions mainly targeted at the individual are doing their job? The answer is clearly 'no'! In a country like the USA where self-regulation and self-responsibility is a leading principle, interventions to drive down overweight and obesity have failed. And also in a country like the Netherlands, where there are relatively speaking lower population levels of overweight and obesity and higher population levels of PA, overweight and obesity creep up exponentially. This points to the need for more Draconic action, along the lines of a systems, and perhaps a 'Nanny State' like, approach to these problems. Such a systems approach can be easiest executed in settings where there is a captive audience, i.e. schools and the workplace. When doing so, one should be aware of the legal and ethical boundaries of such an approach (Mello and Rosenthal, 2008).

2.6. REFERENCES.

Backx, F.J.G., 1991, *Sports injuries and youth. Etiology and prevention* (doctoral thesis. University of Utrecht, the Netherlands).

Bartholomew, L.K., Parcel, G.S., Kok, G., Gottlieb, N.H. and Fernández, M.E., 2011, *Planning Health Promotion Programs; An Intervention Mapping Approach*, 3rd edition. (San Franciso: Jossey-Bass)

Baxter-Jones, A.D.G., Maffulli, N. and Helms, P., 1993, Low injury rates in elite athletes. *Archives of Disease in Childhood*, **68**, pp. 130-132.

Cavill, N., Kahlmeier, S. and Racioppi, F., 2006, Physical activity and health in Europe: Evidence for action, (*WHO Library Cataloguing in Publication Data*).

Collard, D.C.M., Verhagen, E.A.L.M., Chinapaw, M.J.M., Knol, D.L. and van Mechelen, W., 2010, Effectiveness of a school-based physical activity injury prevention program: A cluster randomized controlled trial. *Archives of Pediatrics and Adolescent Medicine*, **164**, pp.145-150.

de Meester, F., van Lenthe, F.J., Spittaels, H., Lien, N. and de Bourdeaudhuij, I., 2009, Interventions for promoting physical activity among European teenagers: A systematic review. *International Journal of Behavioral Nutrition and Physical Activity*, **6**, p. 82.

Dobbins, M., DeCorby, K., Robeson, P., Husson, H. and Tirilis, D., 2009, School-based physical activity programs for promoting physical activity and fitness in children and adolescents aged 6-18. *Cochrane Database of Systematic Reviews*; Issue 1; Art. No.: CD007651.

Gezondheidsraad, Commissie Trends voedselconsumptie, 2002, *Enkele belangrijkeontwikkelingen in de voedselconsumptie.* (Den Haag: Gezondheidsraad, 2002 publicatie nr 2002/12).

Hardeman, W., Griffin, S., Johnston, M., Kinmonth, A.L. and Wareham, N.J., 2000, Interventions to prevent weight gain: A systematic review of psychological models and behaviour change methods. *International Journal of Obesity*, **24**, pp.131-143.

Lobstein, T. and Frelut, M.L., 2003, Prevalence of overweight among children in Europe, *Obesity Reviews*, **4**, pp. 195-200.

Medical Research Council., 1997, *MRC Topic Review.* (London, Medical Research Council. Primary health care).

Mello, M.M. and Rosenthal, M.B., 2008, Wellness programs and lifestyle discrimination – The legal limits. *New England Journal of Medicine*, **359**, pp. 192-199.

Meyers, J.F., 1993, The growing athlete. Sports injuries: Basic principles of prevention and care. *Encyclopaedia of Sports Medicine* Vol. IV, edited by Renstrom, P.O. (Oxford: Blackwell Scientific Publications), pp. 178-193.

Nooyens, A.C., Visscher, T.L., Verschuren, W.M., Schuit, A.J., Boshuizen, H.C., van Mechelen, W. and Seidell, J.C., 2009, Age, period and cohort effects on body weight and body mass index in adults: The Doetinchem Cohort Study. *Public Health Nutrition*, **12**, pp. 862-870.

OECD, 2010, Health at a Glance: Europe 2010 (OECD Publishing, *http://dx.doi.org/10.1787/health_glance-2010-en*).

Olshansky, S.J., Passaro, D.J., Hershow, R.C., Layden, J., Carnes, B.A., Brody, J., Hayflick, L., Butler, R.N., Allison, D.B. and Ludwig, D.S., 2005, A potential decline in life expectancy in the United States in the 21st century. *New England Journal of Medicine*, **352**, pp. 1138-1145.

Parkkari, J., Kujala, U.M. and Kannus, P., 2001, Is it possible to prevent sports injuries? Review of controlled clinical trials and recommendations for future work. *Sports Medicine*, **31**, pp. 985-995.

Raad voor de Gezondheidszorg (RVZ), 2002, Adviesrapport 'Gezondheid en gedrag'. (Zoetermeer: www.rvz.nl, publication no. 02/14).

Singh, A.S., 2008, *Effectiveness of a school-based weight gain prevention programme.* Thesis, (PhD), VU University Amsterdam.

Singh, A.S., Mulder, C., Twisk, J.W., van Mechelen, W. and Chin A. Paw, M.J.M., 2008, Tracking of childhood overweight into adulthood: A systematic review of the literature. *Obesity Reviews*, **9**, pp. 474-488.

Smith, A.D., Andrish, J.T. and Micheli, L.J., 1993, The prevention of sports injuries of children and adolescents. *Medicine and Science in Sports and Exercise*, **25**, pp. 1-7.

Trifiletti, L.B., Gielen, A.C., Sleet, D.A. and Hopkins, K., 2005, Behavioral and social sciences theories and models. Are they used in unintentional injury prevention research? *Health Education Research*, **20**, pp. 298-307.

van Duijvenbode, D.C., Hoozemans, M.J., van Poppel, M.N.M. and Proper K.I., 2009, The relationship between overweight and obesity, and sick leave: A systematic review. *International Journal of Obesity (London)*, **33**, pp. 807-816.

van Sluijs, E.M., McMinn, A.M. and Griffin, S.J., 2007, Effectiveness of interventions to promote physical activity in children and adolescents: Systematic review of controlled trials. *British Medical Journal*, **6,** pp. 335: 703-707.

Verhagen, E.A.L.M., Collard, D.C.M, Chinapaw, M.J.M. and van Mechelen, W., 2009, A prospective cohort study on physical activity and sports-related injuries in 10-12-year-old children. *British Journal of Sports Medicine*, **43**, pp. 1031- 1035.

PHYSICAL ACTIVITY AND EARLY MARKERS OF CARDIOVASCULAR DISEASES IN OBESE CHILDREN

N.J. Farpour-Lambert,
University Hospital of Geneva, Switzerland

3.1 INTRODUCTION

The rising prevalence of childhood obesity represents a major public health crisis, as it is associated with considerable risks to the child's present and future health (Ebbeling *et al.*, 2002). The appearance of pediatric forms of chronic diseases such as hypertension (HTN), early signs of atherosclerosis and glucose intolerance contribute to increased risks in adult life (Srinivasan *et al.*, 2002).

3.1.1 Systemic hypertension

Hypertension is considered as the most important cardiovascular disease (CVD) risk factor worldwide, contributing to one half of the coronary heart disease and approximately two thirds of the cerebrovascular disease burdens (Whitworth, 2003). In children and adolescents, body mass index (BMI) is strongly related to high blood pressure (BP), (Sorof *et al.*, 2002; Paradis *et al.*, 2004) and the prevalence of HTN ranges from 47-62 % in obese pediatric patients (Lurbe *et al.*, 1998; Stabouli *et al.*, 2005; Maggio *et al.*, 2008). Several factors are believed to contribute to increased vascular tone in obese individuals, including activation of the sympathetic nervous system, (Daniels, 1996) insulin resistance, (Kanai, 1990) endothelial and smooth muscle cell dysfunctions (Celermajer, 1992).

3.1.2 Atherosclerosis

Atherosclerosis is a complex multifactorial disease, the earliest stages of which are known to commence in childhood (Berenson *et al.*, 1998). In obese children, impaired function of the endothelial cell has been demonstrated from 6 years of age and this is now considered as the first stage of atherosclerosis that precedes the plaque formation (Aggoun *et al.*, 2005). One of the major pathogenetic mechanisms of atherosclerosis is the recruitment of circulating leucocytes onto the vessel wall and their subsequent migration into the subendothelial space (Price and Loscalzo, 1999). This phenomenon appears to be mediated by cellular adhesion molecules (CAMs), usually expressed on endothelial cells and up regulated in response to pro-inflammatory stimuli. Among the CAMs, the vascular cellular adhesion molecule-1 (VCAM-1), the inter-cellular adhesion molecule-1 (ICAM-1), and E-selectin seem to play a pivotal role in mediating leucocyte transendothelial migration processes (O'Brien *et al.*, 1996).

3.2 ASSESSMENT OF ARTERIAL FUNCTION IN CHILDREN

3.2.1 Arterial wall remodelling

The measurement of carotid artery intima-media thickness (IMT) by high resolution ultrasound is considered as a reasonable tool for CVD risk assessment in asymptomatic individuals at intermediate risk. In adults, the risk of incident coronary heart disease (CHD) events increases in a continuous fashion as carotid IMT increases (Greenland *et al.*, 2010).

In children and adolescents, non-invasive measurements of arterial geometry can be performed with a real time B-mode ultrasound imager using a 10 MHz linear high-resolution vascular probe (Gariepy *et al.*, 1996). Imaging of the intima-media thickness (IMT) is done in the far wall of the right common carotid artery (CCA), 2-3 cm proximal to the bifurcation. Average IMT is calculated as the mean value of a great number of local IMT measurements performed every 100 µm along at least 1 cm of longitudinal length of the CCA.

3.2.2 Arterial function

In a clinical setting, the structure and function of large arteries can be assessed by non-invasive high resolution ultrasound. The measure of the peripheral arterial flow-mediated dilation (FMD) is a reliable tool to study the extent of endothelial dysfunction. In fact, the dilatation response with increased blood flow is mainly mediated by nitric oxide released from the arterial endothelial cells, and endothelial dysfunction is considered as an early marker of atherosclerosis (Aggoun *et al.*, 2005). In adults, FMD is related to coronary artery disease, stroke and cardiovascular mortality later in life (Shechter *et al.*, 2009). However, FMD measure is not used in routine for cardiovascular risk assessment of asymptomatic individuals, because the technique requires a highly skilled sonographer, standardized measurement conditions and must therefore be performed in specialized cardiology centres (Greenland *et al.,* 2010).

In children and adolescents, non-invasive assessment of endothelium-dependent dilation (FMD) of the right brachial artery (RBA) can be performed from approximately 6 years of age (Aggoun *et al.,* 2005). A scan of the RBA is obtained in longitudinal section between 5-10 cm above the elbow by using a 10 MHz linear array transducer. After baseline measure of the RBA diameter, a pneumatic cuff is placed around the forearm just below the elbow and inflated for 4.5 minutes at 300 mmHg, to induce a reactive hypaeremia. The cuff deflation results in increased flow through the brachial artery, which can be quantified, and stimulates endothelial-dependent FMD. The change in brachial artery diameter is measured 1 minute after the cuff release and FMD is calculated as absolute and percentage maximum increase in vessel size from baseline. In addition, smooth muscle cell function can be assessed by measuring the endothelial-independent dilatation after administration of 150 µg sublingual nitroglycerin.

3.2.3 Arterial stiffness

Arterial stiffness is a consequence of arteriosclerosis, the process of arterial wall thickening, and loss of elasticity that occurs with onset of vascular disease. In research settings, adult studies have shown that arterial stiffness may predict CVD or mortality (Greenland *et al.,* 2010).

In children and adolescents, assessment of arterial stiffness can be performed by determining the pulse wave using applanation tonometry (Aggoun *et al.,* 2005). The probe is applied to the surface of the skin overlying the radial artery and the peripheral radial pulse wave is recorded continuously. The mean values of at least 20 pulse waves are used for analyses. Some systems incorporate the pulse recorded at the radial artery and the properties of the transfer function between the aorta and the radial artery to estimate central aortic pressure non-invasively (Chen *et al.,* 1997). The central pulse pressure (PP) is then used to calculate mechanical indices of the CCA. The cross sectional compliance (CSC) and cross sectional distensibility (CSD) are determined according to following formulas:

$$CSC = \pi \, (Ds^2 - Dd^2)/4 \cdot PP \; (mm^2 \cdot mm \, Hg^{-1})$$
$$CSD = (Ds^2 - Dd^2) \, / \, (Dd^2 \cdot PP) \; (mm \, Hg^{-1} \cdot 10^{-2})$$

when Ds is systolic diameter and Dd is diastolic diameter. These parameters provide information about the elasticity of the artery as a hollow structure. Finally, the incremental elastic modulus is calculated using the following formula:

Einc = $(3 \cdot (1+ \text{LCSA} \cdot \text{WCSA}^{-1})) \cdot \text{CSD}^{-1}$ (mm Hg$\cdot 10^3$)

This parameter provides information on the properties of the wall material, independent of its geometry, where lumen cross sectional area (LCSA, mm^2) is calculated as π (Dd^2)/4, and wall cross sectional area (WCSA, mm^2) is calculated as π (π Dd/2 +IMT)^2 - π (Dd/2)^2.

3.3 IMPAIRMENT OF VASCULAR FUNCTION IN OBESE CHILDREN

Childhood obesity is associated with the premature development of atherosclerosis. Impaired FMD of the brachial artery and increased IMT of the common carotid artery have been demonstrated in children and adolescents (Celermajer *et al.*, 1992; Tounian *et al.*, 2001; Meyer *et al.*, 2006). We previously reported that abnormal FMD appears even before puberty; in association with systemic hypertension, (Aggoun *et al.*, 2008) while increased intima-media thickness (IMT) develops later during adolescence (Tounian *et al.*, 2001). Arterial stiffness may also be increased early in obese children (Aggoun *et al.*, 2008). The appearance of hypertension and first signs of atherosclerosis in young obese children forecasts a major health burden and a need for early intervention strategies in this high risk group.

3.4 EFFECTS OF PHYSICAL ACTIVITY ON CARDIOVASCULAR HEALTH IN OBESE CHILDREN

The benefits of physical activity in the prevention and treatment of cardiovascular diseases have been very well described in adults (Thompson *et al.*, 2003). On the contrary, low cardiorespiratory fitness is associated with a 1.3- and 2.6-fold increased risk for hypertension in lean and overweight young adults, respectively (Carnethon *et al.*, 2003). In children, a recent population-based study demonstrated that higher levels of physical activity were associated with lower BP, and results suggested that the volume was more important than the intensity (Leary *et al.*, 2008).

Obese children spend usually less time in moderate and vigorous physical activities and have lower cardiorespiratory fitness than their non-obese counterparts (Trost *et al.*, 2001). The treatment usually includes physical activity, dietary and behavioural interventions. However, most randomized controlled trials were designed to assess the effects of combined lifestyle changes in obese youth (Woo *et al.*, 2004; Savoye *et al.*, 2007) and only few authors investigated the impact of exercise alone (Ferguson *et al.*, 1999; Gutin *et al.*, 2002; Kang *et al.*, 2002; Watts *et al.*, 2004; Meyer *et al.*, 2006). In obese adolescents, they reported significant changes in body fat or visceral fat, endothelial function, IMT, parasympathetic nervous activity, lipids profile and insulin resistance indices.

In pre-pubertal obese children, we recently demonstrated that regular physical activity reduced systemic BP, arterial stiffness, and intima-media thickening (Farpour-Lambert *et al.*, 2009). Forty-four pre-pubertal obese children with an average age of 8.9 ($\pm$ 1.5) years and 22 lean children (age 8.5 $\pm$ 1.5 years) were recruited. Obese participants were randomly assigned to either an exercise or a control group, with an equal distribution of girls and boys in each group. For the first 3 months, the obese children in the exercise group had three 60-min training sessions per week whereas children in the control group remained relatively inactive. In the second 3-month period, children in both groups exercised twice per week (modified cross-over design). Changes were assessed at 3 and 6 months in BP, arterial IMT and stiffness, endothelial function, BMI, and cardiorespiratory fitness (VO_2 max). Children assigned to the exercise intervention had good compliance (83 %) and adherence (86 %) to the programme. After 3 months, the exercise group showed significant decreases in systemic BP, ranging from -7 to -12 mmHg for systolic BP and from -2 to -7 mmHg for diastolic BP. Additionally, physical activity was associated with reductions in abdominal fat (-4.2 %) and whole body fat (-3.6 %), and significant increases in fat-free mass ($+4.6$ %) and peak VO_2 ($+6$ %). We observed further changes in the obese children after 6 months, with a significant decrease in arterial stiffness as well as stabilization of the arterial IMT. Furthermore, in the exercise group, the proportion of obese children with hypertension decreased from 50 % at baseline to 37 % at 3 months, and to 29 % at 6 months. Surprisingly, the changes in BP that we observed during the 3-month intervention were not associated with improved endothelial or smooth muscle cell functions. A longer programme might be needed to detect changes at very early stages of atherosclerosis.

3.5 CONCLUSION

First signs of cardiovascular diseases appear early in life in obese children. Systemic hypertension and premature impairment of vascular function have been demonstrated in this population, forecasting a major public health burden. Recent studies, including exercise training alone or combined to dietary/behavioural interventions, showed beneficial changes on systemic blood pressure, endothelial function, arterial wall remodelling and stiffness, as well as total body and abdominal fat mass. In our study, only three 60-minutes sessions of moderate physical activity per week resulted in significant clinical cardiovascular changes in pre-pubertal children. Therefore, schools should provide regular physical education lessons at least three times per week, and sessions should be adapted to encourage the participation of obese children.

As cardiovascular diseases track from childhood to adulthood, physical activity should be encouraged in young obese children to prevent the premature development of hypertension and atherosclerosis. Future research should investigate the volume, intensity and duration of physical activity that is needed to improve endothelial function in obese children before puberty.

3.6 REFERENCES

Aggoun, Y., Farpour-Lambert, N.J., Marchand, L.M., Golay, E., Maggio, A.B. and Beghetti, M., 2008, Impaired endothelial and smooth muscle functions and arterial stiffness appear before puberty in obese children and are associated with elevated ambulatory blood pressure, *European Heart Journal*, **29**, pp. 792-799.

Aggoun, Y., Szezepanski, I., and Bonnet, D., 2005, Noninvasive assessment of arterial stiffness and risk of atherosclerotic events in children, *Pediatric Research*, **58**, pp. 173-178.

Berenson, G.S., Srinivasan, S.R. and Nicklas, T.A., 1998, Atherosclerosis: A nutritional disease of childhood. *American Journal of Cardiology*, **82**, pp. 22T-29T.

Carnethon, M.R., Gidding, S.S., Nehgme, R., Sidney, S., Jacobs, D.R. and Liu, K., 2003, Cardiorespiratory fitness in young adulthood and the development of cardiovascular disease risk factors, *Journal of the American Medical Association*, **290**, pp. 3092-3100.

Celermajer, D.S., Sorensen, K.E., Gooch, V.M., Spiegelhalter, D.J., Miller, O.I., Sullivan, I.D., Lloyd, J.K. and Deanfield, J.E., 1992, Non-invasive detection of endothelial dysfunction in children and adults at risk of atherosclerosis, *Lancet*, **340**, pp. 1111-1115.

Chen, C.H., Nevo, E., Fetics, B., Pak, P.H., Yin, F.C., Maughan, W.L. and Kass, D.A., 1997, Estimation of central aortic pressure waveform by mathematical transformation of radial tonometry pressure. Validation of generalized transfer function, *Circulation*, **95**, pp. 1827-1836.

Daniels, S.R., Kimball, T.R., Khoury, P., Witt, S. and Morrison, J.A., 1996, Correlates of the hemodynamic determinants of blood pressure, *Hypertension*, **28**, pp. 37-41.

Ebbeling, C.B., Pawlak, D.B. and Ludwig, D.S., 2002, Childhood obesity: public-health crisis, common sense cure, *Lancet*, **360**, pp. 473-482.

Farpour-Lambert, N.J., Aggoun, Y., Marchand, L.M., Martin, X.E., Herrmann, F.R. and Beghetti, M., 2009, Physical activity reduces systemic blood pressure and improves early markers of atherosclerosis in pre-pubertal obese children, *Journal of the American College of Cardiology*, **54**, pp. 2396-2406.

Ferguson, M.A., Gutin, B., Le, N.A., Karp, W., Litaker, M., Humphries, M., Okuyama, T., Riggs, S. and Owens, S., 1999, Effects of exercise training and its cessation on components of the insulin resistance syndrome in obese children, *International Journal of Obesity and Related Metabolism Disorders*, **23**, pp. 889-895.

Gariepy, J., Simon, A., Massonneau, M., Linhart, A., Segond, P. and Levenson, J., 1996, Echographic assessment of carotid and femoral arterial structure in men with essential hypertension, *American Journal of Hypertension*, **9**, pp. 126-136.

Greenland, P., Alpert, J.S., Beller, G.A., Benjamin, E.J., Budoff, M.J., Fayad, Z.A., Foster, E., Hlatky, M.A., Hodgson, J.M., Kushner, F.G., Lauer, M.S., Shaw, L.J., Smith, S.C., Jr., Taylor, A.J., Weintraub, W.S., Wenger, N.K. and Jacobs, A.K., 2010, ACCF/AHA guideline for assessment of cardiovascular risk in asymptomatic adults: A report of the American College of Cardiology Foundation/American Heart Association Task Force on Practice Guidelines, *Circulation*, **122**, pp. e584-e636.

Gutin, B., Barbeau, P., Owens, S., Lemmon, C.R., Bauman, M., Allison, J., Kang, H.S. and Litaker, M.S., 2002, Effects of exercise intensity on cardiovascular fitness, total body composition, and visceral adiposity of obese adolescents, *American Journal of Clinical Nutrition*, **75**, pp. 818-826.

Kanai, H., Matsuzawa, Y., Tokunaga, K., Keno, Y., Kobatake, T., Fujioka, S., Nakajima, T. and Tarui, S., 1990, Hypertension in obese children: Fasting serum insulin levels are closely correlated with blood pressure, *International Journal of Obesity*, **14**, pp. 1047-1056.

Kang, H.S., Gutin, B., Barbeau, P., Owens, S., Lemmon, C.R., Allison, J., Litaker, M.S. and Le, N.A., 2002, Physical training improves insulin resistance syndrome markers in obese adolescents, *Medicine and Science in Sports and Exercise*, **34**, pp. 1920-1927.

Leary, S.D., Ness, A.R., Smith, G.D., Mattocks, C., Deere, K., Blair, S.N. and Riddoch, C., 2008, Physical activity and blood pressure in childhood: Findings from a population-based study, *Hypertension*, **51**, pp. 92-98.

Lurbe, E., Alvarez, V., Liao, Y., Tacons, J., Cooper, R., Cremades, B., Torro, I. and Redon, J., 1998, The impact of obesity and body fat distribution on ambulatory blood pressure in children and adolescents, *American Journal of Hypertension*, **11**, pp. 418-424.

Maggio, A.B., Aggoun, Y., Marchand, L.M., Martin, X.E., Herrmann, F., Beghetti, M. and Farpour-Lambert, N.J., 2008, Associations among obesity, blood pressure, and left ventricular mass, *Journal of Pediatrics*, **152**, pp. 489-493.

Meyer, A.A., Kundt, G., Lenschow, U., Schuff-Werner, P. and Kienast, W., 2006, Improvement of early vascular changes and cardiovascular risk factors in obese children after a six-month exercise program, *Journal of the American College of Cardiology*, **48**, pp. 1865-1870.

Meyer, A.A., Kundt, G., Steiner, M., Schuff-Werner, P. and Kienast, W., 2006, Impaired flow-mediated vasodilation, carotid artery intima-media thickening, and elevated endothelial plasma markers in obese children: The impact of cardiovascular risk factors, *Pediatrics*, **117**, pp. 1560-1567.

O'Brien, K.D., McDonald, T.O., Chait, A., Allen, M.D. and Alpers, C.E., 1996, Neovascular expression of E-selectin, intercellular adhesion molecule-1, and vascular cell adhesion molecule-1 in human atherosclerosis and their relation to intimal leukocyte content, *Circulation*, **93**, pp. 672-682.

Paradis, G., Lambert, M., O'Loughlin, J., Lavallee, C., Aubin, J., Delvin, E., Levy, E. and Hanley, J.A., 2004, Blood pressure and adiposity in children and adolescents, *Circulation*, **110**, pp. 1832-1838.

Price, D.T. and Loscalzo, J., 1999, Cellular adhesion molecules and atherogenesis, *American Journal of Medicine*, **107**, pp. 85-97.

Savoye, M., Shaw, M., Dziura, J., Tamborlane, W.V., Rose, P., Guandalini, C., Goldberg-Gell, R., Burgert, T.S., Cali, A.M., Weiss, R. and Caprio, S., 2007, Effects of a weight management program on body composition and metabolic parameters in overweight children: A randomized controlled trial, *Journal of the American Medical Association*, **297**, pp. 2697-2704.

Shechter, M., Issachar, A., Marai, I., Koren-Morag, N., Freinark, D., Shahar, Y., Shechter, A. and Feinberg, M.S., 2009, Long-term association of brachial artery flow-mediated vasodilation and cardiovascular events in middle-aged subjects with no apparent heart disease, *International Journal of Cardiology*, **134**, pp.52-58.

Sorof, J. and Daniels, S., 2002, Obesity hypertension in children: A problem of epidemic proportions, *Hypertension*, **40**, pp. 441-447.

Srinivasan, S.R., Myers, L. and Berenson, G.S., 2002, Predictability of childhood adiposity and insulin for developing insulin resistance syndrome (syndrome X) in young adulthood: The Bogalusa Heart Study, *Diabetes*, **51**, pp. 204-209.

Stabouli, S., Kotsis, V., Papamichael, C., Constantopoulos, A. and Zakopoulos, N., 2005, Adolescent obesity is associated with high ambulatory blood pressure and increased carotid intimal-medial thickness, *Journal of Pediatrics*, **147**, pp. 651-656.

Thompson, P.D., Buchner, D., Pina, I.L., Balady, G.J., Williams, M.A., Marcus, B.H., Berra, K., Blair, S.N., Costa, F., Franklin, B., Fletcher, G.F., Gordon, N.F., Pate, R.R., Rodriguez, B.L., Yancey, A.K. and Wenger, N.K., 2003, Exercise and physical activity in the prevention and treatment of atherosclerotic cardiovascular disease: A statement from the Council on Clinical Cardiology (Subcommittee on Exercise, Rehabilitation, and Prevention) and the Council on Nutrition, Physical Activity, and

Metabolism (Subcommittee on Physical Activity), *Circulation*, **107**, pp. 3109-3116.

Tounian, P., Aggoun, Y., Dubern, B., Varille, V., Guy-Grand, B., Sidi, D., Girardet, J.P. and Bonnet, D., 2001, Presence of increased stiffness of the common carotid artery and endothelial dysfunction in severely obese children: A prospective study, *Lancet*, **358**, pp. 1400-1404.

Trost, S.G., Kerr, L.M., Ward, D.S. and Pate, R.R., 2001, Physical activity and determinants of physical activity in obese and non-obese children, *International Journal of Obesity and Related Metabolism Disorders*, **25**, pp. 822-829.

Watts, K., Beye, P., Siafarikas, A., Davis, E.A., Jones, T.W., O'Driscoll, G. and Green, D.J., 2004, Exercise training normalizes vascular dysfunction and improves central adiposity in obese adolescents, *Journal of the American College of Cardiology*, **43**, pp. 1823-1827.

Whitworth, J.A., 2003, World Health Organization (WHO)/International Society of Hypertension (ISH) statement on management of hypertension. *Journal of Hypertension*, **21**, pp. 1983-1992.

Woo, K.S., Chook, P., Yu, C.W., Sung, R.Y., Qiao, M., Leung, S.S., Lam, C.W. Metreweli, C. and Celermajer, D.S., 2004, Overweight in children is associated with arterial endothelial dysfunction and intima-media thickening, *International Journal of Obesity and Related Metabolism Disorders*, **28**, pp. 852-857.

DIFFERENTIAL MOTOR-ACTIVATION PATTERNS: THE MOST COMPREHENSIVE EXPLANATION FOR CHILD-ADULT PERFORMANCE DIFFERENCES

B. Falk[1] and R. Dotan[2]

[1]Dept of Physical Education and Kinesiology, [2]Faculty of Applied Health Sciences, Brock University, St. Catharines, ON, Canada

4.1 BACKGROUND

Children's maximal volitional muscular force, contractile velocity and muscular power are notoriously lower than adults', especially in males (see Blimkie, 1989 for review). Although many of the observed differences can be attributed to differences in body size, these differences persist even when body size is taken into account (Inbar and Bar-Or, 1986; Grosset *et al.*, 2008). Thus, additional factors, such as muscle fibre composition, or differences in muscle activation pattern must be considered to account for these differences.

Higher agonist-antagonist co-contraction in children can also explain some of the observed performance differences. Some studies have indeed reported greater co-activation in children (Grosset *et al.*, 2008), but others have not (Bassa *et al.*, 2005). Notably, age-related co-contraction differences have been observed mostly in submaximal, multi-joint, or dynamic contractions. However, in maximal isometric contractions, co-contraction is minimal and most studies show no age-related differences (Falk *et al.*, 2009a,b). Thus, while agonist-antagonist co-contraction differences may account for some of the observed differences in dynamic contractions, they cannot explain differences in maximal isometric strength.

A lower percentage of type II muscle fibres in children could explain many of the observed child-adult functional differences. Information on muscle composition in healthy children is rather scant and is derived mainly from biopsies of children with various diseases, or from cadavers. Several studies suggest similar muscle fibre composition in children and adults (Brooke and Engel, 1969), but other studies (Lexell *et al.*, 1992) suggest that the percentage of type I muscle fibres in pre-pubertal children may be higher than adults'. On the other hand, in twitch-stimulation studies, contractile characteristics such as contraction time and half-relaxation time have been shown to be similar across age groups (Belanger and McComas, 1989). Such findings support the notion of a similar fibre composition in children and adults.

The discussion below outlines numerous known child-adult differences in muscle function and metabolism. Some age-related differences in performance and metabolism may be explained by structural factors and others by functional factors. Nevertheless, it is argued that only differential motor-unit activation between children and adults can explain all of the mentioned differences.

4.2 HYPOTHESIS

Erling Asmussen observed that the increase in strength during childhood and adolescence is more than can be expected from the increase in body size. He was the first to propose that children do not activate their muscles to the extent typical of adults (Asmussen and Heebøll-Nielsen, 1955). Subsequently, in view of various supporting evidence (see below), this suggestion has been put forth by others.

The above suggestion implies that children's maximal neuromuscular activation is generally lower. That is, children recruit a smaller percentage of their total motor-units. We endorse Asmussen's idea, but extend it to a more specific hypothesis. Namely, child-adult differences in muscle strength and other functional measures are due to children's inability to utilize *higher-threshold (type II) motor units* to the extent typical of adults. Thus, we specifically point to type II motor-unit utilization as being the compromised portion of children's muscle function.

4.3 SUPPORTING EVIDENCE

We are unaware of an appropriate technique to unequivocally validate the above hypothesis. Such validation would require sufficiently large samples of individual motor-units to be monitored for activation, frequency, and timing patterns. Thus, in view of the unavailability of direct evidence, it is necessary to rely on indirect evidence to support or dismiss the differential motor-unit activation hypothesis.

4.3.1 Volitional vs. Non-volitional force production

Using the interpolated-twitch technique or a modification thereof, the difference (or ratio) between volitional and non-volitional, electrically-evoked force is used as an index of the degree of muscle activation, or the percentage of the motor-unit pool recruited during a given volitional contraction. Using such a technique, numerous studies demonstrated lower overall muscle activation in children, using electrical (Belanger and McComas, 1989; Blimkie, 1989; Grosset *et al.,* 2008) or magnetic (O'Brien *et al.,* 2009) stimulation.

According to the size principle, it is the slower, low-threshold (type I) motor units which are recruited first. To increase force output, faster, higher-threshold (type II) motor units are recruited by increasing motor neuron firing frequency. It might be argued, therefore, that lower overall motor-unit activation, as described above, reflects lower activation of high-threshold motor units because these are typically activated last.

4.3.2 EMG-derived evidence

Much of the evidence supporting child-adult differences in muscle activation has been derived using surface EMG. Since signal amplitude is greatly affected by muscle size and subcutaneous adiposity, only rate- or timing-related parameters are examined.

The initial slope of the rectified surface-EMG trace has been thought of as reflecting the initial rate of muscle activation. The Q_{30} index (area under the curve during the first 30 ms) is used as an indicator of the degree of faster, higher-threshold motor-unit activation.

We have recently demonstrated consistently lower Q_{30} values, as well as lower rates of force development, in boys vs. men (Falk *et al.,* 2009b; Cohen *et al.* 2010). This suggests that children have a smaller initial burst of EMG activity, and therefore a lower rate of muscle activation, which appears to be related to their lower rate of force development. Such findings can explain children's compromised explosive power.

The power spectrum density of the EMG signal describes the relative distribution of EMG frequencies. The mean power frequency is the weighted mean of that distribution and, in adults, it has been shown to be affected by fibre-type distribution (Gerdle *et al.,* 1997) and/or the relative utilization of type II motor units (Gabriel *et al.,* 2001).

Halin *et al.* (2003) demonstrated higher mean power frequency during maximal contraction in men compared with boys. The authors suggested that the child-adult difference may be explained by a higher composition or greater utilization of type II motor units in the adults. Moreover, during a 28 s fatigue test, the men demonstrated a much greater decrease (~50 %) in mean power frequency compared with the boys (~16 %), suggesting greater initial recruitment and subsequent drop-off of type-II motor units. A similar age-difference in the decrease in mean power frequency was demonstrated more recently (Armatas *et al.,* 2010).

4.3.3 Contractile and power-related child-adult differences

Differential motor-unit activation ought to have implications that extend beyond maximal force. That is, a lower utilization of type II motor units should be manifested in various parameters of whole-muscle performance.

Lower rate of force development would be expected in children if their fast-twitch (type II) motor units are employed to a lesser extent than in adults. Indeed, children's lower rate of force or torque development in maximal isometric contractions has been repeatedly demonstrated (Asai and Aoki, 1996; Falk *et al.*, 2009a,b; Cohen *et al.*, 2010). This age-difference persists even when the rate of force development is corrected to maximal force. That is, child-adult differences in the rate of force development are independent of both, the absolute and relative muscle mass.

Lower rates of force development may be a reflection of lower musculo-tendinous stiffness in children (Lambertz *et al.*, 2003). The latter is likely to affect the early phase of force development (<50 ms), but not the later phase (~200 ms) (Andersen and Aagaard, 2006). However, we have recently demonstrated that after correcting for maximal torque, boys' torque kinetics were still considerably slower than men's at both the early and late phases of contraction (Dotan *et al.*, 2010).

If children indeed employ type II motor units to a lesser extent (i.e., more type I), they would then be expected to demonstrate greater muscular endurance, or lower muscle fatigability in repeated contractions. Children have been shown to fatigue less during dynamic (Armatas *et al.*, 2010), as well as sustained (isometric) contractions (Halin *et al.*, 2003). These differences in fatigue cannot be explained by differences in muscle size or in maximal strength, since in the above studies, both task and fatigue were defined relative to maximal strength. Although these findings could be explained by a different muscle composition and metabolic profile (see below), they also conform to expectations from a smaller proportion of activated type-II motor units in children's muscles.

Hill's classic force-velocity curve, demonstrates the inverse, curvilinear relationships between contractile force and velocity. Since 1953, this relationship has been repeatedly demonstrated in adults, but only to a very limited extent in children. In a study by Asai and Akoi (1996), both boys and men exhibited the characteristic curvilinear inverse force-velocity relationship. However, at each relative force level, velocity was considerably lower in the boys. The age-related difference was especially apparent at low-force, high-velocity contractions (~40 %) and decreased progressively as force increased and velocity decreased, thus supporting the differential motor-unit utilization hypothesis.

Maximal isometric or low-velocity force production depends on both, slow- and fast-twitch motor-unit recruitment. High-velocity force production or high power production, on the other hand, must heavily depend on the extent of fast-twitch (type II) motor-unit utilization.

Seger and Thorstensson (2000) longitudinally examined low- to high-velocity torque production in children from 11-16 years of age. Among the boys, the age-related increase in torque was larger with increasing contractile velocity. Girls exhibited similar trends, although differences did not reach statistical significance. These findings support the idea that fast-twitch (type II) motor units are being increasingly employed as children, boys in particular, go from pre-pubescence to adolescence.

Children's size-normalized power output in short-term, supra-maximal exercise (e.g., the Wingate Anaerobic Test), is significantly lower than that of adults (Inbar and Bar-Or, 1986), suggesting that there is more than age-related muscle-mass differences that distinguishes children's short-term performance capacity from that of adults. Likewise, while children may show greater agonist-antagonist co-activation in dynamic, multi-joint contractions, the age-related difference in co-contraction does not seem sufficiently large to account for the observed age differences in external power output. It is therefore justified to assert that, at least in part, children's lower motor-unit activation accounts for the observed child-adult differences in short-term power output.

Children have been repeatedly shown to recover considerably faster than adults from maximal or high-intensity, short-term exercise (Falk and Dotan, 2006). In view of children's much lower lactate response to such exercise (see below), their apparent faster recovery may be attributable to lower utilization of type-II, glycolytic motor units, thereby producing less power and lactate and, consequently, having less to recover from (Falk and Dotan, 2006).

Thus, differences in muscle activation pattern may explain not only child-adult differences in maximal strength, but also in other strength-related performance measures, such as the rate of force development, short-term power, recovery from intense exercise, and muscle fatigue during sustained contractions.

4.3.4 Metabolic evidence

Different muscle substrate and enzyme activity levels have been shown in children and adults (Eriksson *et al.*, 1973). The findings depict a pattern of lower anaerobic/glycolytic capacity and greater oxidative capacity in children. Such differences have typically been attributed to lagging maturation of children's glycolytic metabolic pathway (Ratel *et al.*, 2008). That view may be valid and can partly account for observed performance differences. However, we suggest that children's different metabolic profile is not the underlying *cause* of their lower contractile and anaerobic capacity but rather, the *result* of their under-utilization of fast-twitch, glycolytic motor-units. Below are several examples of apparent child-adult metabolic differences previously attributed to children's "metabolic immaturity", particularly of the anaerobic pathways. We suggest these differences to be largely due to differential motor-unit activation pattern.

While child-adult differences in short-term power output support the idea of children's lesser overall muscle activation, differences in the blood lactate responses to such exertions shed light on the issue of differential motor-unit activation pattern. If boys' lower power output is due to generally lower motor-unit recruitment or utilization, then the corresponding percentage difference in the lactate response would be expected to be similar in magnitude to the difference in power output. However, child-adult differences in lactate response are more than twice as large as the corresponding differences in power output (Dotan et al., 2003), strongly suggesting that men rely more heavily on glycolytic, type II motor units.

Blood lactate response is expected to increase with greater involvement of the glycolytic, type II motor units. If adults indeed utilize more type II motor-units than children at moderate and high exercise intensities, then during progressive exercise, men's blood lactate concentrations would be expected to start rising at lower relative work rates than would be expected of children. In other words, lower utilization of type II motor units in children, would result in a delayed onset (i.e., higher lactate threshold), and in lower general response of blood lactate concentrations. Indeed, several studies have shown that, in adults, the blood lactate threshold, or related criteria, occurs at lower percentages of maximal or peak VO_2 then in children (Tanaka and Shindo, 1985). Similarly, using non-invasive nuclear magnetic resonance spectroscopy (^{31}P), Willcocks et al. (2010) found that the intra-cellular Pi/PCr threshold (inorganic phosphate to phosphocreatine ratio) during progressive exercise of the quadriceps occurred at a ~20 % higher relative (body-mass-normalized) power output in boys compared with men.

Faster PCr recovery following intense muscular exercise is regarded as an indication of a more oxidative or less glycolytic metabolic profile, or a greater relative reliance on oxidative, type I motor units. Using magnetic-resonance spectroscopy, several authors (Ratel et al., 2008; Willcocks et al., 2010) have shown that PCr recovered considerably faster in children (particularly boys) than in adults (particularly men) following intense exercise.

A lower proportional activation of type-II motor units in children should be expected to result in lower carbohydrate and higher fat metabolism. Indeed, a higher reliance on fat as an energy substrate has been shown in children during steady state exercise (Timmons et al., 2003), as well as during progressive exercise.

Following the onset of exercise, phase II of the pulmonary VO_2 kinetics is thought of as closely reflecting the oxygen uptake kinetics of the working muscles (Barstow et al., 1990). At any relative exercise intensity, faster phase II kinetics would be expected in individuals with higher relative aerobic power (peak VO_2), muscle oxidative capacity, or muscle composition of type I, oxidative fibres (Barstow et al., 1996). If indeed children do not utilize their type II motor units to the same extent as adults, then their muscles would be characterized by higher functional composition of type I muscle fibres. Thus, children would be expected to present with faster muscle VO_2 kinetics and consequently demonstrate faster phase II pulmonary VO_2 kinetics, as well. Indeed, in comparison with adults or adolescents of comparable or even somewhat superior aerobic power, children have been repeatedly shown to attain a given percentage of the ultimate VO_2 response faster than adults (Williams et al., 2001).

The above child-adult differences in the metabolic response to exercise may be explained by the traditional view of children's "metabolic immaturity". They can also easily be explained by the differential motor unit activation hypothesis. However, metabolic differences alone cannot explain child-adult differences in maximal force and rate of force development. These might be explained by differential muscle fibre composition but are clearly dependent on innervation, motor-unit recruitment pattern, and the contractile characteristics of the recruited units, rather than on the supply of new ATP. Furthermore, metabolic differences cannot account for the observed child-adult differences in force kinetics and force-velocity relationships, or the EMG differences in Q_{30} and mean power frequency. Thus, while the existence of inherent metabolic differences cannot be dismissed, they are incapable of explaining the full range of child-adult performance differences, as discussed in this review.

4.3.5 Response to resistance training

It may be argued that many of the above mentioned child-adult differences in muscle performance or metabolic response to exercise can be explained by lower type II muscle-fibre composition in children, with no need to resort to the notion of differential motor-unit activation pattern, as proposed in this review.

It has already been noted that differential levels of volitional muscle activation could not be explained on the basis of differential muscle composition. Additional, compelling evidence is the differential response to resistance training. Following resistance training, children have been shown to improve their strength to a proportionately similar extent observed in adults (Sale, 1989). However, while in adults strength gains are typically closely tied to muscular hypertrophy, no hypertrophy could generally be shown in prepubertal children (Blimkie, 1989; Ramsay et al., 1990; Ozmun et al., 1994). Training-induced hypertrophy in pre-pubertal children, if present, is far too small to account for the observed strength gains. Consequently, it is generally agreed that strength gain in prepubertal children is the result of enhanced motor-unit activation (Sale, 1989; Ramsay *et al.,* 1990; Ozmun *et al.,* 1994). The fact that children exhibit similar or even greater relative strength gains with little or no hypertrophy, suggests that they have a considerably larger untapped motor-unit recruitment and utilization capacity.

4.4 CONCLUSION

The presented body of evidence, although extensive, is inconclusive. In the future, innovative electro-myographical techniques and technology may provide novel and more refined evidence. However, the inherent technical limitations and the ethical constraints associated with paediatric testing appear to preclude the attainment of conclusive evidence from this venue. Breakthrough evidence could very well come from the fast-developing area of imaging in general, and nuclear magnetic resonance imaging in particular. Imaging both the muscle and the motor-cortex during exercise will likely cast new light on child-adult differences in the control of muscle and motor-unit activation.

4.5 REFERENCES

Andersen, L.L. and Aagaard, P. 2006, Influence of maximal muscle strength and intrinsic muscle contractile properties on contractile rate of force development. *European Journal of Applied Physiology*, **96**, pp. 46-52.

Armatas, V., Bassa, E., Patikas, D., Kitsas, I., Zangelidis, G. and Kotzamanidis, C. 2010, Neuromuscular differences between men and prepubescent boys during a peak isometric knee extension intermittent fatigue test. *Pediatric Exercise Science*, **22**, pp. 205-217.

Asai, H. and Aoki, J. 1996, Force development of dynamic and static contractions in children and adults. *International Journal of Sports Medicine*, **17**, pp. 170-174.

Asmussen, E. and Heeboll-Nielsen, K. 1955, A dimensional analysis of physical performance and growth in boys. *Journal of Applied Physiology*, **7**, pp. 593-603.

Barstow, T.J., Jones, A.M., Nguyen, P.H. and Casaburi, R. 1996, Influence of muscle fiber type and pedal frequency on oxygen uptake kinetics of heavy exercise. *Journal of Applied Physiology*, **81**, pp. 1642-1650.

Barstow, T.J., Lamarra, N. and Whipp, B.J. 1990, Modulation of muscle and pulmonary O2 uptakes by circulatory dynamics during exercise. *Journal of Applied Physiology*, **68**, pp. 979-989.

Bassa, E., Patikas, D. and Kotzamanidis, C. 2005, Activation of antagonist knee muscles during isokinetic efforts in prepubertal and adult males. *Pediatric Exercise Science*, **17**, pp. 171-181.

Belanger, A.Y. and McComas, A.Y. 1989, Contractile properties of human skeletal muscle in childhood and adolescence. *European Journal of Applied Physiology*, **58**, pp. 563-567.

Blimkie, C.J. 1989, Age- and sex-associated variation in strength during childhood: Anthropometric, morphologic, neurologic, biomechanical, endocrinologic, genetic, and physical activity correlates. In *Youth, Exercise and Sports*, edited by Gisolfi, C.V. and Lamb, D.R. (Indianapolis, IN: Benchmark Press). pp. 99-163.

Brooke, M.H. and Engel, W.K. 1969, The histographic analysis of human muscle biopsies with regard to fiber types. 4. Children's biopsies. *Neurology*, **19**, pp. 591-605.

Cohen, R., Mitchell, C., Dotan, R., Gabriel, D., Klentrou, P. and Falk, B. 2010, Do neuromuscular adaptations occur in endurance-trained boys and men? *Applied Physiology, Nutrition and Metabolism*, **35**, pp. 471-479.

Dotan, R., Mitchell, C., Cohen, R., Gabriel, D., Klentrou, P. and Falk, B. 2010, Child-Adult Differences in the Kinetics of Force Development. The First Wingate Congress of Exercise and Sport Sciences, Wingate Institute, Israel.

Dotan, R., Ohana, S., Bediz, C. and Falk, B. 2003, Blood lactate disappearance dynamics in boys and men following exercise of similar and dissimilar peak-lactate concentrations. *Journal of Pediatric Endocrinology and Metabolism*, **16**, pp. 419-429.

Eriksson, B.O., Gollnick, P.D. and Saltin, B. 1973, Muscle metabolism and enzyme activities after training in boys 11-13 years old. *Acta Physiologica Scandinavica*, **87**, pp. 485-497.

Falk, B., Brunton, L., Dotan, R., Usselman, C., Klentrou, P. and Gabriel, D. 2009a, Muscle strength and contractile kinetics of isometric elbow flexion in girls and women. *Pediatric Exercise Science*, **21**, pp. 354-364.

Falk, B. and Dotan, R. 2006, Child-adult differences in the recovery from high-intensity exercise. *Exercise and Sport Sciences Reviews*, **34**, pp. 107-112.

Falk, B., Usselman, C., Dotan, R., Brunton, L., Klentrou, P., Shaw, J. and Gabriel, D. 2009b, Child-adult differences in muscle strength and activation pattern during isometric elbow flexion and extension. *Applied Physiology, Nutrition and Metabolism*, **34**, pp. 609-615.

Gabriel, D.A., Basford, J.R. and An, K. 2001, Training-related changes in the maximal rate of torque development and EMG activity. *Journal of Electromyography and Kinesiology*, **11**, pp. 123-129.

Gerdle, B., Karlsson, S., Crenshaw, A.G. and Fridén, J. 1997, The relationships between EMG and muscle morphology throughout sustained static knee extension at two submaximal force levels. *Acta Physiologica Scandinavica*, **160**, pp. 341-351.

Grosset, J. F., Mora, I., Lambertz, D. and Pérot, C. 2008, Voluntary activation of the triceps surae in prepubertal children. *Journal of Electromyography and Kinesiology*, **18**, pp. 455-465.

Halin, R., Germain, P., Bercier, S., Kapitaniak, B. and Buttelli, O. 2003, Neuromuscular response of young boys versus men during sustained maximal contraction. *Medicine and Science in Sports and Exercise*, **35**, pp. 1042-1048.

Inbar, O. and Bar-Or, O. 1986, Anaerobic characteristics in male children and adolescents. *Medicine and Science in Sports and Exercise*, **18**, pp. 264-269.

Lambertz, D., Mora, I., Grosset, J.F. and Perot, C. 2003, Evaluation of musculotendinous stiffness in prepubertal children and adults, taking into account muscle activity. *Journal of Applied Physiology*, **95**, pp. 64-72.

Lexell, J., Sjostrom, M., Nordlund, A.S. and Taylor, C.C. 1992, Growth and development of human muscle: A quantitative morphological study of whole vastus lateralis from childhood to adult age. *Muscle ad Nerve*, **15**, pp. 404-409.

O'Brien, T.D., Reeves, N.D., Baltzopoulos, V., Jones, D. A. and Maganaris, C.N. 2009, The effects of agonist and antagonist muscle activation on the knee extension moment-angle relationship in adults and children. *European Journal of Applied Physiology* **106**, pp. 849-856.

Ozmun, J.C., Mikesky, A.E. and Surburg, P.R. 1994, Neuromuscular adaptations following prepubescent strength training. *Medicine and Science in Sports and Exercise*, **26**, pp. 510-514.

Ramsay, J.A., Blimkie, C.J., Smith, K., Garner, S., MacDougall, J.D. and Sale, D.G. 1990, Strength training effects in prepubescent boys. *Medicine and Science in Sports and Exercise*, **22**, pp. 605-614.

Ratel, S., Tonson, A., Le Fur, Y., Cozzone, P. and Bendahan, D. 2008, Comparative analysis of skeletal muscle oxidative capacity in children and adults: A 31P-MRS study. *Applied Physiology, Nutrition and Metabolism*, **33**, pp. 720-727.

Sale, D.G. 1989, Strength training in children. In *Youth, Exercise and Sports*, edited by Gisolfi, C.V. and Lamb, D.R. . (Indianapolis, IN: Benchmark Press), pp. 165-222.

Seger, J.Y. and Thorstensson, A. 2000, Muscle strength and electromyogram in boys and girls followed through puberty. *European Journal of Applied Physiology and Occupational Physiology*, **81**, pp. 54-61.

Tanaka, H. and Shindo, M. 1985, Running velocity at blood lactate threshold of boys aged 6-15 years compared with untrained and trained young males. *International Journal of Sports Medicine*, **6**, pp. 90-94.

Timmons, B.W., Bar-Or, O. and Riddell, M.C. 2003, Oxidation rate of exogenous carbohydrate during exercise is higher in boys than in men. *Journal of Applied Physiology*, **94**, pp. 278-284.

Willcocks, R.J., Williams, C.A., Barker, A.R., Fulford, J. and Armstrong, N. 2010, Age- and sex-related differences in muscle phosphocreatine and oxygenation kinetics during high-intensity exercise in adolescents and adults. *NMR in Biomedicine*, **23**, pp. 569-577.

Williams, C.A., Carter, H., Jones, A.M. and Doust, J.H. 2001, Oxygen uptake kinetics during treadmill running in boys and men. *Journal of Applied Physiology*, **90**, pp. 1700-1706.

UNDERSTANDING THE GENETICS OF BIRTH WEIGHT

R.M. Freathy

Genetics of Complex Traits, Peninsula College of Medicine and Dentistry, University of Exeter, UK

5.1 INTRODUCTION

Fetal growth is a complex process influenced both by genetic (maternal and fetal) and environmental factors. It is important to understand both environmental and genetic determinants of fetal growth (a) for more effective clinical management of pregnancies and (b) because there are well documented associations between lower birth weight and a higher risk of chronic adult diseases, including cardiovascular disease, type 2 diabetes and hypertension (Barker *et al.*, 1993; Jarvelin *et al.*, 2004). The mechanisms underlying these associations are unclear. A clear understanding of the genetic contribution to fetal growth and its links with adult disease is important to inform our understanding of disease processes and thereby allow effective strategies for intervention and prevention.

5.2 THE FETAL INSULIN HYPOTHESIS

The "Fetal Insulin Hypothesis" proposes that common genetic variants influencing insulin secretion or action may explain the association between lower birth weight and type 2 diabetes (Hattersley and Tooke, 1999). The Hypothesis links two key observations. The first is that type 2 diabetes is characterized by insulin resistance and/or pancreatic beta cell dysfunction. The second is that fetal insulin is a key fetal growth factor. Therefore, genetic variants which influence insulin secretion or action may affect both growth *in utero* and the risk of type 2 diabetes 50 or 60 years later.

Evidence for a genetic link between fetal growth and type 2 diabetes has come from three kinds of genetics studies. The first were studies of rare, monogenic forms of diabetes. The very first evidence for the Fetal Insulin Hypothesis came from observations of patients with a heterozygous mutation in the glucokinase (*GCK*) gene. As a result of the mutation, the patients have an impaired ability to sense glucose levels and consequently reduced insulin secretion, which leads to mild, stable fasting hyperglycaemia. They are also, on average, approximately 500 g lighter at birth than unaffected siblings, due to reduced fetal insulin secretion (Hattersley *et al.*, 1998). This observation established that the disparate phenotypes of low birth weight and diabetes may be caused by a single genotype. Severe, rare diabetes-causing mutations in numerous other genes have also been shown to cause low birth weight by reducing fetal insulin secretion, lending further support to this principle (for a detailed review, see Shields *et al.*, 2010).

While the observations of rare types of monogenic diabetes established the principle of a link with low birth weight, they are not common enough to explain associations between lower birth weight and type 2 diabetes in the general population. Studies of genetic variants which predispose to type 2 diabetes provided further evidence that genetics underpins at least part of this association. Genetic variants at over 35 loci across the genome are now known to predispose to type 2 diabetes (Prokopenko *et al.*, 2008; Dupuis *et al.*, 2010, Voight *et al.*, 2010). We have used meta-analyses to combine large collections of participants from birth cohorts to test for associations between some of these predisposing variants and birth weight. We found that the 4 % of European babies who carried four risk alleles for type 2 diabetes at the *CDKAL1* and *HHEX* loci were, on average 80 g (95 % CI 39g–120g) lighter at birth than the 8 % who carried four non-risk alleles (Freathy *et al.*, 2009; Shields *et al.*, 2010). This work was the first direct evidence to support the Fetal Insulin Hypothesis.

Finally, the most recent evidence in support of the Fetal Insulin Hypothesis comes from genome-wide association (GWA) studies of birth weight. A GWA study typically surveys 2.5 million common genetic variants across the genome in one experiment, testing each for association with the disease or trait of interest. We combined six GWA studies in a meta-analysis, totalling 10,623 Europeans from pregnancy/birth cohorts. We followed up two signals of interest in thirteen replication studies ($n = 27,591$). Common genetic variants near the *CCNL1* ($P = 2 \times 10^{-35}$) and *ADCY5* ($P = 7 \times 10^{-15}$) genes were robustly associated with birth weight. The same variant in *ADCY5* is also known to influence susceptibility to type 2 diabetes. To give some scale to the effect size of the associations, the combined impact of both variants on birth weight was similar to that of a mother smoking 4–5 cigarettes per day in the third trimester of pregnancy (Freathy *et al.*, 2010).

5.3 CONCLUSION

To date, we have identified genetic variants at the *ADCY5* and *CDKAL1* loci, which are convincingly associated both with reduced birth weight and with type 2 diabetes. Further efforts to identify more genetic variants are ongoing. These findings promise to provide important insights into early growth processes and their relationship with chronic adult disease.

5.4 REFERENCES

Barker, D.J., Hales, C.N., Fall, C.H., Osmond, C., Phipps, K. and Clark, P.M., 1993, Type 2 (non-insulin-dependent) diabetes mellitus, hypertension and hyperlipidaemia (syndrome X): Relation to reduced fetal growth. *Diabetologia*, **36**, pp. 62-67.

Dupuis, J., Langenberg, C., Prokopenko, I., Saxena, R., Soranzo, N., Jackson, A.U., Wheeler, E., Glazer, N.L., Bouatia-Naji, N., Gloyn, A.L., Lindgren, C.M., Magi, R., Morris, A.P., Randall, J., Johnson, T., Elliott, P., Rybin, D., Thorleifsson, G., Steinthorsdottir, V., Henneman, P., Grallert, H., Dehghan, A., Hottenga, J.J., Franklin, C.S., Navarro, P., Song, K., Goel, A., Perry, J.R., Egan, J.M., Lajunen, T., Grarup, N., Sparso, T., Doney, A., Voight, B.F., Stringham, H.M., Li, M., Kanoni, S., Shrader, P., Cavalcanti-Proenca, C., Kumari, M., Qi, L., Timpson, N.J., Gieger, C., Zabena, C., Rocheleau, G., Ingelsson, E., An, P., O'Connell, J., Luan, J., Elliott, A., McCarroll, S.A., Payne, F., Roccasecca, R.M., Pattou, F., Sethupathy, P., Ardlie, K., Ariyurek, Y., Balkau, B., Barter, P., Beilby, J.P., Ben-Shlomo, Y., Benediktsson, R., Bennett, A.J., Bergmann, S., Bochud, M., Boerwinkle, E., Bonnefond, A., Bonnycastle, L.L., Borch-Johnsen, K., Bottcher, Y., Brunner, E., Bumpstead, S.J., Charpentier, G., Chen, Y.D., Chines, P., Clarke, R., Coin, L.J., Cooper, M.N., Cornelis, M., Crawford, G., Crisponi, L., Day, I.N., de Geus, E.J., Delplanque, J., Dina, C., Erdos, M.R., Fedson, A.C., Fischer-Rosinsky, A., Forouhi, N.G., Fox, C.S., Frants, R., Franzosi, M.G., Galan, P., Goodarzi, M.O., Graessler, J., Groves, C.J., Grundy, S., Gwilliam, R., Gyllensten, U., Hadjadj, S., *et al.*, 2010, New genetic loci implicated in fasting glucose homeostasis and their impact on type 2 diabetes risk. *Nature Genetics*, **42**, pp. 105-116.

Freathy, R.M., Bennett, A.J., Ring, S.M., Shields, B., Groves, C.J., Timpson, N.J., Weedon, M.N., Zeggini, E., Lindgren, C.M., Lango, H., Perry, J.R., Pouta, A., Ruokonen, A., Hypponen, E., Power, C., Elliott, P., Strachan, D.P., Jarvelin, M.R., Smith, G.D., McCarthy, M.I., Frayling, T.M. and Hattersley, A.T., 2009, Type 2 diabetes risk alleles are associated with reduced size at birth. *Diabetes*, **58**, pp. 1428-1433.

Freathy, R.M., Mook-Kanamori, D.O., Sovio, U., Prokopenko, I., Timpson, N.J., Berry, D.J., Warrington, N.M., Widen, E., Hottenga, J.J., Kaakinen, M., Lange, L.A., Bradfield, J.P., Kerkhof, M., Marsh, J.A., Magi, R., Chen, C.M., Lyon, H.N., Kirin, M., Adair, L.S., Aulchenko, Y.S., Bennett, A.J., Borja, J.B., Bouatia-Naji, N., Charoen, P., Coin, L.J., Cousminer, D.L., de Geus, E.J., Deloukas, P., Elliott, P., Evans, D.M., Froguel, P.,

Glaser, B., Groves, C.J., Hartikainen, A.L., Hassanali, N., Hirschhorn, J.N., Hofman, A., Holly, J.M., Hypponen, E., Kanoni, S., Knight, B.A., Laitinen, J., Lindgren, C.M., McArdle, W.L., O'Reilly, P.F., Pennell, C.E., Postma, D.S., Pouta, A., Ramasamy, A., Rayner, N.W., Ring, S.M., Rivadeneira, F., Shields, B.M., Strachan, D.P., Surakka, I., Taanila, A., Tiesler, C., Uitterlinden, A.G., van Duijn, C.M., Wijga, A.H., Willemsen, G., Zhang, H., Zhao, J., Wilson, J.F., Steegers, E.A., Hattersley, A.T., Eriksson, J.G., Peltonen, L., Mohlke, K.L., Grant, S.F., Hakonarson, H., Koppelman, G.H., Dedoussis, G.V., Heinrich, J., Gillman, M.W., Palmer, L.J., Frayling, T.M., Boomsma, D.I., Davey Smith, G., Power, C., Jaddoe, V.W., Jarvelin, M.R. and McCarthy, M.I., 2010, Variants in ADCY5 and near CCNL1 are associated with fetal growth and birth weight. *Nature Genetics*, **42**, pp. 430-435.

Hattersley, A.T., Beards, F., Ballantyne, E., Appleton, M., Harvey, R. and Ellard, S., 1998, Mutations in the glucokinase gene of the fetus result in reduced birth weight. *Nature Genetics,* **19,** pp. 268-270.

Hattersley, A.T. and Tooke, J.E., 1999, The fetal insulin hypothesis: an alternative explanation of the association of low birthweight with diabetes and vascular disease. *Lancet*, **353**, pp. 1789-1792.

Jarvelin, M.R., Sovio, U., King, V., Lauren, L., Xu, B., McCarthy, M.I., Hartikainen, A.L., Laitinen, J., Zitting, P., Rantakallio, P. and Elliott, P., 2004, Early life factors and blood pressure at age 31 years in the 1966 northern Finland birth cohort. *Hypertension*, **44**, pp. 838-846.

Prokopenko, I., McCarthy, M.I. and Lindgren, C.M., 2008, Type 2 diabetes: new genes, new understanding. *Trends in Genetics*, **24**, pp. 613-621.

Shields, B.M., Freathy, R.M. and Hattersley, A.T., 2010, Genetic influences on the association between fetal growth and susceptibility to type 2 diabetes. *Journal of Developmental Origins of Health and Disease*, **1**, pp. 96-105.

Voight, B.F., Scott, L.J., Steinthorsdottir, V., Morris, A.P., Dina, C., Welch, R.P., Zeggini, E., Huth, C., Aulchenko, Y.S., Thorleifsson, G., McCulloch, L.J., Ferreira, T., Grallert, H., Amin, N., Wu, G., Willer, C.J., Raychaudhuri, S., McCarroll, S.A., Langenberg, C., Hofmann, O.M., Dupuis, J., Qi, L., Segre, A.V., van Hoek, M., Navarro, P., Ardlie, K., Balkau, B., Benediktsson, R., Bennett, A.J., Blagieva, R., Boerwinkle, E., Bonnycastle, L.L., Bengtsson Bostrom, K., Bravenboer, B., Bumpstead, S., Burtt, N.P., Charpentier, G., Chines, P.S., Cornelis, M., Couper, D.J., Crawford, G., Doney, A.S., Elliott, A.L., Elliott, K.S., Erdos, M.R., Fox, C.S., Franklin, C.S., Ganser, M., Gieger, C., Grarup, N., Green, T., Griffin, S., Groves, C.J., Guiducci, C., Hadjadj, H., Hassanali, N., Herder, C., Isomaa, B., Jackson, A.U., Johnson, P.R., Jorgensen, T., Kao, W.H., Klopp, N., Kong, A., Kraft, P., Kuusisto, J., Lauritzen, T., Li, M., Lieverse, A., Lindgren, C.M., Lyssenko, V., Marre, M., Meitinger, T., Midthjell, K., Morken, M.A., Narisu, N., Nilsson, P., Owen, K.R., Payne, F., Perry, J.R.,

Petersen, A.K., Platou, C., Proenca, C., Prokopenko, I., Rathmann, W., Rayner, N.W., Robertson, N.R., Rocheleau, G., Roden, M., Sampson, M.J., Saxena, R., Shields, B.M., Shrader, P., Sigurdsson, G., Sparso, T., Strassburger, K., Stringham, H.M., Sun, Q., Swift, A.J., Thorand, B., *et al.*, 2010, Twelve type 2 diabetes susceptibility loci identified through large-scale association analysis. *Nature Genetics*, **42**, pp. 579-589.

Part III

Exercise Physiology

CHILD AND ADOLESCENT DIFFERENCES IN ECONOMY AT VARIOUS SPEEDS ACROSS A TWO-YEAR TIME PERIOD

R.W. Moore[1], T.S. Wenzlick[1], K.A. Pfeiffer[1], and S.G. Trost[2]
[1]Michigan State University, USA, [2]Oregon State University, USA

6.1 INTRODUCTION

Economy of movement is defined as the mass related aerobic demand (VO_2 $mL \cdot kg^{-1} \cdot min^{-1}$) or energy expenditure required to run or walk at a given submaximal speed (Morgan, 2000). It has been well established that children have a lower economy compared to adults (Rowland and Green, 1988; Rowland et al., 1987; Unnithan and Eston, 1990). This means that at any given walking or running speed, children exhibit a higher weight relative VO_2 compared to that of an adult. The difference in economy between children and adults is thought to be due to differences in stride frequency (SF), leg length, body-surface-area to mass ratio (BSA:M), body mass index (BMI), and ventilatory efficiency (Rowland et al., 1987; Rowland and Green, 1988; Unnithan and Eston, 1990).

While many studies have shown a difference in economy between children and adults, limited information is available on how economy changes throughout childhood and adolescence. Waters et al. (1983) compared the aerobic demand of children and adolescents walking over-ground at a self-selected pace. VO_2 was significantly higher for children (15.3 $mL \cdot kg^{-1} \cdot min^{-1}$) compared to adolescents (12.9 $mL \cdot kg^{-1} \cdot min^{-1}$). However, this study was cross-sectional and provides no information regarding change over time.

Morgan et al. (2002) followed children from 6-10 years of age to determine if changes in economy occurred each year, children walked on a treadmill for 5 minutes at six different speeds ranging from 0.67 $m \cdot s^{-1}$ to 1.79 $m \cdot s^{-1}$. Results from this study indicated that improvements in economy could be seen over a 1 year time period. However, children were required to walk at predetermined speeds on a treadmill, which may not reflect their most economical pace. It is unknown whether a change in economy will occur over a short time period when children and adolescents walk or run at a self-selected pace over-ground. The purpose of this study was to determine if economy

59

improved over a 2 year period in children and adolescents at two different walking speeds and one running speed.

6.2 METHODS

Ninety-one participants (39 boys, 52 girls) 6-16 years old took part in this study and were divided into two categories: children (n=52) 6-11 and adolescents (n=39) 12-16 years old. Participants came to the laboratory on two separate occasions (assessment 1). Two years later, participants returned to the laboratory for two additional visits (assessment 2). Anthropometric measurements including stature, body mass, sitting height, and body composition were completed at each assessment. Anthropometric measures were used to calculate BMI ($kg \cdot m^{-2}$), BSA:M, and leg length. Informed consent and participant assent were obtained, and approval was received from the institutional review board at Michigan State University.

6.2.1 Assessments 1 and 2

For assessment 1, each participant self-selected a comfortable walking pace (visit 1) and a brisk walking and running pace (visit 2) that was performed over-ground around a course of known distance. Each trial lasted 5-minutes. Pace was determined after completion of the first lap. A research assistant walked/ran with each participant thereafter to ensure the pace was maintained. Throughout each trial, oxygen uptake (VO_2) was measured breath-by-breath using the Oxycon portable metabolic analyzer (Yorba Linda, CA). Minutes 2:30-4:30 for each trial were used for analysis. Step count was obtained during each trial from minutes 2:30-3:00 and 3:30-4:00 to determine SF.

Each participant returned to the laboratory after a 2 year period for assessment 2. Participants performed the comfortable walk trial (visit 1) and brisk walk and run trials (visit 2). The pace for each trial was the same as that performed previously in assessment 1. A research assistant walked or ran with each participant in order to ensure pace from assessment 1 was maintained.

6.2.2 Statistical analysis

Repeated measures ANOVA was used to compare VO_2 during assessment 1 and assessment 2 for both walking trials and the running trial. Data were analyzed for the total sample, as well as the children and adolescent groups. Post hoc linear regression was used to determine predictors of change in economy for the total sample and two age groups. Predictor variables included change in BMI (kg·m^{-2}), BSA:M, leg length, and SF. Data was analyzed using the PASW 18 software and significance was set at $P<0.05$.

6.3 RESULTS

Descriptive characteristics for assessments 1 and 2 are displayed in Table 6.1. There were no differences in walking speeds and running speeds between assessment 1 and assessment 2 (comfortable walk 3.9 vs. 3.9 km·h^{-1}, brisk walk 5.1 vs. 5.1 km·h^{-1}, running 7.9 vs. 7.9 km·h^{-1}). For the comfortable walk, VO$_2$ significantly decreased from assessment 1 to assessment 2 for the total sample (16.3 vs. 15.0 mL·kg^{-1}·min^{-1}; $P<0.001$) and children (18.2 vs. 15.9 mL·kg^{-1}·min^{-1}; P <0.001) but not adolescents (13.7 vs. 13.6 mL·kg^{-1}·min^{-1}; P >0.05). For brisk walk, there was a significant difference for the total sample (21.5 vs. 19.4 mL·kg^{-1}·min^{-1}; P <0.001), children (23.5 vs. 20.7 mL·kg^{-1}·min^{-1}; P <0.001), and adolescents (18.8 vs. 17.7 mL·kg^{-1}·min^{-1}; P <0.003). For the running trial, there were no significant differences in VO$_2$ for total sample (38.1 vs. 37.8 mL·kg^{-1}·min^{-1}; P >0.05), children (36.7 vs. 37.1 mL·kg^{-1}·min^{-1}; P >0.05), and adolescents (39.2 vs. 38.3 mL·kg^{-1}·min^{-1}; P >0.05).

Change in BSA:M accounted for 25 % of the variance for total sample and 21 % of the variance for children for the comfortable walk. For brisk walk, change in SF and BSA:M accounted for 21 % of the variance for the total sample, and change in SF accounted for 41 % of the variance in adolescents. None of the predictor variables were found to be significant for brisk walk in children.

Table 6.1. Descriptive characteristics for assessments 1 and 2

Mean (SD)	Assess 1	Assess 2
Age (y)	10.8 (2.5)	12.6 (2.5)
Body mass (kg)	42.8 (17.3)	51.1 (17.8)
Stature (cm)	144.7 (15.3)	154.8 (14.7)
Leg Length (cm)	69.8 (7.8)	73.5 (7.8)
SF (steps/30 s)	CW 59 (7)	CW 55 (5)
	BW 67 (6)	BW 63 (5)
	Run 88 (7)	Run 84 (7)
BSA:M	0.032 (0.005)	0.030 (0.004)
BMI (kg·m^{-2})	14.4 (4.4)	16.2 (4.4)

*All comparisons were statistically significant (p<0.001)
CW=comfortable walk, BW=brisk walk

6.4 CONCLUSION

The main findings of this study were: 1) at a comfortable pace, children showed an improvement in economy over the 2 year period, that was not found in adolescents, 2) both children and adolescents became more economical during brisk walk, 3) neither group showed an improvement in economy during running, and 4) change in SF and BSA:M were responsible for change in economy.

Results from this study are similar to those found previously for children during walking. Morgan *et al.* (2002) found that economy significantly improved between ages 6-8 years at six different walking speeds performed on a treadmill. In the current study, although economy was found to improve over a 2 year period at two walking paces in children, change in economy for adolescents was only seen during the brisk walk. Previous literature lacks direct comparison regarding change in economy during adolescence.

Change in BSA:M and SF accounted for the differences in economy. BSA:M has been previously found to account for differences in economy between children and adults (Rowland and Green, 1988), possibly due to children needing to dissipate more heat to maintain body temperature. Additionally, Unnithan and Eston (1990) found a similar oxygen demand per stride between children and adults, suggesting that increased overall oxygen demand for children were due to greater SF. Results from this study support these findings that BSA:M and SF account for the poorer economy seen in children.

Running economy has been found to improve from childhood to adulthood. In the current study, there was no difference in running economy for children and adolescents. Previous studies comparing adults and children have used a treadmill with predetermined speed (Rowland *et al.*, 1987; Rowland and Green, 1988). The lack of difference in economy in this study could be due to self-selected pace or performance over-ground. It is also possible that change in running economy may occur at a later age than that of walking economy.

In conclusion, change in walking economy was likely due to changes induced by growth and maturation. Factors related to change in running economy for children or adolescents are less clear.

6.5 REFERENCES

Morgan D., 2000, Economy of locomotion. In *Paediatric Exercise Science and Medicine*, edited by Armstrong, N. and van Mechelen, W., (Oxford: University Press), pp. 183-190.

Morgan D.W., Tseh W., Caputo J.L., Keefer D.J., Craig I.S., Griffith K.B., Akins, M.B., Griffith G.E. and Martin P.E., 2002, Longitudinal profiles of oxygen uptake during treadmill walking in able-bodied children: The locomotion energy and growth study. *Gait Posture*, **15**, pp. 230-235.

Rowland T.W., Auchinachie J.A., Keenan T.J. and Green G.M., 1987, Physiologic responses to treadmill running in adult and prepubertal males. *International Journal of Sports Medicine*, **8**, pp. 292-297.

Rowland T.W. and Green G.M., 1988, Physiological responses to treadmill exercise in females: Adult-child differences. *Medicine and Science in Sports and Exercise*, **20**, pp. 474-478.

Unnithan V.B. and Eston R.G., 1990, Stride frequency and submaximal treadmill running economy in adults and children. *Pediatric Exercise Science*, **2**, pp. 149-155.

Waters R.L., Hislop H.J., Thomas L. and Campbell J., 1983, Energy cost of walking in normal children and teenagers. *Developmental Medicine and Child Neurology*, **25**, pp. 184-188.

FUEL USE RESPONSES IN YOUNG BOYS AND GIRLS DURING SUBMAXIMAL EXERCISE

A.D. Mahon, L.M. Guth, M.P. Rogowski, and K.A. Craft
Ball State University, USA

7.1 INTRODUCTION

During submaximal exercise under normally fed conditions the primary fuel sources used to resynthesize ATP are fat and carbohydrate. The balance between the use of these two sources is largely dependent upon the intensity and duration of exercise, although other factors such as aerobic fitness, body fatness, acute and chronic alterations in diet, maturation, and prior physical activity will further influence the metabolic response to exercise (Aucouturier *et al.*, 2008).

In adults there is evidence that females rely more on fat and less on carbohydrate compared to males when exercising at similar intensities (Venables *et al.*, 2005; Tarnopolsky, 2008). This may be, at least in part, influenced by hormonal differences between genders, particularly 17-β estradiol concentration (Tarnopolsky, 2008). Given the hormonal factors that may play a role in exercise metabolism, it is thought that fuel use patterns in young boys and girls are similar (Aucouturier *et al.*, 2008). In some support of this Delamarche *et al.* (1994) reported similar concentrations of fatty acids and glycerol and similar levels of non-esterified fatty acid turnover in 10-year-old boys and girls during 60 minutes of exercise at 60 % of peak VO_2. However, these authors also noted that while transient hypoglycaemia occurred at the onset of exercise in both groups, girls had a slightly, but significantly, lower blood glucose concentration at 30 minutes. In addition, Wirth *et al.*, (1978) showed similar blood glucose and fatty acid responses to 15 minutes of exercise at 70 % of peak VO_2 in pre-pubertal, pubertal, and post-pubertal boys and girls. However, there appears to be a void of studies that have matched boys and girls for fitness, fatness, maturation, and carefully controlled pre-exercise diet in order to eliminate these factors from confounding the outcome of fuel use during exercise. Therefore, this study examined the use of carbohydrate and fat in boys and girls matched for age and maturation, peak VO_2, pre-exercise diet, and body fat. Exercise was performed relative to the child's ventilatory threshold (VT), to minimize limitations associated when exercise is performed relative to peak VO_2.

7.2 METHODS

Eight boys (10.5 ± 0.4 y; pubertal stage 1/2) and 9 girls (10.0 ± 1.0 y; pubertal stage 1/2) were participants in this study. Parental permission and child assent were obtained. The children reported to the laboratory on four separate occasions.

During the first visit a physical examination by a physician was performed for the determination of pubertal stage using Tanner indices (1962) for pubic hair development. Age was recorded, and stature and body mass were measured. Skinfold thickness at six sites were assessed and used to calculate body fat percentage (Slaughter et al., 1988). The second visit served to familiarize the child with the exercise protocol and to establish the VO_2-power output relationship across three levels of exercise. On the third visit, a graded exercise test was performed to determine VT and peak VO_2. The test commenced at 20 W for 2 minutes and increased by 10 W·min⁻¹ until a peak effort was obtained. The use of carbohydrate and fat as energy sources was determined on the fourth visit to the laboratory. The children cycled for 6 minutes at each of the following intensities: 60 %, 80 %, 100 %, and 120 % of VT. This trial was performed after a 10-12 hour overnight fast following a prescribed night-before meal; all subjects verbally confirmed.

All exercise bouts were performed on a Lode Excalibur cycle ergometer. A Hans-Rudolph mouthpiece breathing valve and nose clip were used. Inspired pulmonary ventilation was measured using a Parkinson Cowan dry-gas meter. Expired air samples were analyzed for oxygen and carbon dioxide concentrations from a mixing chamber using calibrated gas analyzers. Respiratory gas exchange measures were recorded at 15 s intervals during the graded exercise test and at 30 s intervals during all other exercise bouts using a 60 s rolling average. HR was assessed with a Polar monitor.

VT was defined as the VO_2 at the point when pulmonary ventilation began to increase out of proportion to the increase in VO_2. Peak exercise responses were noted as the highest responses obtained during the graded exercise test. The percentage of fuel used at each submaximal level of exercise was calculated from the average values from the last minute provided the fraction of expired CO_2 which varied by ≤ 0.10 %; if not the last 90 s were used (Stephens et al., 2006). The respiratory exchange ratio (RER) was used to determine the percentage of fat and carbohydrate (McArdle et al., 2010). The fat and carbohydrate utilization rate (mg·kg⁻¹·min⁻¹) was made according to equations used by Timmons et al. (2003).

The physical characteristics and responses at VT and peak VO_2 were compared using an independent t-test. The responses during submaximal exercise were evaluated using a 2-way (group by intensity) ANOVA. A Bonferroni test was used to probe for specific differences in the event of main effect for intensity or a group-by-intensity interaction. Statistical significance was set at $P < 0.05$.

7.3 RESULTS

The age, stature, body mass and percent body fat were 10.5 ($\pm$ 0.4) y, 140.3 ($\pm$ 5.9) cm, 40.3 ($\pm$ 11.8) kg, and 21.2 ($\pm$ 8.5) % in boys and 10.0 ($\pm$ 1.0) y, 135.0 ($\pm$ 4.7) cm, 34.4 ($\pm$ 7.8) kg, and 21.0 ($\pm$ 5.5) % in girls, respectively ($P >$ 0.05). The VO_2 at VT was 0.95 ($\pm$ 0.13) $L \cdot min^{-1}$ (62.3 $\pm$ 5.6 %) in boys and 0.85 $\pm$ 0.11 $L \cdot min^{-1}$ (63.8 $\pm$ 4.3 %) in girls; differences between groups were not significant. At peak exercise VO_2 was 1.54 ($\pm$ 0.27) $L \cdot min^{-1}$ (39.3 $\pm$ 6.0 $mL \cdot kg^{-1} \cdot min^{-1}$) in boys and 1.33 ($\pm$ 0.18) $L \cdot min^{-1}$ (39.6 $\pm$ 5.6 $mL \cdot kg^{-1} \cdot min^{-1}$) in girls. Peak VO_2 ($L \cdot min^{-1}$) tended ($P < 0.10$) to be higher in boys, but there was no group difference ($P > 0.05$) in mass-relative peak VO_2.

During the four submaximal exercise intensities, there was the expected intensity effect ($P < 0.05$) among all the variables. However, there were no group and interaction effects ($P > 0.05$) for any comparison. The exercise intensity targets were achieved. Boys exercised at 59.2 ($\pm$ 3.4) %, 77.7 ($\pm$ 3.3) %, 99.1 ($\pm$ 2.4) % and 119.0($\pm$ 3.9) % of VT whereas girls exercised at 57.6 ($\pm$ 5.5) %, 77.6 ($\pm$ 3.0) %, 99.8 ($\pm$ 2.8) % and 119.8 ($\pm$ 3.5) % of VT. RER values in boys were 0.84 ($\pm$ 0.03), 0.87 ($\pm$ 0.04), 0.92 ($\pm$ 0.04) and 0.94 ($\pm$ 0.04) across the 4 intensity levels, respectively. For girls RER values were 0.84 ($\pm$ 0.04), 0.86 ($\pm$ 0.04), 0.92 ($\pm$ 0.04), 0.97 ($\pm$ 0.05), respectively.

Due to the similar RER response between groups, the percent use of each fuel was also similar. In boys carbohydrate use ranged from 46.3 ($\pm$ 11.8) at 60 % of VT to 78.6 ($\pm$ 9.8) at 120 % of VT. In girls, the range was 46.4 ($\pm$ 13.2) % to 86.4 ($\pm$ 11.8) %. Percent fat use was 53.7 ($\pm$ 11.8) at 60 % of VT and decreased to 21.4 ($\pm$ 9.8) at 120 % of VT in boys and 53.6 ($\pm$ 13.2) at 60 % of VT and decreased to 13.6 ($\pm$ 11.8) at 120 % of VT in girls. In boys the rate of carbohydrate and fat used ranged from 8.5 ($\pm$ 3.3) to 31.3 ($\pm$ 9.4) $mg \cdot kg^{-1} \cdot min^{-1}$ and 4.0 ($\pm$ 1.3) to 3.0 ($\pm$ 1.4) $mg \cdot kg^{-1} \cdot min^{-1}$, respectively. Carbohydrate use in girls varied from 8.8 ($\pm$ 3.4) to 36.7 ($\pm$ 10.4) $mg \cdot kg^{-1} \cdot min^{-1}$ while fat use ranged from 4.0 ($\pm$ 1.2) to 1.8 ($\pm$ 1.6) $mg \cdot kg^{-1} \cdot min^{-1}$.

7.4 CONCLUSION

This study confirms that the relative and actual rate of use of fat and carbohydrate during submaximal exercise does not vary between pre and early pubertal boys and girls when confounding influences are carefully controlled. The specific hormonal and metabolic factors mediating fuel use in children during exercise remain unclear as does the stage of maturation associated with the onset of gender differences in exercise metabolism.

7.5 NOTE

This study was supported with funding from the Gatorade Sports Science Institute.

7.6 REFERENCES

Aucouturier, J., Baker, J.S. and Duche, P., 2008, Fat and carbohydrate metabolism during submaximal exercise in children. *Sports Medicine*, **38**, pp. 213-238.

Delamarche, P., Gratas-Delamarche, A., Monnier, M., Mayet, M.H., Koubi, H.E. and Favier, R., 1994, Glucoregulation and hormonal changes during prolonged exercise in boys and girls. *European Journal of Applied Physiology*, **68**, pp. 3-8.

McArdle, W.D., Katch, F.I. and Katch, V.L., 2010, *Exercise Physiology: Nutrition, Energy, and Human Performance* (7th edition), (Philadelphia: Lippincott Williams and Wilkins).

Slaughter, M.H., Lohman, T.G., Boileau, R.A., Horswill, C.A., Stillman, R.J., van Loan, M.D. and Bemben, D.A., 1988, Skinfold equations for estimation of body fatness in children and youth. *Human Biology*, **60**, pp. 709-723.

Stephens, B.R., Cole, A.S. and Mahon A.D., 2006, The influence of biological maturation on fat and carbohydrate metabolism during exercise in males. *International Journal of Sports Nutrition and Exercise Metabolism*, **16**, pp. 166-179.

Tanner, J.M., 1962, *Growth at Adolescence*, (Oxford: Blackwell Scientific Publications).

Tarnoplosky, M., 2008, Sex difference in exercise metabolism and the role of 17-beta estradiol. *Medicine and Science in Sports and Exercise*, **40**, pp. 648-654.

Timmons, B.W., Bar-Or, O., Riddell, M.C., 2003, Oxidation rate of exogenous carbohydrate during exercise is higher in boys than in men. *Journal of Applied Physiology*, **94**, pp. 278-284.

Venables, M.C., Acten, J. and Jeukendrup, A.E., 2005, Determinants of fat oxidation during exercise in healthy men and women: A cross-sectional study. *Journal of Applied Physiology*, **98**, pp. 160-167.

Wirth, A., Trager, E., Scheele, K., Mayer, D., Diehm, K., Reischle, K. and Weicker, H., 1978, Cardiopulmonary adjustment and metabolic response to maximal and submaximal physical exercise of boys and girls at different stages of maturity. *European Journal of Applied Physiology*, **39**, pp. 229-240.

RER VARIABILITY ANALYSIS BY SAMPLE ENTROPY: COMPARING TRAINED AND UNTRAINED ADOLESCENT FEMALE SOCCER PLAYERS

G.R. Biltz[1], V.B. Unnithan[2], S.R. Brown[1], S. Marwood[3], D.M. Roche[3], M. Garrard[4], and K. Holloway[3]

[1]School of Kinesiology, University of Minnesota, Minneapolis, MN, USA;
[2]Centre for Sport, Health and Exercise Research, Staffordshire University, UK;
[3]Sport and Exercise Physiology Research Team, Liverpool Hope University, UK; [4]Sport and Exercise Science Department, Leeds Metropolitan University, UK

8.1 INTRODUCTION

Time series data for heart rate (HR), blood pressure, breathing frequency and a number of other physiologic variables exhibit moment to moment variability. As a general principle, this increased fine scale variability seems characteristic of healthy, adaptable physiology (West, 2006). The variability within the data contains potential information that is lost in the traditional calculation of a mean value. Variability analysis encompasses a variety of mathematical techniques that have been applied to physiologic time series data such as: time domain analysis, frequency domain analysis, fractal analysis and entropy analysis (Seely and Macklem, 2004). Sample Entropy (SampEn), a nonlinear method for variability analysis of time series data, characterizes the inherent regularity of a data sequence (Richman and Moorman, 2000). A higher entropy score implies decreased predictability of sequential values – less self-similarity in the data.

In a previous study, RER SampEn had a moderately negative correlation with percent body fat (Biltz *et al.*, 2009). Obesity has been described as a state of metabolic inflexibility with a relatively similar ratio of carbohydrate and fat oxidation independent of the feeding or fasting state (Corpeleijn *et al.*, 2009). Conversely, metabolic flexibility is observed in exercise, as RER changes from rest to progressive effort (Goedecke *et al.*, 2000). Endurance training increases fat oxidation and lowers average RER during exercise

(Jeukendrup and Wallis, 2005). The variability of breath by breath RER has not been investigated for potential effects of training. It has been observed that HRV increased during sub-ventilatory threshold exercise in highly trained adolescent triathletes (Cottin *et al.,* 2004). Aerobic training has also been reported to increase heart rate variability (HRV) in pre-pubertal children (Mandigout *et al.,* 2002). The aim of this study was to investigate soccer training effects on RER variability during exercise. Specifically, we hypothesized that soccer training would increase RER variability, as measured by SampEn, during steady state, sub-maximal exercise. Training effects on RER variability would be analogous to previously reported training effects on HRV.

8.2 METHODS

8.2.1 Experimental design

Eleven trained female soccer players (14.6 ± 0.7 y) were recruited from two professional teams in NW England. They regularly engaged in systematic training (10.3 ± 1.4 months$\cdot$y^{-1}, 5.2 ± 2.0 h$\cdot$wk^{-1}) with 5.9 ± 1 y playing competitive soccer. Nine untrained, but recreationally active girls (15.1 ± 0.6 y) volunteered to participate in the study. Tanner staging by self-assessment of breast development ranged from 3-5 for both groups. All subjects performed an initial incremental cycle ergometer test (Lode Excalibur Sport, Groningen, The Netherlands) to volitional exhaustion. The protocol consisted of 3 min stages, with an initial work rate of 35 W and increments of 35 W per stage at a cadence of 60 rpm throughout the test. Cosmed K4b^2 (Rome, Italy) was used to obtain VE, VO_2, VCO_2, peak VO_2, and RER. Ventilatory threshold (VT) was determined for each subject by standard v-slope method conducted independently by two members of the research team. Subjects returned for evaluation of their VO_2 kinetics as part of a larger UK study.

8.2.2 Determination of RER sample entropy

After 3 minutes of baseline pedalling at 10 W, subjects completed a 6 minute square wave transition maintaining 80 % of their predetermined VT work rate. Data intervals for RER SampEn analysis were matched to the data intervals selected for VO_2 kinetics evaluation by the UK research team. SampEn (m,r,N) is effectively a conditional probability: SampEn = -log A/B. Where B is the total number of matches of length m in a data series of length N. A is the total number of matches at length m+1 within the set of matches B. Data points within m and m +1 are said to match if they agree within a pre-selected tolerance r. A common value for r is 0.2(SD) where SD is the standard deviation of N (Richman and Moorman, 2000). Since SampEn is fundamentally a measure of the regularity or self-similarity of a data sequence, it is a measure without units.

8.2.3 Statistical analysis

All SampEn scores were calculated using Kubios HRV version 2 software (University of Kupio, Kupio, Finland). The SampEn analysis feature in Kubios has preset values of m = 2 and r = 0.2 SD. Although developed for heart rate analysis, the non linear analysis features in Kubios can be applied to other time series data as long as it has not been previously detrended (Tarvainen *et al.*, 2008).

Standard t-tests were used to examine mean differences between the trained (n = 11) and untrained (n = 9) for SampEn, average RER, BMI and peak VO_2 using the statistical program R, an open access software. All results are presented as means (SD). An alpha level of $P < 0.05$ was considered to be statistically significant.

8.3 RESULTS

The trained soccer players had significantly higher RER SampEn scores for the six minute steady state pedaling interval compared to the untrained girls (SampEn 0.914 [± 0.433] vs. 0.564 [± 0.139]; $P = 0.026$). For the trained group, SampEn scores ranged from 0.031 to 1.558 demonstrating large inter-individual differences within the trained group. The untrained group RER SampEn scores were more homogeneous ranging from 0.402-0.841.

Trained players had significantly higher peak VO_2 compared to untrained (peak VO_2 2.41 [± 0.37] L·min^{-1} vs. 1.86 [± 0.25] L·min^{-1}; $P < 0.05$).

The average RER during the 6 minute testing interval was calculated for each subject. For trained females the average RER was significantly lower than untrained females (average RER 0.935 [± 0.063] vs. 1.018 [± 0.041]; $P = 0.002$). The average RER during exercise was also heterogeneous within the trained group ranging from 0.856-1.039. The untrained group had a more homogeneous average RER.

There was no significant difference in body mass index (BMI) between the trained and untrained group (BMI 21.80 [± 2.34] vs. 20.45 [± 2.15] kg·m^{-2}; $P = 0.139$). Differences in averaged RER and relative fat oxidation during exercise are not explained by differences in BMI.

8.4 CONCLUSION

Soccer training significantly enhanced RER SampEn scores as predicted. As a group, trained females showed more variability and less self-similarity, in their sequential RER data during exercise. Trained subjects also exhibited higher peak VO_2 and lower average RER while pedalling indicating relatively more fat oxidation at 80 % of VT compared to untrained girls. This is consistent with previously reported effects of training (Jeukendrup and Wallis, 2005).

Yet, there is large inter-individual variability in both RER SampEn score and average RER for trained subjects. The variability in RER SampEn could be interpreted as a sign of poor reliability of this measure for evaluating a training effect. However, a study of trained cyclists showed large inter-individual differences with resting RERs ranging from 0.718-0.927 and the RER diversity remained with increasing exercise intensity (Goedecke $et\ al.$, 2000). Metabolic flexibility with exercise occurs on at least two levels. Within an individual there is metabolic flexibility in the blending of carbohydrate and fats to match intensity of energy expenditure with available substrates. Between individuals, with seemingly similar levels of training and performance, there also appears to be metabolic flexibility. For example, lean body mass, estimated physical activity level, peak VO_2, gender and fat mass together only accounted for 34 % of the variance in peak fat oxidation (Jeukendrup and Wallis, 2005).

The variability found in RER SampEn scores for trained soccer players may reflect dynamic differences in metabolic state or metabolic flexibility. The fine scale variability pattern may be a marker for the underlying complexity occurring in exercise metabolism. RER SampEn may be useful for distinguishing relative metabolic inflexibility and subsets of subjects who may not respond well to training. Future studies will be needed to investigate applications of the potential information in RER SampEn.

8.5 REFERENCES

Biltz, G.R, Harmon, J.H., Dengel, D.R., Unnithan, V.B., and Witten, G., 2009, RER variability analysis by sample entropy. In *Children and Exercise XXIV*, edited by Jurimae, T., Armstrong, N. and Jurimae, J., (Routledge, London, UK), pp. 51-54.

Corpeleijn, E., Saris, W.H.M. and Blaak, E.E., 2009, Metabolic flexibility in the development of insulin resistance in type 2 diabetes: Effects of lifestyle. *Obesity Reviews*, **10**, pp. 178-193.

Cottin, F., Medique, C., Lepretre, P-M., Papalier, Y., Koralsztein, J-P., and Billat, V., 2004, Heart rate variability during exercise performed below and above ventilatory threshold. *Medicine and Science in Sports and Exercise*, **36**, pp. 594-600.

Goedecke, J.H., St Clair Gibson, A., Groblier, L., Collins, M., Noakes, T.D. and Lambert, E.V., 2000, Determinants of the variability in respiratory exchange ratio at rest and during exercise in trained athletes. *American Journal of Physiology, Endrochronology, and Metabolism*, **279**, pp. E1325-E1334.

Jeukendrup, A.E. and Wallis, G.A., 2005, Measurement of substrate oxygen during exercise by means of gas exchange measurements. *International Journal of Sports Medicine*, **26**, pp. S28-S37.

Mandigout, S., Melin, A., Fauchier, L., N'Guyen, L.D., Courteix, D and Obert, P., 2002, Physical training increases heart rate variability in prepubertal children. *European Journal of Clinical Investigation*, **32**, pp. 479-487.

Richman, J.S. and Moorman, J.R., 2000, Physiological time series analysis using approximate entropy and sample entropy. *American Journal of Physiology Heart and Circulatory Physiology*, **278**, pp. H2039- H2049.

Seely, A.J.E. and Macklem, P.T., 2004, Complex systems and the technology of variability analysis. *Critical Care*, **8**, pp. R367-R384.

Tarvainen, M.P., Niskanen, J-P., Lipponen, J.A., Ranta-Aho, P.O. and Karjalainen, P.A., 2008, Kubios HRV – a software for advanced heart rate variability analysis. *IFMBE Proceedings*, **22**, pp. 1022-1025.

West, B. 2006, *Where Medicine Went Wrong: Studies of Nonlinear Phenomena in Life Science*, Vol.11, (Singapore: World Scientific Publishing Co.Pte. Ltd.)

EFFECT OF EXERCISE MODE ON FAT OXIDATION AND 'FATMAX' IN PRE- TO EARLY PUBERTAL GIRLS AND BOYS

K. Tolfrey and J.K. Zakrzewski

Loughborough University, UK

9.1 INTRODUCTION

Fatmax is the exercise intensity (% peak VO_2) that elicits the maximal fat oxidation (MFO) rate (Jeukendrup and Achten, 2001). Higher fat oxidation during treadmill compared with cycling exercise has been found consistently in adults (e.g., Capostagno and Bosch, 2010). However, similar findings in children are sparse (Lafortuna et al., 2010). Exercise mode comparisons of fat oxidation have used a small number of intensities corresponding to the exercise mode-specific peak (Mácek et al., 1976). However, peak VO_2 is typically 7 to 10 % higher for treadmill (TM) compared with cycling exercise (CE) in untrained individuals (Mácek et al., 1976). The higher absolute VO_2 during treadmill exercise may explain differences in fat oxidation between exercise modes. Therefore, a comparision of fat oxidation over a wide range of both relative and absolute exercise intensities is warranted. Cycling regularly at Fatmax might improve exercise fat oxidation and other health markers in young people (Ben Ounis et al., 2009). Walking or jogging may help to further optimise these effects through the recruitment of a larger active muscle mass and subsequent elevation of fat oxidation. However, we are not aware of studies that have compared Fatmax between treadmill and cycling exercise in children. To our knowledge, only one study has compared fat oxidation over a range of exercise intensities between treadmill and cycling in young people, but this study was limited to obese adolescent boys and Fatmax was not estimated (Lafortuna et al., 2010). Moreover, similar studies involving girls and non-obese children appear to be unavailable and the influence of puberty on fat oxidation must be considered (Riddell, 2008). Therefore, the aim of the present study was to compare fat oxidation and Fatmax over a range of intensities during treadmill and cycling exercise in pre- to early pubertal girls and boys.

9.2 METHODS

Complete data were available for 9 girls and 13 boys (mean (SD) age 9.9 ±0.8 y). Informed consent was provided for all participants. A self-assessment of pubic hair was used to estimate maturation. Following habituation, treadmill and cycling mode specific peak VO_2 and Fatmax (Zakrzewski and Tolfrey, 2011) were determined in a counter-balanced order. Respiratory gas exchange was measured continuously in all tests (Cortex Metalyzer 3B) and Fatmax was estimated after a 12 h overnight fast using standard respiratory gas exchange stoichiometric equations ($\leq$80 % peak VO_2; Romijn *et al.,* 1992). Diet and physical activity were replicated 24 h prior to each measurement. Fatmax (% peak VO_2), MFO (mg·min^{1}) and the 5 % Fatmax zone (range of intensities where fat oxidation rates were within 5 % of MFO) were estimated using individual 2nd order polynomial curves of fat oxidation rate against % peak VO_2. The HR corresponding to Fatmax was calculated using the relationship between % peak VO_2 and HR. Mean(SD) r^2 values for the polynomial curves of fat oxidation vs. % peak VO_2 were 0.74 (0.21) for TM and 0.71 (0.17) for CE.

9.2.1 Statistical analyses

SPSS software version 16.0 for Windows (SPSS Inc, Chicago, IL, USA) was used for all statistical analyses. Shapiro-Wilk tests and Levene's tests confirmed normal distribution and homogeneity of variance respectively. Separate 2 x 2 (mode by sex) mixed measures analysis of variance (ANOVA) repeated for mode were used to examine the data for fat oxidation, Fatmax, and Fatmax zone. Student's independent t-tests were used to compare anthropometric characteristics by sex. Pearson's product moment correlation analyses were used to examine bivariate relationships between Fatmax, MFO, Fatmax zone, peak VO_2 and anthropometric measures. Values are expressed as mean (SD) and effect sizes (ES) complement standard probability values where $P\leq0.05$ was considered to be statistically significant.

9.3 RESULTS

According to the self-assessment of pubic hair, five girls, but only three boys had entered puberty (Tanner stage 2) ($P=0.15$, ES 0.37). Treadmill peak VO_2 (mL·kg^{-1}·min^{-1}) was ~15 % higher than CE (ES 0.87), but this difference was independent of sex (ES 0.14). The boys' peak VO_2 values were higher than the girls by the same margin as the mode-related differences although the effect size was smaller (ES 0.53). Fat oxidation was higher for TM compared with CE at the same absolute ($P=0.01$, ES 0.54) and relative ($P<0.005$, ES 0.59 - Figure

9.1) exercise intensities. These exercise mode differences in fat oxidation were proportional to exercise intensity ($P<0.005$), but independent of sex ($P\geq0.50$).

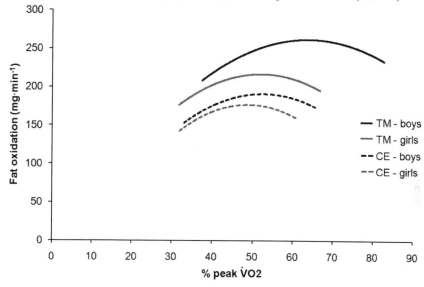

Figure 9.1. Fat oxidation was higher for boys compared with girls at the same relative ($P=0.04$, ES 0.45), but not absolute ($P=0.18$, ES 0.29) exercise intensities. Group mean values for parameters corresponding to Fatmax and maximal fat oxidation are in Table 9.1.

Table 9.1. Group comparisons of Fatmax and maximal fat oxidation for TM and CE

	Girls (n=9)		Boys (n=13)	
Fatmax	**TM**	**CE**	**TM**	**CE**
% peak VO$_2$ [a,b]	52(13)	49(8)	64(10)	53(5)
% HR max [a,c]	70(11)	67(8)	79(8)	67(6)
TM speed (km·h^{-1}) [b]	5.6(1.3)		7.2(1.4)	
CE work rate (W)		31(11)		40(10)
RPE [a]	12(3)	12(2)	12(3)	10(2)
5% Fatmax zone (%peakVO$_2$) [a,b]	20(6)	17(6)	26(6)	19(4)
MFO (mg·min^{-1}) [a]	217(60)	176(36)	262(61)	191(55)
MFO (mg·kgFFM^{-1}·min^{-1}) [a]	7.9(2.5)	6.4(1.6)	9.3(2.3)	6.9(2.4)

[a] between mode significant difference; [b] between sex significant difference; [c] sex by mode interaction ($P\leq0.05$). TM – treadmill, CE – cycle ergometer.

Fatmax (% peak VO_2) was higher for TM compared with CE (P=0.01, ES 0.57), but was independent of sex (P=0.12, ES 0.34). Fatmax was higher in the boys compared with girls (P=0.02, ES 0.50) and the difference was marked for TM (12 % peak VO_2) compared with CE (4 % peak VO_2). The RPE at Fatmax was higher for TM compared with CE (P=0.03, ES 0.47). Peak VO_2 explained 44 % of the variation in Fatmax for TM (r^2=0.44), but only 4 % for CE (r^2=0.04). The relationship between TM Fatmax and absolute MFO was strong (r^2=0.53), but only moderate for CE (r^2=0.28).

The 5 % Fatmax zone was wider for TM compared with CE ($P \leq 0.005$, ES 0.62) and the sex by exercise mode interaction was not meaningful (P=0.25, ES 0.25). The 5 % Fatmax zone extended over a greater range of exercise intensities in the boys compared with the girls (P=0.02, ES 0.49). There was a moderate correlation between Fatmax zone and peak VO_2 for TM (r^2=0.20), but not CE (r^2=0.03).

9.4 CONCLUSION

The main finding from the present study was that fat oxidation was higher during treadmill compared with cycling exercise over a range of absolute and relative exercise intensities in pre- to early pubertal girls and boys. This indicates that the higher fat oxidation during TM exercise was not due to a higher absolute VO_2 during this exercise mode. We also reported that the higher fat oxidation during treadmill compared with cycling exercise was more pronounced at higher exercise intensities, a finding that is also in agreement with previous work in adults (Achten et al., 2003), but appears to be a novel finding in young people. Furthermore, fat oxidation remained high (within 5 % of MFO) over a wider range of intensities for treadmill exercise and Fatmax was higher for treadmill compared with cycling exercise. Collectively, this suggests that walking or jogging exercise is preferential for fat oxidation in pre- to early pubertal children.

9.5 REFERENCES

Achten, J., Venables, M.C. and Jeukendrup, A.E., 2003, Fat oxidation rates are higher during running compared with cycling over a wide range of intensities. *Metabolism*, **52**, pp. 747-752.

Ben Ounis, O., Elloumi, M., Amri, M., Trabelsi, Y., Lac, G. and Tabka, Z., 2009, Impact of training and hypocaloric diet on fat oxidation and body composition in obese adolescents. *Science in Sports*, **24**, pp. 178-185.

Capostagno, B. and Bosch, A., 2010, Higher fat oxidation in running than cycling at the same exercise intensities. *International Journal of Sport Nutrition and Exercise Metabolism*, **20**, pp. 44-55.

Jeukendrup, A.E. and Achten, J., 2001, Fatmax: A new concept to optimize fat oxidation during exercise? *European Journal of Sport Science*, **1**, pp. 1-5.

Lafortuna, C.L., Lazzer, S., Agosti, F., Busti, C., Galli, R., Mazzilli, G. and Sartorio, A., 2010, Metabolic responses to submaximal treadmill walking and cycle ergometer pedalling in obese adolescents. *Scandinavian Journal of Medicine and Science in Sports*, **20**, pp. 630-637.

Mácek, M., Vávra, J. and Novosadová, J., 1976, Prolonged exercise in prepubertal boys. I. Cardiovascular and metabolic adjustment. *European Journal of Applied Physiology and Occupational Physiology*, **35**, pp. 291-298.

Riddell, M.C., 2008, The endocrine response and substrate utilization during exercise in children and adolescents. *Journal of Applied Physiology*, **105**, pp. 725-733.

Romijn, J.A., Coyle, E.F., Hibbert, J. and Wolfe, R.R., 1992, Comparison of indirect calorimetry and a new breath 13C/12C ratio method during strenuous exercise. *American Journal of Physiology*, **263**, pp. E64-E71.

Zakrzewski, J.K. and Tolfrey, K., 2011, Exercise protocols to estimate fatmax and maximal fat oxidation in children. *Pediatric Exercise Science*, **23**, pp. 122-135.

PREFRONTAL CORTEX OXYGENATION AND MUSCLE OXYGENATION DURING INCREMENTAL EXERCISE IN CHILDREN: A NEAR-INFRARED SPECTROSCOPY STUDY

M. Luszczyk[1], S. Kujach[1], R.A. Olek[2], R. Laskowski[1], and A. Szczesna-Kaczmarek[1]

[1]Department of Physiology, [2]Department of Biochemistry, Jedrzej Sniadecki Academy of Physical Education and Sport in Gdansk, Poland

10.1 INTRODUCTION

Cerebral function depends on an uninterrupted oxygen (O_2) delivery. The cerebral O_2 reserve is low as illustrated by the immediate loss of consciousness with arrested cerebral blood flow (CBF) since the effect cannot be explained by depletion of intermediary metabolites. The exercise would improve brain function by increasing cerebral blood volume, however, the exact mechanisms are still unknown (Rasmussen *et al.*, 2007). The advances in neuroimaging techniques have made it possible to investigate changes in the brain. It brought more understanding about cerebral activation processes, due to the close coupling of neural activity and brain metabolism, which accompany changes in cerebral blood flow (Timinkul *et al.*, 2008).

The prefrontal lobe was chosen as it has been previously studied during exercise (Bhambhani *et al.*, 2007), and has shown a linear relationship between frontal lobe oxygenation and exercise intensity in healthy subjects (Ide and Secher, 2000). Exhaustive exercise provoked cerebral deoxygenating, metabolic changes and indices of fatigue similar to those observed during exercise in hypoxia indicating that reduced cerebral oxygenation may play a role in the development of central fatigue and may be an exercise capacity limiting factor (Rasmussen *et al.*, 2010). To date, several studies have used near-infrared spectroscopy (NIRS) to examine alterations in cerebral oxygenation (Bhambhani *et al.*, 2007) and muscle oxygenation (Binzoni *et al.*, 2010) during incremental exercise. Timinkul *et al.* (2008) mention that during incremental cycling, cerebral oxygenation showed a non-linear behaviour with its threshold (CBVT) existing at a mild exercise intensity prior to the lactate threshold (LT). Their presented results suggest that cerebral blood volume (CBV) of the frontal cortex could be increased even with exercise below the LT, which with further investigation might be available in exercise prescription targeting brain haemodynamic improvement. Bhambhani *et al.* (2007) reported that the systemic decline in cerebral oxygenation measured by NIRS above the respiratory compensation threshold (RCT-NIRS) with high correlation to end-tidal carbon dioxide pressure ($PETCO_2$), could limit maximal exercise capacity by reducing neuronal activation. NIRS data has shown a correlation between muscle deoxygenation and blood lactate concentration and it has previously been suggested that NIRS can be used to determine the LT (Beaver *et al.*, 1986).

By identifying particular trends in the rate and extent of muscle deoxygenation these authors have shown a correlation with gas exchange methods of measuring the LT. One possibility of the physiological basis underpinning the increased rate of deoxygenation correspondents to the LT is that this is the point where the blood pH falls and the Bohr Effect causes the further release of oxygen from haemoglobin. This would mean that there was a physiological mechanism underpinning the correlation between the NIRS and the invasive blood lactate measurements of the anaerobic threshold, giving one confidence that the method might be applicable to a wide range of individuals of differing fitness levels (Angus *et al.*, 1999). The formal comparison of NIRS-derived oxygenation indexes and blood lactate concentration [La_b] or with some other parameters often employed to determine the LT has been performed during incremental exercise in adults. There are very few published data on the issue in healthy paediatric populations (Moalla *et al.*, 2005; Leclair *et al.*, 2010).

The aim of this study was to fill this gap. More specifically, we intended to evaluate whether, during a standard incremental exercise conducted on a cycle ergometer, indices of prefrontal cortex oxygenation and muscle oxygenation obtained by NIRS were associated with often employed parameters to determine the LT. Furthermore, we tested the hypothesis that the cerebral blood volume threshold (CBVT) and muscle blood volume threshold (MBVT) predicted the ventilatory anaerobic threshold (VAT).

To address this issue, we used a graded exercise protocol where healthy subjects pedalled a cycle ergometer with incrementally increasing intensity until volitional fatigue, simultaneously monitoring respired air, cerebral oxygenation in the prefrontal area and changes in muscle oxygenation patterns with respect to VAT in response to the graded cycling exercise.

10.2 METHODS

10.2.1 Subjects

Ten healthy right-handed boys (mean SD: 15.9 ± 1.39 y old; 13.7 ± 8.47 % FAT; 53.7 ± 10.6 kg FFM^{-1}; 62.1 ± 9.42 kg body mass; 1.75 ± 9.43 m stature; 49.3 ± 8.88 $mL \cdot min^{-1} \cdot kg^{-1}$ peak VO_2) volunteered and gave informed written consent to participate in this study. All subjects were well-trained competitive table tennis players (7.9 ± 1.1 y of training, 4.7 $h \cdot wk^{-1}$), had no history of cardiovascular, respiratory, endocrinological, musculoskeletal or neurological disorders, and were free of medication. Subjects were requested to refrain from training for the 12 h preceding the test on the 2 days prior to testing. Before the beginning of the study, ethical approval of procedures and the informed consent of both the children and their parents were obtained.

10.2.2 Study protocol

All testing was performed on an electrically braked cycle ergometer (Jaeger VIAsprintTM 150P/200P, Germany). The test aimed to determine maximal oxygen uptake (VO_{2max}) and VAT. The participants were allowed to sit quietly on the cycle ergometer for a while to relax prior to a 2 min resting period to collect baseline cardiorespiratory and NIRS measurements. Subjects performed a 5 min warm-up at 1.5 $W \cdot kg^{-1}$. The test consisted of a ramp exercise test to exhaustion to determine their VO_{2max} using a ramp rate of 25 $W \cdot min^{-1}$. During all tests, the children were instructed to maintain a cycling cadence of 55 rpm. Subjects were rested in sitting position during 5 min of recovery period. Oxygen uptake was determined on-line from breath-by-breath ventilation and metabolic gas exchange measurements (Oxycon Pro Jaeger, Viasys, Germany) and averaged in 20 s intervals using customized STATISTICA 9 software. Heart rate was monitored continuously by telemetry (Polar Monitors, Electro, Kempele, Finland).

10.2.3 Criteria for establishing ventilatory anaerobic threshold (VAT)

The estimated VAT was determined as the VO_2 at which CO_2 production (VCO_2) began to increase out of proportion in relation to VO_2, along with a systematic rise in the $VE \cdot VO_2^{-1}$ ratio and $P_{ET}O_2$, whereas $VE \cdot VCO_2^{-1}$ and $P_{ET}CO_2$ were stable (Beaver et al., 1986; Amann et al., 2004).

10.2.4 Criteria for establishing VO_{2max}

It was judged that subjects had reached VO_{2max} when three or more of the following criteria were obtained: an inability to maintain the required pedalling cadence, a maximal heart rate > 90 % of predicted maximal heart rate (220-age), a plateau in VO_2 despite increasing power (VO_2 change < 2.0 mL·kg^{-1}·min^{-1}), and a final respiratory exchange ratio (RER) higher than 1.0 (Welsman and Armstrong, 1996).

10.2.5 NIRS measurement and determination of cerebral blood volume threshold (CBVT) and muscle blood volume threshold (MBVT)

A first pair of optodes (a light emitter and a detector) from channel-1 NIRS system (NIRO 200, Hamamatsu Photonics KK, Japan) was placed over the left frontal lobe (1 cm above the eyebrow and 1 cm to the left of the skull centre) (Bhambhani *et al.*, 2007) of the subjects for cerebral hemodynamic monitoring. The second optical source and detector from channel-2 NIRS system were positioned on the medial line of the right vastus lateralis along the vertical axis of the thigh, one third of the distance from the lateral epicondyle to the greater trochanter of the femur (Binzoni *et al.*, 2010). In the present study we set the two differential path length factor (DPF) to measure the haemoglobin concentration and expressed as a change from baseline concentration (arbitrary unit, a.u.). One of them at 5.9 (the average PDF for an adult head, not the precise one) (van der Zee *et al.*, 1992; Timinkul *et al.*, 2008). The second at 4.0 for muscle tissue oxygenation. All detection channels were used with an interoptode distance of L = 4.0 cm. Each of the probes were fixed in place by using a dense black rubber vinyl holder and a piece of black plastic wrap that also eliminated any incidental room light and was held in place using double adhesive tape and a tensor bandage. The sensor was calibrated to zero at rest. Real time data was recorded online at 1 Hz and averaged in 20 s intervals using customized STATISTICA 9 software. To calculate the CBVT and MBVT points, we plotted a graph of the 20 s averaged data and calculated the linear lines. The inflection point in cerebral measurement was considered as CBVT (Timinkul *at al.*, 2008). The inflection point in muscle measurement was considered as MBVT.

10.2.6 Statistical analysis

All data were grouped from all subjects to form a single data set for analysis. Analysis was conducted at five different time points: rest, CBVT, MBVT, VT, and all-out exercise stages. Statistical analysis was performed using data analysis software system STATISTICA 9 (StatSoft Inc., 2009). A one-way analysis of variance was performed to test the difference among the four stages. Student-Newman-Keul's test was utilized to determine when differences occurred. The correlation between variables was tested using Pearson's correlation. The alpha level was set at $P{\leq}0.05$ and data are presented as means and standard deviation (SD).

10.3 RESULTS

The cerebral and muscle haemodynamic parameters, namely, HHb, tHb were all increased with differences in rate and pattern in response to the increasing work rate. Overall responsive cerebral and muscle oxygenation showed a non-linear pattern with three distinct phases of the exercise test. The CBVT and MBVT, an event where rapid oxygenation takes place, occurred at approximately 57 % and 65 % of the VO_{2max}. The CBVT and MBVT preceded the VAT, which was at approximately 79 % of the VO_{2max}. We found a strong positive correlation ($P{<}0.05$) between the three methods for all variables. Correlation coefficient for VO_2 ($r{=}0.77$ CBVT, $r{=}0.85$ MBVT), $PETCO_2$ ($r{=}0.98$ CBVT, $r{=}0.99$ MBVT), VE ($r{=}0.72$ CBVT, $r{=}0.70$ MBVT), $O_2{\cdot}HR^{-1}$ ($r{=}$ 0.96 CBVT and MBVT). Decrease of tissue oxygenation index (TOI) in muscle was significantly higher than in cerebral. Furthermore, there was a negative correlation between muscle TOI and work rate ($r{=}{-}0.79$; $P{\leq}0.05$). The change in HbO_2 during exercise at the prefrontal cortex was positively correlated with work rate ($r{=}0.43$; $P \leq0.05$). However, before all-out exercise, it began to decrease gradually. The systemic decline in cerebral oxygenation could limit maximal exercise capacity by reducing neuronal activation. The change in HbO_2 at the muscle was negatively correlated with work rate ($r{=}{-}0.25$; $P \leq0.05$). There was no change in cerebral and muscle HHb in warm-up period prior to a gradual increase. Where power was systematically increased the HHb systematically increased too. Muscle HHb was reached earlier in comparison to cortex HHb.

10.4 CONCLUSION

Our results confirm that the oxygenation of the prefrontal cortex increases during graded cycling even at exercise intensities below the VAT, suggesting the potential role of mild exercise in enhancing cerebral blood volume.

The correlations obtained between VAT and CBVT, MBVT indicate that the anaerobic metabolism solicitation occurs simultaneously in both respiratory muscles and peripheral muscles as a result of deoxygenation. Furthermore, this investigation showed a close agreement between VAT and

CBVT, MBVT and validates the use of NIRS as a noninvasive tool for the determination of VAT.

10.5 REFERENCES

Amann, M., Subudhi, A.W., Walker, J., Eisenman, P., Shultz, B. and Foster, C., 2004, An evaluation of the predictive validity and reliability of ventilatory threshold. *Medicine and Science in Sports and Exercise*, **36**, pp. 1716-1722.

Angus, C., Welford, D., Sellens, M., Thompson, S. and Cooper, C.E., 1999, Estimation of lactate threshold by near infrared spectroscopy. *Advances in Experimental Medicine and Biology*, **471**, pp. 283-288.

Beaver, W.L., Wasssermann, K. and Whipp, B.J., 1986, A new method for detecting anaerobic threshold by gas exchange. *Journal of Applied Physiology*, **60**, pp. 2020-2027.

Bhambhani, Y., Malik, R., Mookerjee, S. 2007, Cerebral oxygenation declines at exercise intensities above the respiratory compensation threshold. *Respiratory Physiology and Neurobiology*, 156, pp. 196–202.

Binzoni, T., Cooper, C.E., Wittekind, A.L., Beneke, R., Elwell, C.E., Van De Ville, D. and Leung, T.S., 2010, A new method to measure local oxygen consumption in human skeletal muscle during dynamic exercise using near-infrared spectroscopy. *Physiological Measurement*, **31**, pp. 1257-1269.

Ide, K. and Secher, N.H., 2000, Cerebral blood flow and metabolism during exercise. *Progress in Neurobiology*, **61**, pp. 397-414.

Leclair, E., Borel, B., Baquet, G., Berthoin, S., Mucci, P., Thevenet, D. and Reguem, S.C., 2010, Reproducibility of measurement of muscle deoxygenation in children during exercise. *Pediatric Exercise Science*, **22**, pp.183-194.

Moalla, W., Dupont, G., Berthoin, S. and Ahmaidi, S., 2005, Respiratory muscle deoxygenation and ventilatory threshold assessments using near infrared spectroscopy in children. *International Journal of Sports Medicine*, **26**, pp. 576-582.

Rasmussen, P., Dawson, E.A., Nybo, L., van Lieshout, J.J., Secher, N.H. and Gjedde, A., 2007, Capillary-oxygenation-level-dependent near-infrared spectrometry in frontal lobe of humans. *Journal of Cerebral Blood Flow and Metabolism,* **27**, pp. 1082-1093.

Rasmussen, P., Nielsen, J., Overgaard, M., Krogh-Madsen, R., Gjedde, A., Secher, N.H. and Petersen, N.C., 2010, Reduced muscle activation during exercise related to brain oxygenation and metabolism in humans. *Journal of Physiology*, **1588**, pp. 1985-1995.

StatSoft, Inc. 2009, STATISTICA (data analysis software system), version 9.0, www.statsoft.com.

Timinkul, A., Kato, M., Omori, T., Deocaris, C.C., Ito, A., Kizuka, T., Sakairi, Y., Nishijima, T., Asada, T. and Soya, H., 2008, Enhancing effect of cerebral blood volume by mild exercise in healthy young men: A near-infrared spectroscopy study. *Neuroscience Research*, **61**, pp. 242-248.

van der Zee, P., Cope, M., Arridge, S.R., Essenpreis, M., Potter, L.A., Edwards, A.D., Wyatt, J.S., McCormick, D.C., Roth, S.C., Reynolds, E.O. and Delpy, D.T., 1992, Experimentally measured optical pathlengths for the adult head, calf and forearm and the head of the newborn infant as a function of inter optode spacing. *Advances in Experimental Medicine and Biology*, **316**, pp. 143-153.

Welsman, J.R. and Armstrong, N., 1996, The measurement and interpretation of aerobic fitness in children: current issues. *Journal of the Royal Society of Medicine*, **89**, pp. 281–285.

CHAPTER NUMBER 11

COMPARATIVE ANALYSIS OF QUADRICEPS ENDURANCE DURING SUSTAINED SUBMAXIMAL ISOMETRIC CONTRACTIONS IN CHILDREN AND ADULTS

A. Bouchant[1], A. Abdelmoula[1], V. Martin[1], C. Lavet[1],
C.A. Williams[2], and S. Ratel[1]

[1]Laboratory of Exercise Biology (BAPS, EA 3533), UFR STAPS, University of Blaise Pascal, Clermont-Ferrand, France, [2]Children's Health and Exercise Research Centre, University of Exeter, Exeter, UK

11.1 INTRODUCTION

Although it has been previously shown that children's exercise performance improves with age (Ratel *et al.*, 2009), it is still unknown whether this enhanced performance level throughout growth could be ascribed to changes in muscle endurance.

Few studies have investigated endurance abilities and neuromuscular responses during sustained contractions in healthy children as compared with young adults and subsequent results have been found to be controversial. For example, during a sustained isometric plantar flexion exercise for 10 min at 20 % of Maximal Voluntary Contraction (MVC), Hatzikotoulas *et al.* (2009) showed that boys displayed the same levels of fatigue as men (*i.e.* the surface electromyogram increased gradually to a similar extent in both groups). In contrast, Halin *et al.* (2003) showed a higher level of fatigue in men compared to boys during a maximal 30 s isometric contraction of *biceps brachii*. Maximal strength and electromyographic signals declined significantly more in men than in boys. These conflicting results could be related to differences in the specificities of the muscles studied and the intensity of exercise.

Therefore, the purpose of this study was to compare quadriceps endurance time during submaximal contractions until exhaustion between children and adults as a function of exercise intensity.

11.2 METHODS

11.2.1 Participants

Twelve boys (8.9 ± 0.8 y) and 24 men (24.2 ± 4.5 y) volunteered to participate in the study. None of participants were involved in any regular or specific competitive training programme.

11.2.2 Protocol

Body mass was measured to the nearest 0.1 kg using a calibrated electronic scale (Seca, model 873 Omega, France) and stature to the nearest 0.01 m using a standing stadiometre (Seca, model 720, Hamburg, Germany). Triceps and subscapular skinfolds thickness were measured in order to estimate body fat (%) using the equations of Slaughter *et al.* (1988).

All participants were tested on a home-built ergometer dedicated to measure isometric strength of the dominant quadriceps. After a standardized warm-up, all participants completed three isometric MVC separated by a passive 3-min rest. The isometric MVC was determined as the best trial among three reproducible measurements. Force output was measured using a calibrated force transducer (0- to 100-daN force range, Scaime Company, France) connected to an ankle cuff and transmitted to a PC using an analog/digital converter (Phoenix contact Typ UEGM). Afterwards, the participants performed sustained isometric contractions until exhaustion at 25 %, 50 % and 75 % MVC. Trials were presented in a randomized order and separated by a passive 20-min rest. The time to task failure (TTF) was recorded for each trial. Verbal encouragement and visual feedback were provided throughout each exercise to promote maximal efforts.

11.2.3 EMG data

Electromyographic signals (EMG) of the superficial heads of quadriceps (*vastus lateralis, vastus medialis* and *rectus femoris*) were recorded during the maximal voluntary contractions and throughout each time trial. EMG was quantified in the time and frequency domains using the Root Mean Square (RMS) value and the Mean Power Frequency (MPF), respectively. Maximal RMS value (RMS_{max}) was recorded during MVC trials. Furthermore, all the RMS values recorded during submaximal contractions were normalized as a percentage of RMS_{max} of the best MVC trial for each muscle.

11.2.4 Statistical analysis

All values are reported as mean (SD). Data were analysed using Statview Software (StatView SE+ Graphics®, Abacus Concepts, Inc.). Unpaired samples t-tests were used to compare the anthropometrical measures and TTF values between children and adults. The time course of EMG signals during each test was analysed as a function of age using a repeated measures ANOVA. When ANOVA were significant, comparisons between groups were made with a *post-hoc* Tukey-Kramer test. The limit for statistical significance was set a priori at $P<0.05$.

11.3 RESULTS

The men were significantly taller and heavier than the boys (176.8 ± 6.7 cm vs. 133.5 ± 6.1 cm; 74.7 ± 9.4 kg vs. 29.4 ± 4.9 kg, respectively; $P<0.001$). However, the percentage of body fat was similar in boys and men (15.5 ± 3.6 % vs. 15.2 ± 3.7 %, respectively). MVC torque was lower in boys as compared to men (83.9 ± 24.0 N·m *vs.* 368.2 ± 76.0 N·m, respectively; $P<0.001$). No significant difference was observed in TTF values at 25, 50 and 75 % MVC between boys and men (Fig. 11.1a). However, it is worth noting that the mean TTF of boys at 25 % MVC was 43 seconds higher than men's, which represented 28 % of men's TTF and 22 % of boys' (Fig. 11.1b). Overall, data variability was higher in boys.

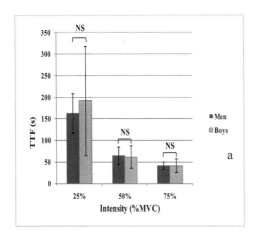 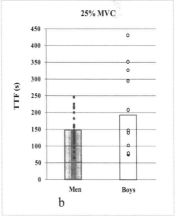

Figure 11.1. Comparison of time to task failure (TTF) values between children and adults **(a)**, and individual TTF values distribution at 25 % MVC in both groups **(b)**.

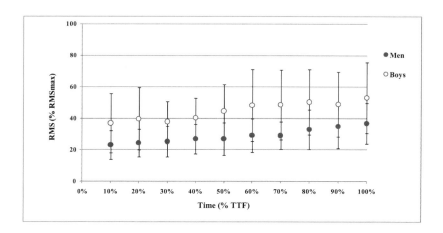

Figure 11.2. Time course of RMS values at 25 % MVC in boys and men for the *vastus medialis*

Similar EMG changes were observed throughout each time trial in both groups. Whilst a significant decline in MPF was associated with a significant increase in RMS for *vastii* (see Fig. 11.2 for the *vastus medialis* at 25 % MVC), no significant change in EMG signals was observed for the *rectus femoris*.

11.4 CONCLUSION

The results of the present study show that 1) muscle endurance during sustained isometric tasks did not differ between children and adults, whatever the intensity of exercise; 2) fatigue-induced changes in muscle activation patterns are independent of age.

On this basis, it could be suggested that muscle endurance may not be a limiting factor in the children's lower exercise performance in the low-to-moderate intensity domain as compared to adults. However, it is worth noting that the time to task failure at 25 % MVC tended to be longer in the boys than in the men and the variability of the individual measurements was larger in the boys. This finding could be attributed to psychological factors, such as motivation, and/or differences in the implication of central factors during sustained low-intensity exercises between children and adults.

Further research with a larger cohort of children is therefore required to ascertain whether or not muscle endurance is similar during exhausting low-intensity contractions between children and adults. Furthermore, additional measurements of muscle oxygenation by near-infrared spectroscopy should be made as a function of exercise intensity to ascertain to what extent the level of ischaemia induced by contraction intensity could account for muscle endurance in children and adults.

11.5 REFERENCES

Halin, R., Germain, P., Bercier, S., Kapitaniak, B., and Buttelli, O., 2003, Neuromuscular response of young boys versus men during sustained maximal contraction. *Medicine and Science in Sports and Exercise*, **35**, pp. 1042-1048.

Hatzikotoulas, K., Patikas, D., Bassa, E., Hadjileontiadis, L., Koutedakis, Y., and Kotzamanidis, C., 2009, Submaximal fatigue and recovery in boys and men. *International Journal of Sports Medicine*, **30**, pp. 741-746.

Ratel, S., Duché, P., and Williams, C.A., 2009, Muscle fatigue in children. In *Human Muscle Fatigue*, edited by Williams, C.A., and Ratel, S. (London: Routledge), pp. 79-102.

Slaughter, M. H., Lohman, T. G., Boileau, R. A., Horswill, C. A., Stillman, R. J., Van Loan, M. D., and Bemben, D. A., 1988, Skinfold equations for estimation of body fatness in children and youth. *Human Biology*, **60**, pp. 709-723.

HEAT SENSATION OF OBESE AND NON-OBESE PUBESCENT BOYS DURING CYCLING AND RECOVERY IN THE HEAT

P.L. Sehl, G.T. Leites, J.B. Martins, G.S. Cunha, and F. Meyer
Federal University of Rio Grande do Sul, UFRGS, Porto Alegre, Brazil

12.1 INTRODUCTION

Adherence to physical activity programmes for obese children is consensual and therefore their perceptual responses during and after physical activities in warm environments should be elucidated to ensure their enjoyment, well-being, and safety.

Few studies (Haymes *et al.,* 1974, 1975; Dougherty *et al.,* 2009, 2010) have investigated the responses of obese children and adolescents during exercise in the heat. Dougherty *et al.* (2009, 2010) showed that obese boys who live in temperate climate had higher heat sensation and ratings of perceived exertion (RPE) compared to their non-obese peers when they exercised at similar relative intensities (% VO_{2max}). But, in these studies the obese group also had lower aerobic fitness. To clarify whether adiposity is related to perceptual responses during exercise in the heat, it is necessary to compare obese and non-obese groups with similar aerobic conditioning. It is also unknown if the heat sensation difference is only during exercise or if it persists during the recovery period. Another aspect to consider is the level of heat acclimatization of the children and whether responses would be affected by the fact that the children already live in a tropical and predominantly warm environment.

The purpose of this study was to compare heat sensation and RPE between obese and non-obese pubescent boys during cycling and heat sensation after cycling in the same warm conditions.

12.2 METHODS

Seventeen obese (BMI=29.4 ± 4.3 $kg \cdot m^{-2}$) and 16 non-obese (BMI=16.8 ± 1.7 $kg \cdot m^{-2}$), boys classified according to BMI percentile as ≥95th and <85th respectively by Centers for Disease Control and Prevention (Kuczmarski *et al.,* 2000) participated in this study. Each subject gave his verbal consent and a parent/guardian signed the written consent. The study was approved by the University Ethics Committee. Experiments took place during the warm months of January through April in the South of Brazil (28-42°C and 40-95 % relative humidity (RH)). All boys performed at least 400 min of outdoors activities per week (i.e. cycling, soccer, basketball and athletics) apart from their regular school physical education classes.

12.2.1 Preliminary session

The boys came to the laboratory for the following evaluations: 1) health history, 2) physical activity practices, 3) maturational stage (self-reported, according to Tanner), 4) anthropometry (stature, body mass), and 5) peak VO_2 using the McMaster protocol (Bar-Or and Rowland, 2004) and indirect calorimetry (open circuit O_2 and CO_2 analyser Medigraphics CPX/D, breath by breath). Peak VO_2 was also expressed using allometry (Armstrong and Welsman, 2000).

12.2.2 Experimental session

Approximately 24-72 h after the preliminary session, the boys cycled (ERGO FIT 167, Spain, 5 W) in the heat (35°C, 40-45 % RH) in an environmental chamber (Russells, Holland) for 30 min at 50-60 % of their peak VO_2. The boys were instructed to keep the cadence of 60-70 rpm during the session. The mean pedaling work rate (in watts) was similar (P=0.15) between the obese (86.7 ± 21.9) and non-obese (76.6 ± 16.2) groups. To check the target exercise intensity, VO_2 was measured (Medigraphics model CPX/D) for 3 min from the 15th to 18th min of cycling. After cycling, they were observed sitting at rest in the chamber for 30 min at the same environmental conditions.

Heat sensation was measured at the start (minute zero), at the middle (minute 15) and at the end (minute 30) of exercise and at minutes 15 and 30 of recovery. We used a horizontal 10 cm analog scale with anchor points zero (not hot), middle point 5 (hot), and 10 (extremely hot). RPE (6-20 scale; Borg, 1970) was recorded every 5 min of cycling and HR (Polar model S610) was recorded every 5 min during cycling and recovery. The cycling lasted 30 min or less if one of these termination criteria was reached: HR>195 b·min^{-1}; symptoms of nausea, headache, dizziness; or if two of the following criteria were present: request to stop, failure to keep cadence (≤50 rpm), and RPE>19.

12.2.3 Statistical analysis

Data showed normal distribution and results were described as mean (SD). Two way ANOVA was used to compare heat sensation, RPE and HR between the groups over the time, and independent t test to compare groups at specific moments. When there was an interaction group $vs.$ time, ANOVA of repeated measures (1 factor) and Bonferroni post hoc was used to locate intragroup differences. The level of significance was set at $P<0.05$.

12.3 RESULTS

Of all 33 pubescent boys, 12 obese and 12 non-obese were in Tanner stage 2, five obese were in stage 3, and 4 non-obese in stage 4. Obese and non-obese were similar in age (12.7 ± 1.6 and 13.0 ± 1.4 y, respectively; $P=0.545$) and stature (158.2 ± 8.4 and 153 ± 10.7 cm, respectively; $P=0.131$). Peak VO_2 was similar between groups (295.2 ± 48.9 and 313 ± 36.52 mL·kg^{-050}·min^{-1}; $P=0.247$), as well as maximal work rate (182 ± 55 and 161 ± 44.6 W; $P=0.231$) and HR$_{max}$ (185 ± 13.1 and 185 ± 10.8 b·min^{-1}; $P=0.914$).

Two obese boys (Tanner stage 2) stopped pedalling at the 10th min of cycling: one was feeling dizzy and reached HR>195 b·min^{-1}; and the other requested to stop due to a headache and they were excluded from analyses. The % allometric VO_2 measured in the middle of the 30 min-cycling was similar ($P=0.230$) in the obese (51.6 ± 3 %) and non-obese (53.3 ± 4 %) boys.

Heat sensation was higher in obese than non-obese boys at the start (3.6 ± 2.7 $vs.$ 1.3 ± 1.4 cm; $P=0.008$), at the middle (6.7 ± 1.2 $vs.$ 4.1 ± 1.5 cm; $P=0.001$) and at the end (7.6 ± 2 $vs.$ 5.2 ± 2.2 cm; $P=0.003$) of exercise. The increased rate (or magnitude) over time did not differ between groups ($F_{(2,28)}=0.051$; $P=0.950$; Power=0.057). During recovery, heat sensation was similar between obese and non-obese at each 5 min (minutes $0 = 5.7 \pm 2.9$ and 5.2 ± 2.2 cm, $P=0.651$; $15 = 1.9 \pm 1.5$ and 2.2 ± 1.2 cm, $P=0.570$; and $30 = 1.2 \pm 1.5$ and 1.9 ± 1.6 cm, $P=0.571$) and over the 30 min ($F_{(2,27)}=0.689$; $P =0.511$).

During cycling, there was no interaction between group and time in RPE ($F_{(6,24)}=1.036$; $P=0.427$), being similar in obese and non-obese boys in minute 5 (10 ± 1 and 9 ± 2), minute 10 (12 ± 1.5 and 11 ± 3) minute 15 (14 ± 2 and 12 ± 3) and minute 20 (15 ± 2 and 13 ± 3). Nevertheless, RPE was higher in the obese boys at minutes 25 (17 ± 2 vs. 14 ± 3; $P=0.040$) and 30 (17 ± 3 vs. 15 ± 3; $P=0.019$).

The initial and final HR was similar ($P=0.226$ and $P=0.680$) in obese (93 ± 9 and 169 ± 14 b·min^{-1}) and non-obese (87 ± 16 to 167 ± 13 b·min^{-1}) boys. During cycling, HR responses showed interaction between group and time ($F_{(6,23)}=3.481$; $P=0.014$; Power=0.870). Until the 15th minute of cycling, the magnitude of HR increase was not so high in the obese compared to the non-obese boys, and thereafter it became more prominent. However, HR was similar at each 5 min of measurement. Both groups showed similar reductions in HR along the 30 min recovery ($F_{(6, 23)}=1.125$; $P=0.379$; Power=0.352).

12.4 CONCLUSION

In the present study, the higher heat sensation of the obese boys was restricted to the exercise period, and RPE was also higher in the obese towards the end of the exercise.

Therefore, checking obese boys for their heat sensation while they exercise in the heat may be useful to ensure their enjoyment and well-being, which are key factors for adherence to a physical activity programme. These responses apply to heat-acclimatized obese boys who practice physical activities in the heat, and might have even more impact to those who are not-acclimatized and/or sedentary. Further investigations should clarify whether a higher heat sensation of obese boys during exercise is related to thermoregulatory factors.

12.5 REFERENCES

Armstrong, N. and Welsman, J.R., 2000, Development of aerobic fitness during childhood and adolescence. *Pediatric Exercise Science*, **12**, pp.128-149.

Bar-Or, O. and Rowland, T.W., 2004, *Pediatric Exercise Medicine: From Physiologic Principles to Health Care Application*. (Champaign, IL: Human Kinetics), pp.69-101.

Borg, G., 1970, Perceived exertion as an indicator of somatic stress, *Journal of Rehabilitation Medicine*, **2**, pp.92-98.

Dougherty, K.A., Chow, M. and Kenney, L., 2009, Responses of lean and obese boys to repeated summer exercise in the heat bouts. *Medicine and Science in Sports and Exercise*, **41**, pp.279-289.

Dougherty, K.A., Chow, M. and Kenney, W.L., 2010, Critical environmental limits for exercising heat-acclimated lean and obese boys. *European Journal of Applied Physiology*, **108**, pp.779-789.

Haymes, E.M., Buskirk, E.R., Hodgson, J.L., Lundegren H.M. and Nicholas, W.C., 1974, Heat tolerance of exercising lean and heavy prepubertal girls. *Journal of Applied Physiology*, **36**, pp.566-571.

Haymes, E.M., McCormick, R.J. and Bursirk, E.R., 1975, Heat tolerance of exercising lean and heavy prepubertal boys. *Journal of Applied Physiology*, **39**, pp.457-461.

Kuczmarski, R.J., Ogden C.L., Grummer-Strawn, L.M., Flegal, K.M., Guo, S.S., Wei, R., Mei, Z., Curtin, L.R., Roche, A.F. and Johnson, C.L., 2000, CDC growth charts: United States. *Advances in Data*, **8**, pp.1-27.

ABILITY OF MILK TO REPLACE FLUID LOSSES IN CHILDREN AFTER EXERCISE IN THE HEAT

K. Volterman, J. Obeid, B. Wilk, and B.W. Timmons
Child Health and Exercise Medicine Program
Department of Pediatrics, McMaster University, Canada

13.1 INTRODUCTION

The promotion of physical activity among Canadian youth is of great importance in today's society; however, it is important to understand how to get the most out of exercise during the growing years, as well as the associated risks of physical activity. One long recognized risk for children has been exercising in the heat and the associated sweat-induced dehydration that occurs (Maughan and Noakes, 1996; Maughan *et al.,* 1997), posing negative effects on cardiovascular function, thermoregulation, and exercise performance (Cheuvront *et al.*, 2003; Coyle, 2004).

When fluid intake does not sufficiently match sweat rate during exercise, the importance of post-exercise restoration of fluid losses becomes apparent. Strategies to maintain body fluid balance while exercising in the heat have often focused on sport drinks which contain minimal nutrient value needed for the growing child. Therefore, it is critical to identify a more complete rehydration beverage for active children. Recently, the use of low-fat milk (a nutrient and sodium-rich beverage) as a safe and effective post-exercise rehydration beverage has been investigated in the adult population (reviewed by Roy, 2008). Original research in this area has shown that skim milk allowed for the greatest amount of beverage retained in the body over a 4 h period after exercising in the heat, compared to water or a carbohydrate-electrolyte solution (CES) (Shirreffs *et al.,* 2007), and that when matched for energy density, fat content and electrolyte content, the addition of milk-protein to a CES is more effective at retaining fluid than a CES alone (James *et al.,* 2011). There are, however, no studies that demonstrate milk's potential to rehydrate children.

Given the known growth-related differences in thermoregulation (Falk, 1998) and electrolyte losses (Meyer and Bar-Or, 1994) during exercise, it is plausible that children may have less to gain from milk than do adults. Since it has been found that children lose ~60 % less sodium in their sweat during exercise compared with adults (Meyer *et al.,* 1992), and one property of a rehydration beverage is to replenish sweat sodium, the sodium in a CES alone could be sufficient to meet this loss.

Consequently, a thorough understanding of the effectiveness of milk to replace body fluid losses after exercise in the heat in active children needs to be explored. The purpose of this study was to test the hypothesis that, due to higher sodium content, milk will be more effective than both water and a CES in replacing body fluid losses in children following exercise in the heat.

13.2 METHODS

13.2.1 Experimental design

Eight 8-10 y old heat-acclimated children (5 girls, 3 boys) performed three exercise trials, separated by 7 days, in a warm environment (35°C, 50 % relative humidity). A mechanically-braked cycle ergometer (Fleisch-Metabo, Geneva, Switzerland) was used for all testing. Exercise trials consisted of two 20 min cycling bouts at 60 % peak VO_2 with 10 min seated rest between bouts. Participants then consumed either water (W), CES, or skim milk (SM) in a volume equal to 100 % of their dehydration, beginning immediately after exercise. Urine samples were collected before, during, and immediately after exercise, as well as during a 2 h recovery period following drink consumption.

13.2.2 Statistical analysis

Statistical analysis was performed using STATISTICA software (STATISTICA for Windows 5.0, Statsoft, Tulsa, Oklahoma). Boys' and girls' data were grouped (n=8), forming a single data set for analysis. The experimental values are expressed as mean (SD). A one-way analysis of variance (ANOVA) and Tukey *post hoc* test were used to examine the differences between beverage trials. Data are expressed as mean (SD). Statistical significance was set at $P<0.05$.

13.3 RESULTS

Initial body mass of the subjects (29.3 ± 4.4 kg (W), 29.4 ± 4.3 kg (CES), 29.4 ± 4.1 kg (SM)) were not different between trials ($P=0.71$), indicating subjects were equally hydrated beginning each drink trial. Similarly, body mass loss throughout the exercise induced dehydration protocol (0.41 ± 0.13 kg (W), 0.43 ± 0.13 kg (CES), 0.39 ± 0.14 kg (SM)) was not different between trial ($P=0.63$).

As a result, subjects ingested similar volumes of drinks among trials (406 ± 125 mL).

Over the three trials, the mean body loss of 0.4 ± 0.1 kg represented a mean dehydration of 1.4 ± 0.4 % from pre-exercise values. At the end of the 2 h recovery period, all eight subjects experienced a loss in body mass compared to initial body mass (0.34 ± 0.21 kg (W), 0.37 ± 0.13 kg (CES), 0.26 ± 0.11 kg (SM)), suggesting that all participants were in a hypohydrated state (1.1 ± 0.6 % (W), 1.4 ± 0.6 % (CES), 0.8 ± 0.4 % (SM) dehydration) at the end of each trial.

After 2 h of recovery, the difference in cumulative urine output observed throughout the recovery period (226 ± 192 mL (W), 172 ± 104 mL (CES), 95 ± 78 mL (SM)) approached significance ($P=0.056$). The fraction of the ingested drink retained at 2 h was 53 (± 29) % (W), 60 (± 20) % (CES), and 77 (± 18 %) (SM). There was a significant main effect of the trial ($P<0.05$) on the fraction of the ingested drink retained at 2 h. *Post hoc* analysis revealed a significant difference between trials SM and W ($P<0.05$); however, no differences were seen between CES and W ($P=0.63$) or CES and SM ($P=0.12$). Results are presented in Figure 13.1.

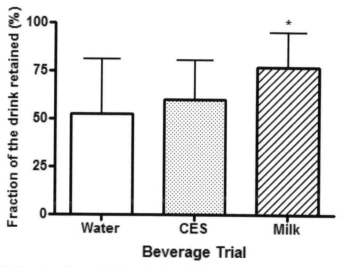

Figure 13.1. Fraction of ingested drink retained at 2 h of recovery after ingestion of either water, CES or skim milk. *Significantly different from water ($P<0.05$).

13.4 CONCLUSION

These preliminary findings indicate that, in healthy, active children, skim milk is more effective than water and similar to a typical sports drink at replacing fluid losses after exercise-induced dehydration in the heat. Water and a carbohydrate-electrolyte solution tended to increase urine production over the 2 h recovery period compared to milk, resulting in a significantly higher fraction of the ingested drink retained in the milk trial compared with water.

Evidence suggests that a volume equal to 150 % of body mass loss is needed to ensure complete restoration of fluid losses (Shirreffs *et al.*, 1996). The fact that none of the subjects in the current study maintained euhydration might be due to the fact that a volume equal to 100 % body mass loss was consumed.

Though further research is needed, the results from the current study suggest that milk is a safe and effective rehydration beverage in the paediatric population and should be considered as an additional strategy to help children beat the heat.

13.5 NOTE

This study was supported by a Grant from Dairy Farmers of Canada, Agriculture and Agri-Food of Canada and the Canadian Dairy Commission.

13.6 REFERENCES

Cheuvront, S., Carter, R., and Sawka, M.N., 2003, Fluid balance and endurance exercise performance. *Current Sports Medicine Reports*, **2**, pp. 202-208.

Coyle, E.F., 2004, Fluid and fuel intake during exercise. *Journal of Sports Sciences*, **22**, pp. 39-55.

Falk, B., 1998, Effects of thermal stress during rest and exercise in the pediatric population. *Sports Medicine*, **25**, pp. 221-240.

James, L.J., Clayton, D., and Evans, G.H., 2011, Effect of milk protein addition to a carbohydrate-electrolyte rehydration solution ingested after exercise in the heat. *British Journal of Nutrition*, **105**, pp. 393-399.

Maughan, R.J., and Noakes, T.D., 1996, Fluid replacement and exercise stress. A brief review of studies on fluid replacement and some guidelines for the athlete. *Sports Medicine*, **12**, pp. 16-31.

Maughan, R.J., Leiper, J.B., and Shirreffs, S.M., 1997, Factors influencing the restoration of fluid and electrolyte balance after exercise in the heat. *British Journal of Sports Medicine*, **31**, pp. 175-182.

Meyer, F., and Bar-Or, O., 1994, Fluid and electrolyte loss during exercise. The pediatric angle. *Sports Medicine*, **18**, pp. 4-9.

Meyer, F., Bar-Or, O., MacDougall, D., Heigenhauser, G.J.F., 1992, Sweat electrolyte loss during exercise in the heat: effects of gender and maturation. *Medicine and Science in Sports and Exercise*, **24**, pp. 776-781.

Roy, B.D., 2008, Milk: the new sports drink? A review. *Journal of the International Society of Sports Nutrition*, **5**, p. 15.

Shirreffs, S.M., Taylor, A.J., Leiper, J.B., and Maughan, R.J., 1996, Post-exercise rehydration in man: effects of volume consumed and drink sodium content. *Medicine and Science in Sports and Exercise*, **28**, pp. 1260-1271.

Shirreffs, S.M., Watson, P., and Maughan, R.J., 2007, Milk as an effective post-exercise rehydration drink. *British Journal of Nutrition*, **91**, pp. 173-180.

Part IV

Physical Activity and Health

RELATIONSHIPS BETWEEN CARDIOMETABOLIC RISK FACTORS AND AEROBIC FITNESS: A FRESH LOOK

R.G. McMurray[1], C. Lehman[1], P.A. Hosick[1], and A. Bugge[2]
[1]University of North Carolina, Chapel Hill, NC, USA, and [2]University of Southern Denmark, Odense, DK

14.1 INTRODUCTION

The measurement of maximal oxygen uptake (VO_2max) is commonly used to describe aerobic fitness/power. In youth, VO_2max has been scaled per kilogramme body mass ($mL \cdot kg^{-1}$), per kilogramme fat free mass ($mL \cdot kgFFM^{-1}$), or allometrically scaled ($mL \cdot kg^{0.67-0.75}$). Studies, summarized by McMurray and Andersen (2010), have shown a relationship between VO_2max and cardiometabolic risk factors (CMRF), including blood pressure, blood levels of total cholesterol, HDL cholesterol, or triglycerides, and insulin resistance. The majority of these studies have scaled VO_2max per kilogramme body mass. Body mass can be compartmentalized into fat free mass (FFM), which contains the metabolically active tissue, and fat mass, which contributes to energy demand, but not energy production. Furthermore, fat mass is independently related to the CMRF; thus, scaling VO_2max per kilogramme body mass may be confounding metabolic capacity and fatness.

Research has questioned the relationship between the CMRF and fitness, noting that when VO_2max is expressed per kg FFM, little relationship exists (Ondrak *et al.*, 2007), but children with large FFM may have VO_2max overestimated when using this method (Toth *et al.*, 1993). Allometric scaling allows for size-related changes in physiological function and the disproportionate increase in muscle mass with increasing body size (Welsman *et al.*, 1996; Malina *et al.*, 2004). Curiously, the relationship between allometric scaled VO_2max and CMRFs has not been explored. Thus this study sought to clarify the relationship between the CMRFs and aerobic power scaled in different units and to determine how sex, age and body fat influence the relationships.

14.2 METHODS

Subjects for this study were 931 girls and 853 boys (n = 1784), ages 8-16 y, from the CHIC III data base. Informed assent was obtained from the youth and consent from his/her parent before participation. The study was approved by the University of North Carolina Institutional Review Board. All trials were completed at the participant's school.

A venous blood sample was obtained from each child after a verified overnight fast. At a separate session each child had their seated blood pressure taken twice after a 5 minute rest, triceps and subscapular skinfolds measured twice and used to estimate body fat, and completed a multi-stage submaximal cycle ergometry test to predict VO$_2$max.

The blood samples were analyzed for total cholesterol, HDL-cholesterol (HDL-C) and triglycerides using automated coupled-enzymatic procedures, glucose using an automated chemistry system, and insulin using radioimmuno-assay technique. The HOMA-IR was calculated to indicate insulin resistance.

The relationships between CMRF and VO$_2$max units were analyzed using regression in two steps: unadjusted r^2 and then adjusting the r^2 for sex, age and body fat.

14.3 RESULTS

There were wide ranges in physical characteristics and VO$_2$max values. The girls and boys were similar in stature and body mass, but the girls, compared to the boys, had higher BMI (22.3 ± 5.8 vs. 21.4 ± 5.5 kg·m^{-2}) and body fat (28.5 ± 7.8 vs. 18.4 ± 9.8 %), and 11-17 % lower VO$_2$max values, regardless of scaling ($P \leq$ 0.001). Blood pressures and lipids were similar between the sexes ($P > 0.05$) and the HOMA-IR value were lower for the boys than the girls (3.6 ± 2.8 vs. 4.4 ± 3.2; P=0.0001).

Table 14.1. The r^2 values for the relationships between the CMRF and the scaled units for VO$_2$max. The unadjusted values (UA) and values adjusted for sex, age, and body fat (A) are presented. * $P = 0.0001$

Risk Factor		$mL \cdot kg^{-1}$	$mL \cdot kg^{-1} \cdot min^{-1}$	$mL \cdot kg_{FFM}^{-1} \cdot min^{-1}$	$mL \cdot kg^{0.67}$
BPsys	UA	0.149*	0.041*	0.012	0.001
	A	0.032*	0.006	0.007	<0.001
BPdia	UA	0.043*	0.047*	0.035*	0.015*
	A	<0.001	0.026*	0.027*	0.012
HOMA-IR	UA	0.044*	0.085*	0.009	0.015*
	A	0.003	<0.001	<0.001	0.003
Cholesterol	UA	0.012	0.008	<0.001	0.009
	A	0.003	<0.001	0.001	<0.001
HDL-C	UA	0.043*	0.026*	0.002	<0.001
	A	0.012	<0.001	<0.001	<0.001
Triglyceride	UA	0.014*	0.018*	0.001	0.002
	A	0.005	<0.001	<0.001	0.001

The relationships between the CMRF and the scaled units for VO$_2$max are presented in Table 14.1. Unadjusted relationships between VO$_2$max and CMRF were generally weak but significant, particularly for $mL \cdot min^{-1}$ or $mL \cdot kg^{-1}$ scaling ($P = 0.001$). Adjusting these relationships for sex, age and body fat, caused a reduction in the variance accounted for by any scaling of VO$_2$max, with the only significant associations remaining were between $mL \cdot kg^{-1}$ or $mL \cdot kg^{-1}$ and blood pressure or HOMA-IR ($r^2 \sim$3-8 %).

14.4 DISCUSSION

If aerobic power is influencing the CMRF then muscle must be the active components. Individuals with high aerobic power have increased oxidative capacity of the muscle, improved insulin sensitivity, and improved capacity to produce HDL-cholesterol. Thus, any measure of aerobic power should focus on the metabolic capacity *per unit* of muscle mass and be minimally influenced by the *total* amount of muscle or fat mass.

Absolute VO$_2$max was related to total kg FFM ($r \sim 0.77$) and minimally related to body fat ($r \sim 0.03$). So, absolute VO$_2$max was influenced by the *total* muscle mass, rather than the oxidative capacity *per unit* of muscle mass. Thus, relationships between CMRF and absolute VO$_2$max are probably not related to aerobic fitness. Scaling of VO$_2$max in mL·kg^{-1} is the most common method (McMurray and Andersen, 2010). However, Dencker *et al.* (2010) have shown that scaling in mL·kg^{-1} had a strong association with percent body fat. These correlations suggested that the use of mL·kg^{-1}·min^{-1} may not be a good indication of the metabolic capacity of the muscles.

Scaling VO$_2$max to FFM eliminates fat mass and focuses more on the metabolically active tissue (Ondrak *et al.*, 2007; Dencker *et al.*, 2010). However, scaling for FFM includes other tissues like bone and organs which increase in mass disproportionally as youth age (Malina *et al.*, 2004). Also, FFM may not address the issue of gender differences in the development of muscle mass during adolescence (Janz *et al.*, 1998) and may over-estimate VO$_2$max for individuals with a large amount of FFM (Toth *et al.*, 1993). Thus, VO$_2$max scaled per unit FFM, maybe our best indirect estimate of the maximal metabolic capacity of the muscle, although not ideal. Like scaling for body mass, allometric scaling also appears to be influenced by fat (Dencker *et al.*, 2010). In addition, controversy exists regarding the appropriate exponent for the scaling (Welsman *et al.*, 1996; Dencker *et al.*, 2010). Thus, allometric scaling may not be the best method when relating to CMRF to VO$_2$max.

Regardless of the scaling for VO$_2$max the most consistent finding was a relationship with systolic pressure. A relationship between VO$_2$max and blood pressure appears equivocal (Janz *et al.*, 2000, 2002; Hurtig-Wennlof *et al.*, 2007). In the same way the relationship between VO$_2$max and lipids or HOMA is also inconsistent (Hurtig-Wennlof *et al.*, 2007; Ondrak *et al.*, 2007; Jago *et al.*, 2010). One difference between these studies is the units of scaling VO$_2$max; some using mL·kg^{-1}·min^{-1} scaling (Hurtig-Wennlof *et al.*, 2007), others allometric (Janz *et al.*, 2002), or FFM scaling (Ondrak *et al.*, 2007). Jago *et al.* (2010) used laps completed for a multistage shuttle run and found a significant association between lipids and laps completed.

Although our data are cross-sectional and should not be interpreted to say that exercise training can impact CMRF (Janz *et al.*, 2002), our results suggest that any relationship between VO$_2$max and cardiometabolic risk factors in youth is highly dependent upon sex, age and body fat. Thus, any study that attempts to relate VO$_2$max to CMRF should take into consideration these characteristics. An alternative approach could be to avoid VO$_2$max scaling and use a surrogate for aerobic power, like time or distance completed on a standardized performance protocol, or number of laps completed (20 metre shuttle run).

14.5 REFERENCES

Dencker, M., Bugge, A., Hermansen, B. and Andersen, L.B., 2010, Aerobic fitness in prepubertal children according to level of body fat. *Acta Paediatrica*, **99**, pp. 1854-1860.

Hurtig-Wennlof, A., Ruiz, J.R., Harrod, M. and Sjostroma, M., 2007, Cardiorespiratory fitness relates more strongly than physical activity to cardiovascular disease risk factors in healthy children and adolescents: the European Youth Heart Study. *European Journal of Cardiovascular Prevention and Rehabilitation*, **14**, pp. 575-581.

Jago, R., Drews, K.L., McMurray, R.G., Thompson, D., Volpe, S.L., Moe, E.L., Jakicic, J.M., Phang, T.H., Bruecker, S., Blackshear, T.B. and Yin, Z, 2010, Fatness, fitness, and cardiometabolic risk factors among sixth grade youth. *Medicine and Science in Sports and Exercise*, **42**, pp. 1502-1510.

Janz, K.F., Burns, T.D., Witt, J.D. and Mahoney, L.T., 1998, Longitudinal analysis of scaling VO$_2$ for differences in body size during puberty: The Muscatine Study. *Medicine and Science in Sports and Exercise*, **30**, pp. 1436-1444.

Janz K.F, Dawson, J.D. and Mahoney, L.T., 2000, Predicting heart growth during puberty: The Muscatine Study. *Pediatrics*, **105**, E63.

Janz, K.F., Dawson, J.D. and Mahoney, L.T., 2002, Increases in physical fitness during childhood improves cardiovascular health during adolescence: The Muscatine Study. *International Journal of Sport Medicine*, **23**, pp. S15-S21.

Malina, R.M., Bouchard, C. and Bar-Or, O., 2004, *Growth, Maturation, and Physical Activity*. (Champaign, IL: Human Kinetics), pp. 41-116.

McMurray, R.G., and Andersen, L.B., 2010, The influence of exercise on metabolic syndrome in youth: A review. *American Journal of Lifestyle Medicine*, **4**, pp. 176-186.

Ondrak, K.S., McMurray, R.G., Bangdiwala, S.I. and Harrell, J.S., 2007, The influence of aerobic power and percent body fat on cardiovascular disease risk in youth. *Journal of Adolescent Health*, **41**, pp. 146-152.

Rowland, T.W. and Cunningham, L.N., 1992, Oxygen uptake plateau during maximal treadmill exercise in children. *Chest*, **101**, pp. 485-489.

Toth, M.J., Goran, M., Ades, P.A., Howard, B.B. and Poehlamn, E.T., 1993, Examination of data normalization procedures for expressing peak VO$_2$ data. *Journal of Applied Physiology.* **75**, pp. 2288-2292.

Welsman, J.R., Armstrong, N., Nevill, A.M., Winter, E.M. and Kirby, B.J., 1996, Scaling peak VO$_2$ for differences in body size. *Medicine and Science in Sports and Exercise*, **28**, pp. 259-265.

EFFECTS OF A SCHOOL-BASED CROSS-CURRICULAR PHYSICAL ACTIVITY INTERVENTION ON CARDIOVASCULAR DISEASE RISK FACTORS IN 11-14 YEAR OLDS

G.J. Knox[1], J.S. Baker[2], B. Davies[3], A. Rees[1], K. Morgan[4],
and N.E. Thomas[4]

[1]University of Wales Institute Cardiff, UK, [2]University of the West of Scotland, UK, [3]University of Glamorgan, UK., [4]Swansea University, UK

15.1 INTRODUCTION

Cardiovascular disease (CVD) is considered the leading cause of premature death (<75 years) in the United Kingdom (British Heart Foundation, 2010). It is widely accepted that the underlying mechanism to CVD, namely atherosclerosis, has its genesis in childhood (Berenson et al., 1998). A number of risk factors have been identified for the early detection of CVD, many of which are thought to be influenced by physical activity (PA) (Strong et al., 2005).

Researchers have attempted to manipulate childhood physical activity (PA) behaviour by implementing school-based interventions; some of these have resulted in modest improvements to CVD risk factor status (Brown and Summerbell, 2009). PA interventions have typically involved strategies to improve current physical education (PE) curricula or introduce activities out of regular school hours. Recently, Reed et al. (2008) demonstrated improved blood pressure and aerobic fitness (AF) in primary school children following the introduction of PA into normally sedentary curriculum subjects. No effect was observed for adiposity, lipid and lipoprotein variables which may be attributed to the short time allocation provided for the daily activity sessions (15 min). This strategy may prove effective in reducing CVD risk status by targeting all school children.

This study investigated the impact on adolescent CVD risk factor profiles following the introduction of brisk walking into two normally classroom-based (sedentary) curriculum lessons (60 min duration) per week over 18 weeks.

15.2 METHODS

15.2.1 Study design and measurements

A quasi-experimental design was employed. An intervention group (INT) consisted of 115 participants from year eight (12.4±0.5 y), whereas 77 maturation matched participants from years seven and nine (12.1±1.1 y) formed a control (CON) group. CVD risk factors were assessed over a 3 week period prior to commencement of the intervention; these measurements were repeated post-intervention. Anthropometric assessments included measures of body mass index (BMI), waist (WC), hip circumference (HC), and skinfold thickness assessed at the biceps, triceps, subscapular, and suprailiac sites. Physical and physiological parameters included systolic (SBP) and diastolic blood pressure (DBP). AF was assessed using the 20 m multistage fitness test, and PA behaviour was determined by use of the physical activity questionnaire for adolescents (PAQ-A). Fasting blood samples from the antecubital vein were analysed for total cholesterol (TC), low-density lipoprotein cholesterol (LDL-C), high-density lipoprotein cholesterol (HDL-C), triglycerides, glucose, insulin, high-sensitivity C-reactive protein (hs-CRP), and high molecular weight adiponectin (HMW-adip).

15.2.2 Intervention

A secondary school-based, cross-curricular PA intervention was implemented. The intervention increased school-time PA by an additional 2 h per week. For 18 weeks, INT participants briskly walked 3,200 m during what would normally be classroom-based lessons (60 min). This occurred twice a week and took place within the school grounds. Metronomes were used to set a pace at 130 b min^{-1}, so that one beat equalled one step. These sessions were in addition to two weekly PE lessons. Intervention lessons were administered on separate days to PE lessons, ensuring that participants engaged in PA for a minimum of 4 days a week. Crucially, stations were set up every 400 m or 800 m for participants to complete academic tasks relevant to the subject being taught. Each station lasted approximately 1 minute. Tasks were designed by teachers and monitored by the local education authority to ensure that appropriate curriculum content and standards were maintained. All academic subjects, except PE, took it in turn to participate. Each subject delivered four intervention lessons during the 18 week period.

15.2.3 Statistical analysis

Independent t tests were employed to detect significant differences between INT and CON for mean change following intervention. Dependent t tests were utilised to discover significant changes in CVD risk factors from baseline to post-intervention. A Dunn-Sidak correction was implemented to account for type I error. Significance was set at $P \leq 0.002$. Prevalence of elevated BMI, WC, SBP, DBP, TC, LDL-C, TG and glucose, as well as reduced HDL-C were determined using published, child-specific cut-off values (Cole *et al.*, 2000; Kavey *et al.*, 2003; International Diabetes Federation, 2007).

15.3 RESULTS

For all variables, mean change was not significantly different between INT and CON (P>0.002). Body mass index significantly increased for INT (0.53 ± 0.96 kg·m^2, P=0.000) and CON (0.46 ± 1.07 kg·m^{-2}, P=0.001). Despite no significant change in WC for both groups, a reduction in the prevalence of elevated WC was observed for INT (9.8 vs. 6.9 %), whereas CON remained unchanged (10.8%). Prevalence of elevated SBP decreased in INT (3.3 vs. 0 %), and increased for CON (1.7 vs. 5.1 %).

Following intervention, TC, LDL-C, HDL-C, and non-HDL-C were significantly reduced for INT (-0.5 ± 0.4, -0.3 ± 0.3, -0.1 ± 0.2, -0.3 ± 0.3 mmol·L^{-1}, respectively, $P \leq 0.002$) and CON (-0.3 ± 0.4, -0.3 ± 0.3, -0.1 ± 0.2, -0.2 ± 0.4 mmol·L^{-1}, respectively, $P \leq 0.002$). A significant increase in HDL-C/TC ratio was observed for INT (2 ± 4 %, P=0.001), but not CON. Glucose was significantly reduced for INT (-0.1 ± 0.4 mmol·L^{-1}, P=0.002), yet remained unchanged for CON. HMW-adip significantly increased for INT (-1042 ± 2506 ng·mL^{-1}, P=0.000) and CON (-1130 ± 2313ng·mL^{-1}, P=0.000). Prevalence of reduced HDL-C and elevated TG were increased for CON (5.4 vs. 7.1 % and 0 vs. 7.1 %, respectively), whereas reductions were observed for INT (3.7 vs. 2.7 % and 2.5 vs. 1.2 %, respectively).

AF and PA behaviour did not significantly change between baseline and post-intervention for INT and CON (P>0.002).

15.4 CONCLUSION

Cross-curricular PA was successfully implemented into a school environment increasing activity time by an additional 2 hours per week. This pilot study led to a reduction in prevalence of adverse levels of WC, SBP, HDL-C and TG in INT participants. Despite no attempt to alter dietary behaviour, small, but favourable changes in HDL-C/TC ratio and glucose were evident for INT. Combining this intervention with a strategy to improve saturated fat and sugar intake may evoke additional benefits to lipid, lipoprotein and glucose metabolism.

One hour of PA most days of the week is recommended for children and adolescence (Strong *et al.*, 2005). Our intervention may prove to be a sustainable, effective and cost-effective strategy to engage all school children in PA on a daily basis.

15.5 REFERENCES

Berenson, G.S., Srinivasan, S.R., Bao, W., Newman, W.P., Tracy, R.E. and Wattigney, W.A., 1998, Association between multiple cardiovascular risk factors and atherosclerosis in children and young adults. *New England Journal of Medicine*, **338**, pp. 1650-1656.

British Heart Foundation Health Promotion Research Group, 2010, *UK Coronary Heart Disease Statistics 2009-10*, (London: British Heart Foundation).

Brown, T. and Summerbell, C., 2009, Systematic review of school-based interventions that focus on changing dietary intake and physical activity levels to prevent childhood obesity: An update to the obesity guidance produced by the National Institute for Health and Clinical Excellence. *Obesity Reviews*, **10**, pp. 110-141.

Cole, T.J., Bellizzi, M.C., Flegal, K.M. and Dietz, W.H., 2000, Establishing a standard definition for child overweight and obesity worldwide: International survey. *British Medical Journal*, **320**, pp. 1-6.

International Diabetes Federation, 2007, *The IDF consensus definition of the metabolic syndrome in children and adolescents*, (Brussels: International Diabestes Federation), pp.1-24.

Kavey, R-E.W., Daniels, S.R., Lauer, R.M., Atkins, D.L., Hayman, L.L. and Taubert, K., 2003, American Heart Association guidelines for primary prevention of atherosclerotic cardiovascular disease beginning in childhood. *Circulation*, **107**, pp. 1562-1566.

Reed, K.E., Warburton, D.E.R., Macdonald, H.M., Naylor, P.J. and McKay, H.A., 2008, Action schools! BC: A school-based physical activity intervention designed to decrease cardiovascular disease risk factors in children. *Preventive Medicine*, **46**, pp. 525-531.

Strong, W.B., Malina, R.M., Blimkie, C.J.R., Daniels, S.R., Dishman, R.K., Gutin, B., Hergenroeder, A.C., Must, A., Nixon, P.A., Pivarnik, J.M., Rowland, T., Trost, S. and Trudeau, F., 2005, Evidence based physical activity for school-age youth. *Journal of Pediatrics*, **146**, pp. 732-737.

IMPACT OF CHANGES IN SCREEN TIME ON BLOOD PROFILES AND BLOOD PRESSURE IN ADOLESCENTS OVER A TWO YEAR PERIOD

D.R. Dengel, M.O. Hearst, J.H. Harmon, and L.A. Lytle
University of Minnesota, Minneapolis, Minnesota, USA

16.1 INTRODUCTION

Cardiovascular and metabolic diseases are the main causes of morbidity and mortality (Kannel *et al.,* 1984; Lloyd-Jones *et al.,* 2009). Evidence exists that many of these diseases begin in childhood (Enos *et al.,* 1953; McNamara *et al.,* 1971). It has been suggested that the increasing prevalence of cardiovascular and metabolic risk factors in adolescents may be due in part to increasing trends in adolescent obesity and physical inactivity (Wang and Lobstein, 2006).

Although physical inactivity and sedentary behaviours are often thought of as similar and are often categorized together, studies in adolescents have shown that time spent in sedentary behaviours should be considered independently from physical inactivity (Taveras *et al.,* 2007). Television (TV) viewing is a well-known sedentary behaviour that has been linked with obesity and other cardiovascular and metabolic risk factors (American Academy of Pediatrics, 2001). With growth of other types of screen media (i.e., computer, DVD, video games) adolescents have a wealth of new technology that encourages sedentary behaviours.

In an attempt to understand the effect of these new technologies on cardiovascular and metabolic health in adolescents, we examined the effect of longitudinal changes in daily screen time (i.e., watching TV; playing video games; time spent on computer and/or internet) on biological markers of cardiovascular and metabolic disease in adolescents over a 2 year period.

16.2 METHODS

16.2.1 Experimental design

This research was conducted using data from two aetiological studies of adolescent obesity in the Twin Cities Metropolitan Area from 2006-2009 (Lytle, 2009). For both samples, a parent/child dyad was enrolled. Parent/child dyads were excluded from eligibility if they planned to move from the area in the next 3 years, had a medical condition that affected their growth, or had difficulty comprehending English. Both studies were approved by the University of Minnesota Institutional Review Board. Data were collected at two time points for a total of 646 adolescents. Of those, there were 217 (105 males and 112 females) who participated at both baseline and 24 months with an optional blood draw (34 %). There were no significant differences in screen time, change in screen time, race, age, or puberty between those who completed the blood draw and those who did not at the follow-up appointment. Participants in this longitudinal study had a mean (SEM) age of 14.6 ± 0.1 y at baseline.

16.2.2 Measurements

Stature was measured without shoes using a Shorr Height Board (Shorr Productions, Olney, MD, USA) and body mass was assessed using a digital scale (Tanita TBF-300A, Tanita Corporation, Tokyo, Japan). Blood pressure was measured using an automated sphygmomanometry (Dinamap 8100, GE Healthcare, Piscataway, NJ) after a minimum of 5 minutes of seated rest. Three measurements of blood pressure were made and averaged. Self-report data on demographics were obtained at the initial clinic visit from both adolescents and parents. Pubertal status was assessed in all youth participants by the self-report Pubertal Development Scale (PDS) (Petersen *et al.*, 1988).

During a second clinic visit, a 12 hour fasting blood sample was obtained by venipuncture from the anticubital vein into chilled tubes containing ethylene diamine tetraacetic acid (EDTA) at the University of Minnesota General Clinical Research Center. Plasma samples were measured for glucose and insulin, adiponectin, C-reactive protein, tumor necrosis factor-alpha, triglycerides, total cholesterol, low-density lipoproteins and high-density lipoproteins. Homeostasis model assessment for insulin resistance (HOMA-IR) was calculated as: (fasting glucose*fasting insulin)/22.5 (Matthews *et al.*, 1985).

At the second clinic visit, the participant filled out a questionnaire to assess their off screen time behaviour included weekdays and weekends. As part of the self-report survey, weekday screen time behaviour was assessed asking: "On a typical weekday (Monday-Friday), how many hours do you spend watching TV?" The same question was asked for watching DVDs or videos,

Nintendo/PlayStation/computer games and internet/computers. A similar question was used to assess weekend (Saturday-Sunday) screen time behaviour. Six response options ranged from 'none' to "6+ hours" per day. Response categories were set at the mid-range, weighted for weekday versus weekend, summed and divided by seven resulting in the number of daily minutes of screen time behaviour.

16.2.3 Statistical analysis

Descriptive statistics were calculated and tested for differences ($P<0.05$) by baseline and follow-up measurement using a paired t-test. Distribution of the biological measures was assessed and log transformed if skewness factor was greater than 2.0. Change in screen time behaviour was calculated, subtracting follow-up daily minutes from baseline daily minutes and modelled as the primary independent variable. Each biomarker was modelled independently for the full sample as the dependent variable, and adjusted for baseline values of the biomarker. Fully adjusted models included baseline gender, puberty, age, and race. All models used PROC GENMOD in SAS version 9.1 (SAS Institute, Cary, NC), accounting for clustering at the school level. All values are present as the mean and standard error of the means (SEM).

16.3 RESULTS

In the present study, we did not observe any significant changes in mean values in the minutes of daily screen time (299.4 ± 14.1 vs. 218.0 ± 21.8 min, $P=0.18$), high-density lipoproteins (1.29 ± 0.02 vs. 1.29 ± 0.02 mmol·L^{-1}, $P=0.75$), C-reactive protein (1.29 ± 0.20 vs. 1.88 ± 0.28 mg·L^{-1}, $P=0.07$), tumor necrosis factor-alpha (1.58 ± 0.25 vs. 1.69 ± 0.30 pg·mL^{-1}, $P=0.30$), glucose (4.39 ± 0.03 vs. 4.39 ± 0.03 mmol·L^{-1}, $P=0.98$) and systolic blood pressure (114 ± 1 vs. 113 ± 1 mmHg, P=0.34). We did observe a significant increase in mean values of low-density lipoproteins (2.22 ± 0.04 vs. 2.32 ± 0,04 mmol·L^{-1}, $P=0.001$), total cholesterol (3.91 ± 0.05 vs. 4.06 ± 0.05 mmol·L^{-1}, $P<0.001$), and triglycerides (0.87 ± 0.03 vs. 0.98 ± 0.03 mmol·L^{-1}, $P=0.004$), and a significant mean decrease in insulin (57.3±2.2 vs. 49.2±2.5 pmol·L^{-1}, $P=0.001$), HOMA-IR (1.63 ± 0.07 vs. 1.40 ± 0.07, $P=0.002$), adiponectin (22.47 ± 1.73 vs. 19.84 ± 1.34 mg·L^{-1}, $P=0.03$) and diastolic blood pressure (54 ± 1 vs. 53 ± 1 mmHg, P=0.01). From the adjusted regression models, we also observed that as the amount of daily minutes of screen time increased there was an increase in adiponectin ($\beta=0.0002$, $P=0.08$), insulin ($\beta=0.003$, $P=0.02$), glucose ($\beta=0.01$, $P=0.04$), total cholesterol ($\beta=0.01$, $P=0.03$), and HOMA-IR ($\beta=0.001$, $P=0.02$).

16.4 CONCLUSION

Previously, we have utilized cross-sectional study designs to demonstrate the effects of both the built and home environments on biological markers of cardiovascular and metabolic health in adolescents (Dengel *et al.,* 2009, 2010). The results of the present study extend those initial cross-sectional studies by demonstrating that longitudinal changes in sedentary behaviours such as watching TV, playing video games and time spent on computer and/or internet have an impact on biological markers of cardiovascular and metabolic disease in adolescents. As technology advances adolescents are confronted with more devices that promote sedentary behaviours, with potential cardiovascular and metabolic risk effects. Future studies are needed to examine the role of these new technologies on promoting sedentary behaviours in adolescents and their effects on cardiovascular and metabolic disease in this population.

16.5 REFERENCES

American Academy of Pediatrics, 2001, Committee on Public Education: Children, adolescents, and television. *Pediatrics*, **107**, pp. 423-426.

Dengel, D.R., Hearst, M.O., Harmon, J.H., Forsyth, A. and Lytle L.A., 2009, Does the built environment relate to the metabolic syndrome in adolescents? *Health and Place*, **15**, pp. 946-951.

Dengel, D.R., Hearst, M.O., Harmon, J.H., Sirard, J., Heitzler, C.D. and Lytle, LA., 2010, Association of the home environment with cardiovascular and metabolic biomarkers in youth. *Preventive Medicine*, **51**, pp. 259-261.

Enos, W.F., Holmes, R.H. and Beyer, J., 1953, Coronary diseases among United States soldiers killed in action in Korea. *Journal of the American Medical Association*, **152**, pp. 1090-1093.

Kannel, W.B., Doyle, J.T., Ostfeld, A.M., Jenkins, C.D., Kuller, L., Podell, R.N. and Stamler, J., 1984, Optimal resources for primary prevention of atherosclerotic diseases. Atherosclerosis Study Group. *Circulation*, **70**, pp. 155A-205A.

Lloyd-Jones, D., Adams, R., Carnethon, M., De Simone, G., Ferguson, T.B., Flegal, K., Ford, E., Furie, K., Go, A., Greenlund, K., Haase, N., Hailpern. S., Ho, M., Howard, V., Kissela,. B., Kittner, S., Lackland, D., Lisabeth, L., Marelli, A., McDermott. M., Meigs, J., Mozaffarian, D., Nichol, G., O'Donnell, C, Roger, V., Rosamond, W., Sacco, R., Sorlie, P., Stafford, R., Steinberger, J., Thom. T., Wasserthiel-Smoller, S., Wong, N., Wylie-Rosett, J. and Hong Y., 2009, American Heart Association Statistics Committee and Stroke Statistics Subcommittee: Heart disease and stroke statistics-2009 update: A report from the American Heart Association Statistics

Committee and Stroke Statistics Subcommittee. *Circulation*, **119**, pp. e21-181.

Lytle, L.A., 2009, Examining the etiology of childhood obesity: The IDEA Study. *American Journal of Community Psychology*, **44**, pp. 338-349.

Matthews, D.R., Hosker, J.P., Rudenski, A.S., Naylor, B.A., Treacher, D.F., and Turner, R.C., 1985, Homeostasis model assessment: insulin resistance and beta-cell function from fasting plasma glucose and insulin concentrations in man. *Diabetologia*, **28**, pp. 412-419.

McNamara, J.J., Melot, M.A., Stremple, J.F. and Cutting, R.T., 1971, Coronary artery disease in combat casualties in Vietnam. *Journal of the American Medical Association*, **216**, pp. 1185-1187.

Petersen, A., Crockett, L., Richards, M. and Boxer, A. 1988, A self-report measure of pubertal status: Reliability, validity, and initial norms. *Journal of Youth and Adolescence*, **17**, pp. 117-133.

Taveras, E.M., Field, A.E., Berkey, C.S., Rifas-Shiman, S.L., Frazier, A.L., Colditz, G.A., and Gillman, M.W., 2007, Longitudinal relationship between television viewing and leisure-time physical activity during adolescence. *Pediatrics*, **119**, pp. e314-e319.

Wang, Y. and Lobstein, T., 2006, Worldwide trends in childhood overweight and obesity. *International Journal of Pediatric Obesity*, **1**, pp. 11-25.

AEROBIC FITNESS AND PHYSICAL ACTIVITY ARE RELATED TO LEAN BODY MASS AND NOT ADIPOSITY IN PRESCHOOLERS

L. Gabel, N.A. Proudfoot, and B.W. Timmons

Child Health and Exercise Medicine Program, McMaster University, Canada

17.1 INTRODUCTION

Body composition is assessed as a marker for health in children and adults. Children that are overweight at a young age have an increased risk of developing cardiovascular and metabolic conditions later in life (Must and Strauss, 1999; Twisk *et al.*, 2002). Current data from Canada suggest that 21 % of preschoolers are overweight or obese (Shields, 2006). The high prevalence of overweight/obesity has increased public concern regarding potential health implications. Lean body mass also plays an important role in metabolic health; however, it is not as commonly assessed as adiposity with respect to health measures.

In adults, lower aerobic fitness has been linked to an increased risk of cardiovascular disease mortality (Lee *et al.*, 1999). Studies conducted in youth have similarly shown a protective effect of aerobic fitness on metabolic and cardiovascular health (Twisk *et al.*, 2002; Steele *et al.*, 2008). In preschoolers, however, there is paucity of literature characterizing aerobic fitness, along with its relation to other health measures, such as body composition.

Physical activity is an important contributor to daily energy expenditure and long-term energy balance. Longitudinal studies have shown a negative relationship between habitual physical activity and adiposity in preschool children (Moore *et al.*, 1995; Janz *et al.*, 2005). Less frequently has the influence of physical activity been examined with respect to lean body mass.

The aim of this investigation was to explore the cross-sectional relationships between aerobic fitness, physical activity, adiposity and lean body mass in a sample of preschool children (3-5 years).

17.2 METHODS

Thirty-six healthy preschool children (4.6 ± 0.8 y) from the Hamilton, Ontario region were recruited to participate. Participants completed one session consisting of aerobic fitness testing and body composition measurement, followed by one week of physical activity monitoring.

Standard anthropometric measurements of stature using a calibrated stadiometer and mass with light clothing using a digital scale (BWB-800, Tanita Corporation, Japan) were performed. Body composition was assessed by bioelectrical impedance analysis using RJL systems 101A (Miami, FL, USA). Lean body mass (LBM) was calculated using an equation validated in young children (Kriemler et al., 2009). Percent body fat was calculated as [(body mass-LBM)/body mass].

Aerobic fitness was assessed on a treadmill (GE Marquette Series 2000, USA) using the Bruce protocol, with performance based on time to exhaustion. Children were instructed to hold onto handrails for the duration of the test to assist with balance, and a researcher was positioned directly behind the child to ensure safety. The test was terminated when the child could no longer keep up with the increasing grade or slope of the treadmill, or once a heart rate of 195 b·min^{-1} was achieved.

Habitual physical activity was measured using the Actigraph GT3XE accelerometer (Fort Walton Beach, FL, USA). Activity counts were recorded in 3 second epochs. Participants were instructed to wear the accelerometer over their right hip during all waking hours for seven consecutive days, except when engaging in water activities. Parents were given a log to record times that the accelerometer was put on and removed. Only participants who wore the accelerometer for ≥ 5 hours per day on ≥ 4 days, including 1 weekend day, were included in the analyses. Accelerometer data were visually inspected and activity counts during reported times of non-wear were deleted. Physical activity was defined using cut-points from a previous validation study in a similar age group (Pate et al., 2006), with times of physical activity (TPA) indicated as >8 counts/3 s and moderate-to-vigorous activity (MVPA) as >84 counts/3 s. To account for different accelerometer wear times between children (h·day^{-1}), physical activity data (TPA and MVPA) are reported as a percentage of monitoring time and in absolute terms (min·day^{-1}).

All data are presented as mean (SD), unless otherwise noted. Pearson's correlation coefficient was used to assess the relationships between body composition, aerobic fitness, and physical activity. All variables exhibited significant relationships with age; thus, partial correlations were performed controlling for age. All statistics were calculated in SPSS Statistics 18 for Windows (SPSS Inc, Chicago, IL, USA).

17.3 RESULTS

Participants' mean lean body mass was 14.2 (± 2.6) kg with a mean body fat percentage of 23.3 (± 4.8) %. At termination of the aerobic fitness test, the mean heart rate was 190 (± 12.7) b·min^{-1} with a time of 9.2 (± 2.2) min to exhaustion. Children with higher aerobic fitness (longer time to reach exhaustion) had significantly more lean body mass (r=0.37, P<0.03) than those with lower fitness (Figure 17.1). Body fat percentage and aerobic fitness were unrelated (P>0.05).

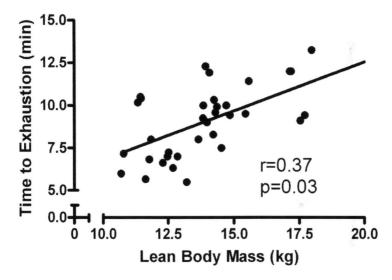

Figure 17.1. Relationship between lean body mass and aerobic fitness.

Participants engaged in 244.8 (± 41.8) min·day^{-1} of physical activity (TPA) or 35.8 (± 5.8) % of accelerometer monitoring time. Preschoolers with higher lean body mass engaged in more TPA, expressed in min·day^{-1} (r=0.59, P<0.001) and as a percent of monitoring time (r=0.49, P=0.005). The mean moderate-to-vigorous activity (MVPA) was 89.7 (± 22.9) min·day^{-1} or 13.1 (± 3.2) % of monitoring time. Preschoolers with higher lean body mass engaged in more MVPA, expressed in (r=0.54, P=0.002) and as a percent of monitoring time (r=0.48, P=0.006). No associations were found between physical activity and body fat percentage (P>0.05).

17.4 CONCLUSION

For the first time, we provide data on the relationship between lean body mass and aerobic fitness in preschool children. Our results indicate that participating preschool children with more lean body mass have higher aerobic fitness. We did not observe an association between aerobic fitness and adiposity.

Preschoolers in our sample with higher lean body mass engaged in more physical activity, expressed in min·day[-1] and as a percent of monitoring time. In contrast to literature indicating a protective effect of physical activity on adiposity (Moore *et al.*, 1995; Janz *et al.*, 2005), we did not observe an association between the two. While all studies used objective measures of physical activity, it is possible that adiposity was not adequately represented in our small cohort. The majority of our participants were of normal weight status, with only 8 % classified as overweight or obese, compared with the national average of 21 %. Nevertheless, our study is ongoing and we hope to confirm or clarify these associations with a larger, more representative cohort.

No relationship was observed between physical activity and aerobic fitness, suggesting both variables independently influence or are influenced by lean body mass. Unfortunately, due to the cross-sectional design of the present study we cannot determine whether greater physical activity causes increased lean body mass or whether higher lean body mass makes movement easier, thus, resulting in increased physical activity. Consequently, we will follow these participants over a number of years to assess the direction of these associations.

This study shows that participating children with more lean body mass have higher aerobic fitness and engage in more physical activity than those with less lean body mass. Adiposity was not related to fitness or physical activity in this small sample of preschoolers.

17.5 NOTE

This study was supported by the Canadian Institute of Health Research.

17.6 REFERENCES

Janz, K.F., Burns, T.L., and Levy, S.M., 2005, Tracking of activity and sedentary behaviours in childhood: The Iowa Bone Development Study. *American Journal of Preventive Medicine*, **29**, pp. 171-178.

Kriemler, S., Puder, J., Zahner, L, Roth, R., Braun-Fahrlander, C. and Bedogni, G., 2009, Cross-validation of bioelectrical impedance analysis for the validation of body composition in a representative sample of 6- to 13-year-old children. *European Journal of Clinical Nutrition*, **63**, pp. 619-626.

Lee, C.D., Blair, S.N., and Jackson, A.S., 1999, Cardiorespiratory fitness, body composition, and all-cause and cardiovascular disease mortality in men. *American Journal of Clinical Nutrition*, **69**, pp. 373-380.

Moore, L.L., Nguyen, U.D.T., Rothman, K.J., Cupples, L.A. and Ellison, R.C., 1995, Preschool physical activity level and change in body fatness in young children: The Framingham Children's Study. *American Journal of Epidemiology*, **142**, pp. 982-988.

Must, A., and Strauss, R.S., 1999, Risks and consequences of childhood and adolescent obesity. *International Journal of Obesity*, **23**(S2), pp. S2-S11.

Pate, R.R., Almeida, M.J., Pfeiffer, K.A., and Dowda, M., 2006, Validation and calibration of an accelerometer in preschool children. *Obesity*, **14**, pp. 2000-2006.

Shields, M., 2006, Overweight and obesity among children and youth. *Statistics Canada Health Reports*, **17**, pp. 27-42.

Steele, R.M., Brage, S., Corder, K., Wareham, N.J., and Ekelund, U., 2008, Physical activity, cardiorespiratory fitness, and the metabolic syndrome in youth. *Journal of Applied Physiology*, **105**, pp. 342-351.

Twisk, J.W.R., Kemper, H.C.G., and van Mechelen, W., 2002, Prediction of cardiovascular disease risk factors later in life by physical activity and fitness in youth: General comments and conclusions. *International Journal of Sports Medicine*, **23**(S1), pp. S44-S49.

VALIDATION OF THE GENEA WAVEFORM ACCELEROMETER FOR ASSESSMENT OF CHILDREN'S PHYSICAL ACTIVITY

L.R.S. Phillips, A.V. Rowlands, and C.G. Parfitt
University of Exeter, UK

18.1 INTRODUCTION

Although many physical activity measures exist, the majority prove unsuitable for examining habitual physical activity within a child population; this has led to an increase in the use of movement sensors, such as accelerometers, to undertake such tasks (Puyau *et al.*, 2004). The advantages of this method include minimal burden to the user (Rowlands *et al.*, 2004), while their small size allows for easy use with children (Freedson *et al.*, 2005). Several accelerometers, e.g. the Actical (Mini Mitter, Bend, Oregon, USA), the ActiGraph GT1M (ActiGraph, Pensacola, Florida, USA) and the RT3 (Stayhealthy Inc., Monrovia, California, USA), have been validated for use with both adults and children. However, lack of compliance with the wearing protocol when using these accelerometers can lead to a reduction in participant numbers. For example, Van Coevering *et al.* (2005) found that only 50 % of students were compliant for the full 7 day measurement period where as 92 % of students were compliant for ≥ 3 days. The issue of non compliance may be exacerbated by the necessity to remove the monitor when changing clothes (as most are worn on the hip) and when partaking in water-based activities (due to the lack of waterproofing). In an attempt to overcome these problems, the GENEA waveform triaxial accelerometer was developed (Unilever Discover, Colworth, UK, manufactured and distributed by Activinsights Ltd, Kimbolton, Cambridge, UK).

The GENEA is designed to be worn on the wrist and is waterproof, therefore essentially negating the need for the monitor to be removed during the day and potentially leading to greater compliance from participants. The GENEA also has an extended battery life and memory capacity enabling it to record data in three axes (vertical, anteroposterior and mediolateral) at 80 Hz for 7 days.

The GENEA has recently been found to demonstrate good technical reliability and validity (Esliger *et al.*, 2010), and has been found to be a valid tool for measuring adult physical activity when worn at the wrist or the hip (Esliger *et al.*, 2010). The aim of the current study was to validate the GENEA for the assessment of activity in children and establish the GENEA as peer to the ActiGraph.

18.2 METHODS

18.2.1 Experimental design

Forty-four apparently healthy children (n = 26 females, n = 18 males) aged between 8 and 14 years (Mean = 10.9 ± 1.9 y) undertook eight activities designed to represent a range of everyday childhood movements. The activities included lying, sitting, DVD viewing, active computer games, slow walking, brisk walking, slow running and medium running. With the exception of the lying condition (performed for 10 minutes) all activities were undertaken for 3 minutes, followed by a 2 minute rest period. Participants wore GENEA monitors at three locations (left wrist, right wrist and right hip), along with an ActiGraph GT1M worn adjacent to the hip-mounted GENEA in order for concurrent validity to be established. Participants also wore a portable gas analyser (Cosmed K4b2, Cosmed, Rome, Italy) throughout the activities in order to measure oxygen uptake.

18.2.2 Data analysis

To assess the criterion referenced validity, correlations between each monitor (GENEA at each of the three sites and the ActiGraph GT1M) and steady state VO_2 were calculated for each participant. The Pearson's r values were transformed into Fisher's Zr values, the mean calculated, then converted back to Pearson's r values. The same method was used to assess the concurrent validity for the GENEA at each of the three sites relative to the ActiGraph GT1M.

18.3 RESULTS

Table 18.1. Pearson's *r* values for criterion and concurrent validity

	GENEA			ActiGraph
	Left Wrist	**Right Wrist**	**Hip**	**Hip**
Criterion Validity (VO$_2$)	0.910	0.900	0.965	0.970
Concurrent Validity (GT1M)	0.845	0.830	0.985	N/A

As Table 18.1 shows, the wrist mounted GENEA monitors demonstrated good criterion and concurrent validity; however the hip-mounted monitor yielded significantly higher validity scores for both criterion and concurrent measures ($P < 0.05$).

Due to the large age range of the participants, criterion and concurrent validity of all GENEA monitors were also assessed across different age groups (group 1 = 8–10 years; group 2 = 11–12 years; group 3 = 13–14 years). Table 18.2 shows that criterion validity fluctuates slightly across location and age range, with the hip-mounted GENEA consistently demonstrating the highest validity across position and age groups ($P<0.05$). Similar results were also seen with regard to the concurrent validity (Table 18.3), again, with the hip-mounted GENEA reporting significantly higher concurrent validity than the wrist-worn monitors, for each group ($P<0.05$).

Table 18.2. Criterion validity by age groups

	Criterion validity			
Group	**GENEA Right Wrist**	**GENEA Left Wrist**	**GENEA Hip**	**GT1M Hip**
1	0.910	0.910	0.970	0.970
2	0.890	0.880	0.965	0.965
3	0.900	0.925	0.965	0.975

Table 18.3. Concurrent validity by age groups

	Concurrent validity		
Group	**GENEA Right Wrist**	**GENEA Left Wrist**	**GENEA Hip**
1	0.830	0.860	0.990
2	0.795	0.800	0.985
3	0.845	0.870	0.975

18.4 DISCUSSION

The aim of the current study was to establish both criterion and concurrent validity for the new GENEA waveform triaxial accelerometer. Irrespective of body location, the GENEA monitor showed good criterion validity, however, the hip monitor demonstrated a significantly higher value than the wrist monitors. The same pattern of results was evident when data were broken down by age group. Despite this, the slightly lower validity of the wrist monitors may be compensated for by the potential increase in compliance with wear protocols.

Similar results were found with regard to the concurrent validity of the GENEA; each monitor demonstrated good concurrent validity when compared to the ActiGraph GT1M, with the monitors worn on the hip performing significantly better than both wrist-worn monitors. As output depends on body location (Mathie *et al.*, 2004), the weaker concurrent validities of the wrist-worn monitors relative to the hip-mounted ActiGraph GT1M are not surprising.

Although this is the first study to establish validity for the use of the GENEA with children, similar results were found during the validation of the GENEA with adults (Esliger *et al.*, 2010); monitors at each body location showed good criterion referenced validity, with values being similar across all locations. However, the criterion validity scores reported for the adult population were lower than those reported in the present study with children.

18.5 CONCLUSION

The GENEA has been found to be a valid tool for measuring children's physical activity when worn on either wrist or at the hip. It has also been established as peer to the ActiGraph GT1M. However, further research is warranted, in order to cross validate the monitors with an independent sample of children, and establish activity intensity cut-points for both wrist- and hip-mounted GENEA monitors.

18.6 REFERENCES

Esliger, D.W., Rowlands, A.V., Hurst, T.L., Catt, M., and Eston, R.G., 2010, Validation of the GENEA accelerometer. *Medicine and Science in Sports and Exercise*, **43**, pp. 1085-1093.

Freedson, P., Pober, D., and Janz, K.F., 2005, Calibration of accelerometer output for children. *Medicine and Science in Sports and Exercise*, **37**, pp. S523–S530.

Mathie, M.J., Coster, A.C.F., Lovell, N.H., and Celler, B.G., 2004, Accelerometery: Providing an integrated, practical method for long term, ambulatory monitoring of human movement. *Physiological Measurement*, **25**, pp. R1–R20.

Puyau, M.R., Adolph, A.L., Vohra, F.A., Zakeri, I., and Butte, N.F., 2004, Prediction of activity energy expenditure using accelerometers in children. *Medicine and Science in Sports and Exercise*, **36**, pp. 1625–1631.

Rowlands, A.V., Thomas, P.W.M., Eston, R.G. and Topping, R., 2004, Validation of the RT3 triaxial accelerometer for the assessment of physical activity. *Medicine and Science in Sports and Exercise*, **36**, pp. 518–524.

Van Coevering, P., Harnack, L., Schmitz, K., Fulton, J.E., Galuska, D.A. and Gao, S. 2005, Feasibility of using accelerometers to measure physical activity in young adolescents. *Medicine and Science in Sports and Exercise*, **37**, pp. 867–871.

ENERGY COST OF PLAYING ACTIVITY VIDEO GAMES: A COMPARISON BETWEEN CHILDREN WITH OBESITY AND NORMAL WEIGHT CONTROLS

C. O'Donovan and J. Hussey
Trinity College Dublin, Ireland

19.1 INTRODUCTION

It is recommended that children accumulate at least 60 minutes of moderate to vigorous intensity exercise a day (Strong *et al.*, 2005). An accepted description for moderate intensity exercise is that which results in an energy expenditure of between 3 and 6 METs or a heart rate reserve (HRR) of greater than 50 % (ACSM, 2006). Despite these recommendations, low activity levels are seen in children today, and have been implicated in the increase in obesity (Tremblay and Willms, 2003). Children with obesity have been shown to be less likely than their healthy peers to participate in traditional exercise or sports (Dowda *et al.*, 2001), and spend more time in sedentary activities such as television viewing and computer gaming (Hoos *et al.*, 2003). The World Health Organisation recommends reducing inactivity in obese children (Branca *et al.*, 2007). However, children value screen time (Epstein *et al.*, 1998), and the popularity of video games is increasing (Rideout *et al.*, 2010).

With the recent production of active video games (AVGs), computer gaming has the potential to become a more active pastime (Tremblay and Willms, 2003). One such AVG console is the Wii, (Nintendo Co Ltd, Tokyo, Japan). The Wii is operated through hand-held wireless controllers which enable players to move during gaming. Theoretically, the invention of AVGs could lead to increased physical activity levels or reduced sedentary behaviour.

To date, studies examining energy expended playing AVGs have grouped children who are overweight and obese together, disabling a comparison between those with obesity and those of a healthy weight (Unnithan *et al.*, 2006; Penko and Barkley, 2010). In children with obesity the relative intensity of games played on the Wii is likely to be higher due to lower fitness levels

(Zanconato *et al.*, 1989). Furthermore games necessitating lower limb movement require greater energy expenditure in obese compared to lean children (Maffeis *et al.*, 1993).

The aim of this study was to measure the energy cost of playing an upper limb controlled and a lower limb controlled AVG in children with obesity, and healthy weight children. A secondary aim was to examine the effect of body composition and fitness on the energy expended.

19.2 METHODS

Twenty-seven children with obesity (7 male, mean age 12 ± 3 y) and 27 age and gender matched lean children completed this study. Those who were overweight according to the WHO BMI for age z scores were excluded from participation.

Stature was measured with a Seca stadiometer and body mass was measured with a Seca balance beam scale. Lean body mass was estimated from skin fold measurements using an accepted equation (Durnin and Womersley, 1974). Subjects also completed the 6 minute walk test (6MWT, Morinder *et al.*, 2009).

Oxygen consumption (VO_2), kilocalories expended (kcal), and heart rate (HR) were measured at rest and while playing AVGs with an indirect calorimeter (Oxycon Mobile) and Polar HR monitor. For the purpose of this study Wii Sports boxing and Wii Fit free jogging (hereafter referred to as boxing and jogging respectively) were used. Each game was played for 15 minutes with a 5 minute seated rest between games.

19.2.1 Statistical analysis

METs were calculated for each individual as gaming VO_2 divided by resting VO_2. Age-related predicted maximal HR was calculated as $208 - (0.7*age)$, (Mahon *et al.*, 2010). Paired t tests were conducted within groups to determine if variables differed between conditions. Differences between groups were assessed using independent t tests.

19.3 RESULTS

Participant characteristics and their cardiovascular response to rest and playing activity video games are detailed in Table 19.1.

Table 19.1. Mean (±) of participant characteristics and cardiovascular response to rest and activity video game play. *Indicates a statistically significant difference between groups.

Variables	Obese	Lean	*P* Value
Age, y	12 ± 3	12 ± 3	0.892
BMI, $kg \cdot m^{-2}$ *	30 ± 5	19 ± 2	<0.0001
Lean Body Mass, kg *	48 ± 13	32 ± 10	<0.0001
6MWT distance, m *	491 ± 84	550 ± 77	0.013
Rest			
VO_2, $mL \cdot min^{-1} \cdot kg^{-1}$ *	4.0 ± 0.8	6.0 ± 1.6	<0.0001
$kcal \cdot 15\ min^{-1}$ *	20.8 ± 4.8	14.8 ± 5.7	0.0001
$VO_2\ mL \cdot min^{-1} \cdot FFM^{-1}$	6.3 ± 2.2	7.5 ± 2.0	0.051
Boxing			
HRR, % *	39 ± 12	53 ± 21	0.005
VO_2, $mL \cdot min^{-1} \cdot kg^{-1}$*	10.9 ± 3.4	17.8 ± 6.6	<0.0001
METs	2.7 ± 0.7	3.1 ± 1.0	0.184
$kcal \cdot 15\ min^{-1}$ *	51.2 ± 16.5	41.2 ± 14.6	0.024
$VO_2\ mL \cdot min^{-1} \cdot FFM^{-1}$ *	16.8 ± 6.0	22.7 ± 7.6	0.004
Jogging			
HRR, %	64 ± 14	62 ± 13	0.543
VO_2, $mL \cdot min^{-1} \cdot kg^{-1}$ *	21.8 ± 4.3	27.8 ± 6.6	<0.0001
METs	5.4 ± 1.6	4.9 ± 1.4	0.194
$kcal \cdot 15\ min^{-1}$ *	108.9 ± 30.6	66.5 ± 24.6	<0.0001
$VO_2\ mL \cdot min^{-1} \cdot FFM^{-1}$	32.8 ± 8.2	35.4 ± 8.3	0.265

19.3.1 Comparisons between obese and lean children

When VO_2 was corrected for fat free mass there was no difference in energy expenditure between groups for rest or jogging conditions. Those with obesity expended significantly less energy per kg fat free mass during boxing. Similar trends were seen with HR data, as those with obesity reached a significantly lower % HRR while boxing than lean participants. There was no association between the energy cost of activities and distance covered during the 6 minute walk test.

Participants with obesity reached a light intensity of activity while engaging in Wii Sports boxing, while control children reached moderate levels. Both groups reached moderate levels while playing Wii Fit free jogging.

19.3.2 Comparison between conditions

VO_2 (in $mL \cdot kg^{-1} \cdot min^{-1}$) and kcal expended were significantly higher during boxing than rest, and during jogging than boxing for both groups. Among lean participants HR was higher during boxing and jogging than rest, but there was no significant difference in HR between boxing and jogging. Among those with obesity boxing HR was significantly greater than resting, and significantly lower than jogging.

19.4 CONCLUSION

Wii Fit free jogging can be recommended as a moderate form of aerobic exercise to obese and healthy weight children. Caution should be exercised in recommending Wii Sports boxing to children with obesity as they may not reach the same exercise intensities during play as their healthy peers.

It is unknown why those with obesity did not reach a HR as high as lean participants during Wii Sports boxing. The distribution of lean muscle mass or physiological differences in the upper limb muscles of those with obesity (Ara *et al.*, 2010) may explain the differences between groups seen during boxing which were not evident during jogging.

19.5 REFERENCES

American College of Sports Medicine, 2006, *ACSM's Guidelines for Exercise Testing and Prescription*. Philadelphia, edited by Whaley, M.H., Brubaker, P.H., Otto, R.M. (Baltimore: Lippincott Williams and Wilkins).

Ara, I., Larsen, S., Stallknecht, B., Guerra, B., Morales-Alamo, D., Andersen, J.L., Ponce-González, J.G., Guadalupe-Grau, A., Galbo, H., Calbet, J.A. and Helge, J.W., 2011, Normal mitochondrial function and increased fat oxidation capacity in leg and arm muscles in obese humans. *International Journal of Obesity*, **35**, pp. 99-108.

Branca, F., Nikogosian, H. and Lobstein, T., 2007, *The challenge of obesity in the WHO European Region and the strategies for response*. Geneva, edited by Branca, F., Nigogosian, H., Lobstein, T. (Copenhagen WHO: Europe).

Dowda, M., Ainsworth, B.E., Addy, C.L., Saunders, R. and Riner, W., 2001, Environmental influences, physical activity, and weight status in 8- to 16-year-olds. *Archives of Pediatric and Adolescent Medicine*, **155**, pp. 711-717.

Durnin, J.V. and Womersley, J. 1974, Body fat assessed from total body density and its estimation from skinfold thickness: Measurements on 481 men and women aged from 16 to 72 years. *British Journal of Nutrition*, **32**, pp. 77-97.

Epstein, L.H., Myers, M.D., Raynor, H.A. and Saelens, B.E., 1998, Treatment of pediatric obesity. *Pediatrics*, **101**, pp. 554-570.

Hoos, M.B., Plasqui, G., Gerver, W.J. and Westerterp, K.R., 2003, Physical activity level measured by doubly labeled water and accelerometry in children. *European Journal of Applied Physiology*, **89**, pp. 624-626.

Maffeis, C., Schutz, Y., Schena, F., Zaffanello, M. and Pinelli, L., 1993, Energy expenditure during walking and running in obese and nonobese prepubertal children. *The Journal of Pediatrics*, **123**, pp. 193-199.

Mahon, A.D., Marjerrison, A.D., Lee, J.D., Woodruff, M.E. and Hanna, L.E., 2010, Evaluating the prediction of maximal heart rate in children and adolescents. *Research Quarterly for Exercise and Sport*, **81**, pp. 466-471.

Morinder, G., Mattsson, E., Sollander, C., Marcus, C. and Larsson, U.E., 2009, Six-minute walk test in obese children and adolescents: Reproducibility and validity. *Physiotherapy Research International*, **14**, pp. 91-104.

Penko, A.L. and Barkley, J.E., 2010, Motivation and physiological responses of playing a physically interactive video game relative to a sedentary alternative in children. *Annals of Behavioural Medicine*, **39**, pp. 162-169.

Rideout, V.J., Foehr, U.G. and Roberts, D.F., 2010, *Generation M2 Media in the Lives of 8-to-18-Year-Olds*, edited by Rideout, V.J., (California: The Henry J. Kaiser Family Foundation).

Strong, W.B., Malina, R.M., Blimkie, C.J., Daniels, S.R., Dishman, R.K., Gutin, B., Hergenroeder, A.C., Must, A., Nixon, P.A., Pivarnik, J.M., Rowland, T., Trost, S. and Trudeau, F., 2005, Evidence based physical activity for school-age youth. *The Journal of Pediatrics*, **146**, pp. 732-737.

Tremblay, M.S. and Willms, J.D., 2003, Is the Canadian childhood obesity epidemic related to physical inactivity? *International Journal for Obesity and Related Metabolic Disorders*, **27**, pp. 1100-1105.

Unnithan, V.B., Houser, W. and Fernhall, B., 2006, Evaluation of the energy cost of playing a dance simulation video game in overweight and non-overweight children and adolescents. *International Journal of Sports Medicine*, **27**, pp. 804-809.

Zanconato, S., Baraldi, E., Santuz, P., Rigon, F., Vido, L., Da Dalt, L. and Zacchello, F., 1989, Gas exchange during exercise in obese children. *European Journal of Pediatrics*, **148**, pp. 614-617.

CONTRIBUTION OF ORGANIZED SPORTS TO ESTIMATED ENERGY EXPENDITURE IN FEMALE ADOLESCENTS

I.S. Rêgo[1], A.M. Rodrigues[1], H.M. Carvalho[1], E. Ronque[2], E. Cyrino[2], and M. Coelho-e-Silva[1]

[1]Faculty of Sport Science and Physical Education, University of Coimbra, Portugal; [2]State University of Londrina, Brazil

20.1 INTRODUCTION

Studies of energy expenditure are valuable in understanding the cause of childhood obesity. Children and adolescents with overweight and obesity are at an increased risk of co-morbidities including type 2 diabetes, endocrine and orthopaedic disorders, and low health-related quality of life (Cumming and Riddoch, 2008). Dietary energy requirements and recommendations for youth are usually predicted from estimation of daily energy expenditure. Sport is probably one of the most relevant forms of physical activity in young people and the determination of the amount of energy that adolescents are expending in different contexts of sport participation is of interest to public health. The contribution of organized sport to daily physical activity and energy expenditure is not clear and may be culturally specific. Previous studies were performed in the US (Katzmarzyk and Malina, 1998; Wickel and Eisenmann, 2007) and considered attendees of a mid-Michigan junior high school and participants from youth basketball, soccer and flag football programmes sponsored by recreation departments. The purpose of this study was to examine the contribution of participation in institutionalized and adult-supervised sports to estimated daily energy expenditure in female adolescents aged 12-16 years.

20.2 METHODS

The scientific committee of *University of Coimbra* and *Portuguese Foundation for Science and Technology* approved the procedure of this study. Adolescents were informed about the aim and design of the study. Signed informed consent was obtained prior to data collection. The sample was composed of 100 female adolescents aged 12-16 years.

20.2.1 Variables

Stature was measured with a portable stadiometer (Harpenden model 98.603, Holtain Ltd, Crosswell, UK) to the nearest 0.1 cm. Body mass (BM) was measured with a portable balance (Seca model 770, Hanover, MD, USA) to the nearest 0.1 kg. The 3 day diary created by Bouchard *et al.* (1983) was used to estimate the total daily energy expenditure (TDEE). The protocol partitioned each day into 96 periods and the respondent was asked to mention the dominant activity for each 15 min period throughout the day, so that energy expenditure estimates could be calculated adopting the following equivalents in $kcal \cdot kg^{-1} \cdot min^{-1}$: [code 1] sleeping: 0.26; [code 2] sitting: 0.38; [code 3] light activity standing: 0.57; [code 4] slow walking ~ 4 $km \cdot h^{-1}$: 0.69; [code 5] light manual tasks: 0.84; [code 6] light activities: 1.2; [code 7] manual tasks at a moderate pace: 1.4; [code 8] activities of higher intensity: 1.5; [code 9] very intensive activities: 2.0. In addition, adolescents were instructed to mark the cells that corresponded to organized sports defined as a practice performed at an institution under the supervision of an adult (school sport club or community sport club), so that energy expenditure estimates specific to organized sport programmes could also be derived.

20.2.2 Statistical analysis

Analysis of variance was used to compare youth who participated (group P) in adult-supervised sport programme and those who did not (group NP). Dependent variables were chronological age (CA), body size, TDEE (categories 1-9), AEE (categories 2-9) and MVEE (categories 6-9). The significance level was set at $P<0.05$.

20.3 RESULTS

Participant and non-participant adolescents did not differ in CA ($F=1.15$, n.s.), stature ($F=0.04$, n.s.), body mass ($F=2.83$ n.s.), absolute TDEE (NP: 2388 kcal; P: 2406 kcal; $F=0.01$, n.s.), absolute AEE (NP: 1674 kcal; P: 1756 kcal; $F=0.39$, n.s.). Differences between groups were significant for MVEE expressed in kcal (NP: 424 kcal; P: 657 kcal; $F=4.65$, $P<0.05$) and also when the expenditure is expressed in $kcal \cdot kg^{-1}$ (NP: 6.7 $kcal \cdot kg^{-1}$; P: 11.9 $kcal \cdot kg^{-1}$; $F=7.66$, $P<0.01$). When the estimates of TDEE and AEE were expressed in $kcal \cdot kg^{-1}$ differences were significant as presented in Table 20.1. Female adolescents who participated in organized sport programmes presented, in average, 51.4 minutes per day in those activities. Figure 20.1 shows the contribution of organized sports to TDEE and its portions: 12.5 % of TDEE, 17.4 % of AEE and 58.4 % of MVEE (only for participants, n=70).

Table 20.1. Descriptive statistics of female adolescents who participate in institutionalized organized sports and those who did not and results of ANOVA.

Group	Non-Participants (n=30)	Participants (n=70)	F (p)
Chron. Age, y	14.32 ± 0.98	14.12 ± 0.88	1.15 (0.31)
Stature, cm	159.3 ± 5.2	158.9 ± 7.4	0.04 (0.84)
Body mass, kg	60.33 ± 15.4	55.6 ± 11.7	2.83 (0.10)
TDEE, kcal·day^{-1}	2388 ± 762	2406 ± 633	0.01 (0.91)
TDEE, kcal·kg^{-1}·day^{-1}	39.3 ± 5.0	43.4 ± 7.8	6.77 (0.01)
AEE, kcal·day^{-1}	1674 ± 684	1756 ± 565	0.39 (0.54)
AEE, kcal·kg^{-1}·day^{-1}	27.4 ± 5.9	31.7 ± 8.9	6.05 (0.02)
MVEE, kcal·day^{-1}	424 ± 434	657 ± 519	4.65 (0.03)
MVEE, kcal·kg^{-1}·day^{-1}	6.7 ± 6.1	11.9 ± 9.4	7.66 (0.01)

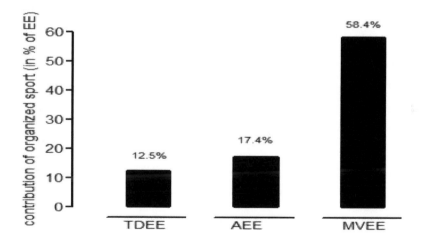

Figure 20.1. Contribution of institutionalized and adult-supervised sport programmes to total daily energy expenditure (TDEE), activity energy expenditure (AEE) and moderate-to-vigorous energy expenditure (MVEE).

20.4 CONCLUSION

In summary, institutionalized programmes of youth sports appeared as a relevant component of energy expenditure among female adolescents. It corresponded to a substantial portion of energy expenditure at moderate-to-vigorous intensity level that is considered relevant for the development of cardiorespiratory fitness. In parallel, additional research modelling energy expenditure for body mass and lean body mass is needed to compare participants and non-participants.

20.5 REFERENCES

Bouchard, C., Tremblay, A., Leblanc, C., Lortie, G., Savard, R., and Theriault, G., 1983, A method to assess energy expenditure in children and adults. *American Journal of Clinical Nutrition*, **37**, pp. 461-467.

Cumming, S.P., and Riddoch, C., 2008, Physical activity, physical fitness and health: Current concepts. In *Paediatric Exercise Science and Medicine*, edited by Armstrong, N. and van Mechelen, W. (Oxford: Oxford University Press), pp. 327-338.

Katzmarzyk, P.T., and Malina, R.M., 1998, Contribution of organized sports participation to estimated daily energy expenditure in youth. *Pediatric Exercise Science*, **10**, pp. 378-386.

Wickel, E.E., and Eisenmann, J.C., 2007, Contribution of youth sport to total daily physical activity among 6- to 12-yr-old boys. *Medicine and Science in Sports and Exercise*, **39**, pp. 1493-1500.

THE EFFECT OF A 6 WEEK SCHOOL BASED ACTIVE PLAY INTERVENTION ON PRE-SCHOOL PHYSICAL ACTIVITY AND SEDENTARY BEHAVIOUR

M.V. O'Dwyer[1], Z. Knowles[1], S.J. Fairclough[1], N.D. Ridgers[2], L. Foweather[1], and G. Stratton[1]

[1] The REACH Group, Liverpool John Moores University, UK
[2] Centre for Physical Activity and Nutrition Research, Deakin University, Australia

21.1 INTRODUCTION

Regular physical activity (PA) may benefit health (Anderssen *et al.*, 2007), aid social development (Sawyers, 1994), and improve psychological welfare (Ekelund *et al.,* 2004). Yet, few interventions have significantly increased PA in pre-school children. This study aimed to investigate the effectiveness of a 6 week Active Play intervention on pre-school children's PA levels.

21.2 METHODS

21.2.1 Participants and settings

Participants (n=240; 52 % male, age=4.4 ± 0.6 y) were recruited from 12 schools based in a city in England following ethical approval from the Liverpool John Moores University Ethics Committee. Each school was randomly assigned to an intervention or comparison group. An overview of the intervention is described elsewhere (O'Dwyer *et al.,* 2011).

21.3 MEASURES

Habitual PA was measured using 5 s epochs over 7 days using the GT1M Actigraph uniaxial accelerometer (Pensacola, FL), which is a valid measure of PA in pre-school children (Sirard et al., 2005).

21.3.1 Analyses

PA was defined using age specific cut-points (Sirard et al., 2005). Participants were required to have worn the monitors on 3 days, including one weekend day (Penpraze et al., 2006). For a day to be included, it was necessary that the monitor was worn for a minimum period of time (Catellier et al., 2005). The minimum wear time was defined separately for weekdays and weekend days. The final sample consisted of 154 children during the weekday and 73 children during the weekend.

A mixed between-within subject's ANOVA assessed the effectiveness of intervention on time spent in sedentary and active behaviours. The level of significance was set at 0.05.

21.4 RESULTS

At baseline, pre-school children spent 6.9 % (mean: 41.7 minutes) of the weekday in moderate-to-vigorous physical activity (MVPA) while 81.5 % (mean: 642.5 minutes) of time was spent being sedentary. Thirteen % of the participants achieved 60 minutes of MVPA per day during weekdays. Table 21.1 shows that there was no significant interaction between intervention type and time spent being sedentary or in any other PA intensity.

Table 21.2 shows that weekend sedentary time also decreased in both groups (mean decrease: 31.2 minutes) although not significant ($P=0.6$). Nineteen % of the participants achieved 60 minutes of MVPA per day during the weekend. There was no significant group differences recorded for any of the intensities.

21.5 DISCUSSION

Results indicate that the intervention was not successful in increasing PA or decreasing sedentary time in either group.

Low levels of baseline PA on weekdays emphasise the potential of the school environment to increase PA engagement. However, the interventions evaluated in this study were not effective in increasing the engagement in PA.

Our findings are consistent with Reilly *et al.* (2006), who concluded that three 30 minute sessions lasting 24 weeks were an inadequate dose of PA to impact on PA levels. Six weeks is thus too short to expect a change in behaviour. The absence of significant others (parents and siblings) may contribute to the lack of change. Bronfenbrenners Ecological Model (Bronfenbrenner, 1989) proposes that for a pre-school child, the two main influencing factors are parents and teachers. Future research may include the involvement of these people.

Table 21.1. Mean (SD) weekday group differences with respect to physical activity variables

	Weekday							
	Sedentary min		Light min		Moderate min		Vigorous min	
	Pre	Post	Pre	Post	Pre	Post	Pre	Post
Total (n=154)	642.5 (59.4)	599.9 (81.3)	72.0 (14.6)	69.9 (16.0)	27.6 (12.8)	26.4 (14.7)	14.1 (11.1)	14.4 (7.0)
Intervention (n=70)	655.6 (61.1)	604.4 (79.2)	70.3 (15.8)	69.2 (16.1)	26.0 (12.1)	25.1 (17.2)	13.2 (6.2)	13.6 (6.4)
Comparison (n=84)	631.6 (59.4)	596.0 (83.3)	73.4 (13.5)	70.5 (15.8)	28.9 (13.2)	27.5 (12.2)	14.8 (7.3)	15.0 (7.3)
P-value for group effect	0.06		0.58		0.38		0.33	

Table 21.2. Mean (SD) weekend day group differences with respect to physical activity variables

	Weekend day							
	Sedentary min		Light min		Moderate min		Vigorous min	
	Pre	Post	Pre	Post	Pre	Post	Pre	Post
Total (n=73)	649.8 (71.6)	618.8 (105.1)	71.4 (18.7)	71.4 (23.9)	29.8 (15.1)	27.3 (15.7)	17.4 (25.2)	14.8 (9.0)
Intervention (n=31)	657.5 (74.5)	618.2 (96.7)	75.1 (19.6)	71.8 (26.1)	31.0 (18.8)	26.4 (13.7)	15.6 (8.5)	13.1 (5.8)
Comparison (n=42)	644.2 (69.9)	619.3 (112.1)	68.6 (17.8)	71.1 (22.4)	28.8 (15.1)	27.9 (17.1)	18.6 (32.6)	16.0 (10.8)
P-value for group effect	0.65		0.30		0.68		0.45	

A second limitation concerns the PA cut-points used. According to Cliff *et al.* (2007), more research is needed to reach a greater consensus on the most appropriate cut-points to use. Evidence from high quality calibration studies in children is fairly consistent in suggesting that the most appropriate cut-point for MVPA lies in the 3000–3600 CPM range (Reilly *et al.,* 2008). In this study the age specific cut-points of Sirard *et al.* (2005) were used, which are specific for 5 second measurement intervals. However, when multiplying these cut-points by 12, they are in the suggested range for only 4- and 5-year olds, therefore underestimating MVPA for 3-year olds. Other limitations to this study include the statistical analysis used. Ideally multi-level analyses should be used to take into account the clustering of children within schools. Strengths of this study include the use of an objective measure of PA and a medium sized representative sample.

21.6 REFERENCES

Anderssen, S.A., Cooper, A.R., Riddoch, C., Sardinha, L.B., Harro, M., Brage, S. and Andersen, L.B., 2007, Low cardiorespiratory fitness is a strong predictor for clustering of cardiovascular disease risk factors in children independent of country, age and sex. *European Journal of Cardiovascular Prevention and Rehabilitation*, **14**, pp. 526-531.

Bronfenbrenner, U., 1989, Ecological system theories. *Annals of Child Development*, **6**, pp. 187-251.

Catellier, D.J., Hannan, P.J., Murray, D.H., Addy, C.L., Conway, T.L. and Yang, S., 2005, Imputation of missing data when measuring physical activity by accelerometry. *Medicine and Science in Sports and Exercise*, **37**, pp. 555–562.

Cliff, D.P. and Okeley, A.D., 2007, Comparison of two sets of accelerometer cut-off points for calculating moderate-to-vigorous physical activity in young children. *Journal of Physical Activity and Health*, **4**, pp. 509–513.

Ekeland, E., Heian, F., Hagen, K.B., Abbott, J.M. and Nordheim, L., 2004, Exercise to improve self-esteem in children and young people. *Cochrane Database Systematic Reviews*, 1, CD003683.

O'Dwyer, M.V., Foweather, L, Stratton, G. and Ridgers, N.D., 2011, Physical activity in non-overweight and overweight UK preschool children: Preliminary findings and methods of the Active Play Project. *Science and Sports*, (in press).

Penpraze, V., Reilly, J.J., MacLean, C.M., Montgomery, C., Kelly, L.A. and Paton, J.Y., 2006, Monitoring of physical activity in young children: How much is enough? *Pediatric Exercise Science*, **18**, pp. 483-491.

Reilly, J.J., Kelly, L., Montgomery, C., Williamson, A., Fisher, A., McColl, J.H and Grant, S., 2006, Physical activity to prevent obesity in young children:

Cluster randomised controlled trial. *British Medical Journal*, **333**, pp. 1041-1045.

Reilly, J.J., Penpraze, V., Hislop, J., Davies, G., Grant, S. and Paton J.Y., 2008, Objective measurement of physical activity and sedentary behavior: Review with new data. *Archives of Disease in Childhood*, **93**, pp. 614-619.

Sawyers, J.K., 2004, The preschool playground: Developing skills through outdoor play. *The Journal of Physical Education, Recreation and Dance*, **65**, pp. 31-34.

Sirard, J.R., Trost, S.G., Pfeiffer, K.A., Dowda, M. and Pate, R.R., 2005, Calibration and evaluation of an objective measure of physical activity in preschool children. *Journal of Physical Activity and Health*, **3**, pp. 345-357.

RELATIONSHIPS BETWEEN BONE MINERAL DENSITY AND JUMPING HEIGHT IN PREPUBERTAL GIRLS WITH DIFFERENT PHYSICAL ACTIVITY PATTERNS

A.-L. Parm[1,2], J. Jürimäe[1], M. Saar[1], K. Pärna[1], V. Tillmann[1], K. Maasalu[1], I. Neissaar[1], and T. Jürimäe[1]

[1]University of Tartu, Estonia; [2]Tartu Health Care College, Estonia

22.1 INTRODUCTION

Better bone mineral density (BMD) in childhood might prevent osteoporosis in later life (Baxter-Jones *et al.*, 2008). Recent studies show that high impact loading (such as rhythmic gymnastics) is the most effective type of bone-building activity in pubertal years (Gruodyté *et al.*, 2010), because high-impact activity, for example jumping, seems to be even more osteogenic than calcium or protein intake (Iuliano-Burns *et al.*, 2005). In girls, with regard to physical activity, greater emphasis should also be placed on prepubertal period (Bass *et al.*, 1998), when half of lumbar adult peak bone mass is acquired (Sabatier *et al.*, 1999).

Jumping ability seems to correlate well with the different bone values. Different vertical jumps have been used to evaluate jumping ability in young athletes. Maximum vertical jump performed from the standing position with a countermovement (CMJ) as well as rebound jumps for 15 (RJ15s) and 30 (RJ30s) seconds reflect well the jumping abilities in young athletes (Gruodyté *et al.*, 2009). For example, Gruodyté *et al.* (2009) have demonstrated some background information on the relationship between vertical jumping height and areal BMD values in pubertal girls with different physical activity patterns. However, there has been very little information available about the relationships between different BMD measures and jumping ability in prepubertal girls participating in different sport disciplines. The aim of the study was to investigate the relationship between jumping height and bone mineral density in prepubertal girls with different physical activity patterns. For this purpose, single (CMJ) and continuous (RJ15s) jumping tests were used. It was hypothesized that jumping height of both these tests is related to total and areal BMD values already in prepubertal years at least in the rhythmic gymnasts group.

22.2 METHODS

The participants were 89 prepubertal girls aged 7-9 years comprising two groups: rhythmic gymnastics (n=46) and controls (n=43). Gymnasts had practiced rhythmic gymnastics and ballet lessons 6-12 h per week for the last 1-3 years. Controls had only 2-3 times a week compulsory physical education lessons at school. All participants were free from present or past diseases known to affect skeletal metabolism, and none of the girls were receiving medications known to affect bone. The study was approved by the Medical Ethics Committee of the University of Tartu (Estonia).

Stature (cm) and body mass (BM, kg) were measured and body mass index (BMI, $kg \cdot m^{-2}$) was calculated. Body composition (body fat %, fat mass [FM], and fat free mass [FFM]) and BMD ($g \cdot cm^{-2}$) from whole body (WB), lumbar spine (LS, L2-L4) and femoral neck (FN) were measured by dual energy X-ray absorptiometry. DXA measurements and results were evaluated by the same examiner. Bone age was assessed with an X-ray of the left hand and determined according to the method of Greulich and Pyle (1959).

The maximal height of two-footed hands-on-the-hips vertical jumps was measured using contact mat (Newtest OY, Finland) which was connected to a digital recorder that calculated the flight height. All the participants performed at first a single countermovement jump (CMJ) from a standing position with a preliminary countermovement, followed by the rebound jump with continuous countermovement jumps for 15 s (RJ15s). The girls were instructed and verbally encouraged to jump as high and as rapidly as they could. The hands remained on waist throughout all jumping tests to avoid upper extremeties contribution to the jump height.

The Statistical Package for the Social Sciences (SPSS) version 16.0 (SPSS Inc, Chicago, USA) was used. Mean and standard deviation (SD) were calculated. Differences between groups were calculated using an independent t-test, Pearson product movement correlation coefficients were computed to identify relationships between measured variables. Stepwise multiple regression analysis was performed to determine the possible independent effect of body composition (FM, FFM and BMI) and vertical jumps (CMJ, RJ15s) parameters on measured BMD values. The level of significance was set at $P \leq 0.05$ for all statistical analysis.

22.3 RESULTS

There were no differences ($P>0.05$) between gymnasts and controls regarding to age or body composition values, only body fat % and FM values were significantly lower ($P<0.05$) in gymnasts compared with controls. The measured total and areal (LS and FN) BMD and also vertical jumps (CMJ and RJ15s) tests were higher ($P<0.05$) in gymnasts compared with controls.

Whole-body BMD was significantly correlated to BM and FM, LS BMD was significantly related to height and FN BMD to chronological age in gymnasts (Table 22.1). Whole-body and LS BMD values were significantly correlated with chronological age, bone age, height, BM, BMI, body fat %, FM and FFM in controls. Body composition parameters correlated with jumping height (CMJ and RJ15s) only in controls. Interestingly FN BMD was significantly correlated with height of RJ15s jumping test only in gymnasts and LS BMD and WB BMD were significantly correlated with RJ15s only in controls (Table 22.1).

In gymnasts, stepwise multiple regression analysis revealed a significant association between WB BMD and FM, where FM explained 11.3 % of the variability in WB BMD. In controls, FFM was the most significant predictor of WB and LS BMD, explaining 40.9 % and 55.6 % of the variability in WB and LS BMD values, respectively. In addition, stepwise multiple regression analysis demonstrated that the height of CJ15s was the most significant predictor of FN BMD, explaining 8.7 % of the variability in gymnasts.

Table 22.1. Correlation coefficients between bone mineral density with measured body composition and jumping height characteristics in prepubertal rhythmic gymnasts and controls (* Statistically significant: $P<0.05$).

Variable	Whole body BMD ($g \cdot cm^{-2}$)		Lumbar spine BMD ($g \cdot cm^{-2}$)		Femoral neck BMD ($g \cdot cm^{-2}$)	
	Gymnast	Control	Gymnast	Control	Gymnast	Control
Age (y)	0.122	0.454*	0.093	0.375*	0.373*	0.032
Bone age (y)	0.013	0.578*	0.131	0.541*	0.290	0.233
Stature (cm)	0.264	0.535*	0.310*	0.599*	-0.287	0.014
Body mass (kg)	0.343*	0.617*	0.202	0.721*	-0.190	0.044
BMI ($kg \cdot m^{-2}$)	0.242	0.487*	0.003	0.583*	0.013	0.078
Body fat (%)	0.277	0.367*	0.051	0.437*	-0.064	0.064
Fat mass (kg)	0.337*	0.490*	0.115	0.584*	-0.119	0.050
Fat free mass (kg)	0.208	0.640*	0.209	0.746*	-0.168	0.036
CMJ (cm)	0.160	-0.185	-0.011	-0.237	-0.079	0.116
RJ15s (cm)	0.101	-0.373*	0.213	-0.348*	-0.294*	0.033

22.4 CONCLUSION

Better bone parameters in adolescent rhythmic gymnasts compared to controls is found several times (Courteix *et al.*, 2007; Gruodyté *et al.*, 2009). The results of the present investigation demonstrated that gymnastics as high-impact activity has an osteogenic effect already in prepubertal years. We confirmed that already pre-pubertal gymnasts present higher total and areal BMD and jumping height values compared with relatively inactive controls.

Single maximum jumping height is not related with total or areal BMD values in prepubertal girls. Repeated jumps (RJ15s) better characterize BMD values in prepubertal girls. Femoral neck seems to be more sensitive to the specific physical activity patterns in prepubertal years compared to the BMD at the LS and WB, because from BMD values only FN BMD correlated with RJ15s in gymnasts. Gruodyté *et al.* (2009) found similar results in their adolescent gymnasts group. Differently from Gruodyté *et al.* (2009) we did not find significant correlation between LS BMD and RJ15s in gymnasts, but it may occur later in adolescent years.

In conclusion, the present study demonstrated that 1) continuous high-impact physical activity has beneficial effects on the development of areal and total BMD in prepubertal girls; 2) FN BMD is more sensitive to the mechanical loading than LS BMD or WB BMD; and 3) repeated jumps test characterize bone development better than single maximal jump.

We acknowledge some limitations of our study, the first stemming from the cross-sectional design and secondly, from the relatively small groups of subjects. Thirdly, there was no experimental group of the same-age girls who exercised using non weight-bearing exercises (for example swimming).

22.5 REFERENCES

Bass, S., Pearce, G., Bradney, M., Hendrich, E., Delmas, P.D., Harding, A. And Seeman, E., 1998, Exercise before puberty may confer residual benefits in bone density in adulthood: Studies in active prepubertal and retired female gymnasts. *Journal of Bone and Mineral Research*, **13**, pp. 500-507.

Baxter-Jones, A.D.G., Kontulainen, S.A., Faulkner, R.A., and Bailey, D.A. 2008, A longitudinal study of the relationship of physical activity to bone mineral accrual from adolescence to young adulthood. *Bone*, **43**, pp. 1101-1107.

Courteix, D., Rieth, N., Thomas, T., Van Praagh, E., Benhamou, C.L., Collomp, K., Lespessailles, E. and Jaffré, C., 2007, Preserved bone health in adolescent elite rhythmic gymnasts despite hypoleptinemia. *Hormone Research*, **68**, pp. 20-27.

Greulish, W.W. and Pyle, S.I., 1959, *Radiographics atlas of skeletal development of hand and wrist*. 2nd ed. Stanford, CA, USA: Stanford University Press.

Gruodyté, R., Jürimäe, J., Saar, M., Maasalu, K. and Jürimäe, T., 2009, Relationships between areal bone mineral density and jumping height in pubertal girls with different physical activity patterns. *Journal of Sports and Physical Fitness*, **49**, pp. 474-479.

Gruodyté, R., Jürimäe, J., Cicchella, A., Stefanelli, C., Passariello, C. And Jürimäe, T., 2010, Adipocytokines and bone mineral density in adolescent female athletes. *Acta Paediatricia*, **99**, pp. 1879-1884.

Iuliano-Burns, S., Stone, J., Hopper, J.L. and Seeman, E., 2005, Diet and exercise during growth have site-specific skeletal effects: A co-twin control study. *Osteoporosis International*, **16**, pp. 1225-1232.

Sabatier, J.P., Guaydier-Souquieres, G., Benmalek, A. and Marcelli, C., 1999, Evolution of lumbar bone mineral content during adolescence and adulthood: A longitudinal study in 395 healthy females 10-24 years of age and 206 pre-menopausal women. *Osteoporosis International*, **9**, pp. 476-488.

CHAPTER NUMBER 23

BODY STRUCTURE, PHYSICAL ACTIVITY AND QUANTITATIVE ULTRASOUND MEASUREMENTS IN PREPUBERTAL BOYS

M. Szmodis, E. Bosnyák, G. Szőts, E. Trájer, M. Tóth,
and A. Farkas
Semmelweis University, Budapest, Hungary

23.1 INTRODUCTION

Osteopenia and osteoporosis are common diseases in the world. It is well known that bone degeneration can be prevented or decreased by regular physical activity.

High-impact exercise, like football has been shown to be associated with higher bone mass. Football involves running, kicking, jumping, tackling, turning, sprinting. During these movements the lower extremities are loaded with high-impact forces (Tarakçi and Oral, 2009).

A quantitative ultrasound measurement is a relatively inexpensive, portable, non-invasive and radiation-free method of evaluating bone status. The main aim of this pilot study was to analyze the relationships between different physical activity levels, anthropometric and bone parameters in prepubertal boys.

23.2 SUBJECTS AND METHODS

The subjects were non-athletic (n=34) and soccer player prepubertal boys (n=76), grouped also as younger (9-10 y, n=64) and older (11-12 y, n=46). Subjects had 1.5 to 4 years sport-related experience. Anthropometric measurements were taken by the suggestion of the IBP (Weiner and Lourie, 1969), including estimated body fat percentage (Pařižková, 1961) and physique was characterised by Conrad's growth type (1963). Biological age was assessed by anthropometric measurements using the method of Mészáros and Mohácsi (1983).

161

Calcaneal quantitative ultrasound parameters were registered by a Sonost 3000 bone densitometer. The analysis included speed of sound (SOS, m·s⁻¹), broadband ultrasound attenuation (BUA, dB/MHz) and the calculated bone quantity index (BQI=αSOS+βBUA, αβ: temperature corrections).

Correlation patterns of anthropometric variables and bone characteristics for total sample and for subgroups were analyzed. Differences between athletic and non-athletic boys were tested by Student t-test; and if the F-test of ANOVA was significant for the respective means (age and physical activity), Tukey's post-hoc test was used at the 5 % level of effective random error.

23.3 RESULTS

Anthropometric measurements of subgroups by physical activity and age are summarised in Table 23.1.

Table 23.1. Basic statistics of the four subgroups

	Morphological age (y)		Fat %		MIX		PLX (cm)	
	mean	SD	mean	SD	mean	SD	mean	SD
Athletes	9.55	1.32	13.92	5.49	-1.53	0.24	64.90	3.86
Non-athletes	11.17	1.51	20.47	7.73	-1.55	0.37	69.96	4.84
Younger	9.19	1.26	14.82	6.49	-1.48	0.28	64.65	4.50
Older	11.18	1.20	17.53	7.33	-1.62	0.29	68.89	4.11

There were moderate significant relationships between age, stature, plastic index and SOS, BUA, BQI for the total sample. In non-athletes, all bone parameters were significantly correlated with age and no significant correlation was found in athletes but for SOS (Table 23.2).

Table 23.2. Correlation pattern of anthropometric and bone parameters; (* denotes significant correlation coefficient, $P<0.05$).

		Age	Stature	Body Weight	Plastic index
Total Sample	BUA	0.26*	0.19*	0.19*	0.20*
	SOS	0.35*	0.26*	0.16	0.20*
	BQI	0.37*	0.29*	0.18	0.22*
Athletes	BUA	0.06	0.02	0.06	0.07
	SOS	0.24*	0.18	0.16	0.16
	BQI	0.20	0.16	0.17	0.19
Non-athletes	BUA	0.75*	0.60*	0.30	0.37*
	SOS	0.50*	0.30	0.01	0.08
	BQI	0.72*	0.51*	0.13	0.20

In comparison of the activity-related subgroups the bone parameters, i.e. SOS in m·s^{-1} (1493.4 ± 10.78 vs. 1497.6 ± 9.57), BUA in dB/MHz (71.92 ± 11.29 vs. 74.38 ± 11.12) and BQI (60.16 ± 11.17 vs. 63.00 ± 10.87) did not differ (Figures 23.1, 23.2, 23.3).

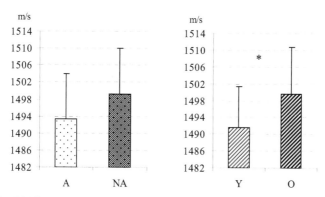

Figure 23.1. SOS in subgroups . Abbr: A = athletes, NA = non-athletes, Y = 9-10y, O = 11-12y. *=*P*<0.05.

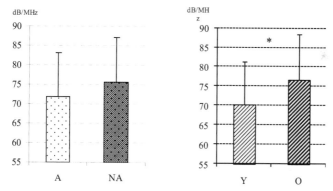

Figure 23.2. BUA in subgroups. Abbr: A = athletes, NA = non-athletes, Y = 9-10y, O = 11-12y. *=*P*<0.05.

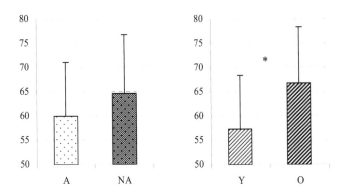

Figure 23.3. BQI in subgroups. Abbr: as in Figure 23.2. *=*P*<0.05

Bone variables differed significantly by age: SOS (1491.59 ± 9.69 vs. 1499.09 ± 10.24), BUA (70.11 ± 10.69 vs. 76.26 ± 11.13) and BQI (57.27 ± 10.05 vs.66.27 ± 10.45) (Figures 23.1-3).

23.4 CONCLUSION

The bone variables did not significantly differ in athletes and in non-athletic prepubertal boys, similar to Cvijetić *et al.* (2003), in contrast to Falk *et al.* (2003) and Mentzel *et al.* (2005).

It seems that quantity bone parameters depend on the chronological as well as the biological age. Although the bone parameters were related with antropometric variables no difference was found at the same age even with various body size. That means that age had the strongest effect on bone parameters in prepubertal boys.

The older boys had larger values, so favourable characteristics of bone in this sample, irrespective to body size.

23.5. REFERENCES

Conrad, K., 1963, *Der Konstitutionstypus* (2. Aufl.) Springer, Berlin.

Cvijetić, S., Barić, I.C., Bolanca, S., Juresa, V. And Ozegović, D.D., 2003, Ultrasound bone measurement in children and adolescents. Correlation with nutrition, puberty, anthropometry, and physical activity. *Journal of Clinical Epidemiology*, **56**, pp. 591-597.

Falk, B., Bronsthein, Z., Constantini, N.W. and Eliakim, A., 2003, Quantitative ultrasound of the tibia and radius in prepubertal and early-pubertal female athletes. *Archives of Pediatric and Adolescent Medicine.* **157**, pp. 139-143.

Mentzel, H.-J., Wünsche, K., Malich, A., Böttcher, J., Vogt, S. and Kaiser, W.A., 2005, Einfluss sportlicher Aktivität von Kindern und Jugendlichen auf den Kalkaneus – Eine Untersuchung mit quantitativem Ultraschall, *Pädiatrische Radiologie*, **177**, pp. 524-552.

Mészáros, J., and Mohácsi, J., 1983, *A biológiai fejlettség meghatározása és a felnõtt termet elõrejelzése a városi fiatalok fejlõdésmenete alapján.* Kandidátusi értekezés, Budapest.

Pařižková, J., 1961, Total body fat and skinfold thickness in children. *Metabolism*, **10**, pp. 794-807.

Tarakçi, D. and Oral, A., 2009, How do contralateral calcaneal quantitative ultrasound measurements in male professional football (soccer) players reflect the effects of high-impact physical activity on bone? *Journal of Sports Medicine and Physical Fitness*, **49**, pp. 78-84.

Weiner J.E.S. and Lourie. J.A., 1969, (Eds) *Human Biology*. A Guide to Field Methods. IBP Handbook, No. 9. Blackwell, Oxford.

THE COMBINED ASSOCIATION OF SELF-EFFICACY AND FATNESS ON PHYSICAL ACTIVITY IN LOW INCOME, MINORITY CHILDREN

K.A. Pfeiffer, D. Suton, J.C. Eisenmann, J.M. Pivarnik, J.J. Carlson, and E. Lamb

Michigan State University and Crim Fitness Foundation, USA

24.1 INTRODUCTION

The prevalence of overweight and obesity in United States children and adolescents was recently reported to be 32 % (Ogden *et al.*, 2010). Researchers believe that low levels of physical activity are at least partially responsible for prevalence rates, since approximately 60 % of U.S. children and adolescents do not meet physical activity recommendations (Troiano *et al.*, 2008). Low income, minority populations in the U.S. experience higher prevalence of obesity and are less physically active compared to their white counterparts (Sallis *et al.*, 2000; Butcher *et al.*, 2008; Flegal *et al.*, 2010). Thus, it is important to address correlates of physical activity (PA) in low income, minority populations in order to determine psychosocial variables upon which to focus physical activity interventions.

Self-efficacy (SE) for PA is an important psychosocial factor related to PA during childhood and adolescence (Sallis *et al.*, 2000). Many previous studies have shown a positive link between SE for PA and PA behaviour (Trost *et al.*, 2001, De Bourdeaudhuij *et al.*, 2005). Additionally, SE for PA has been shown to be a determinant of PA in underserved, minority adolescents (Kitzman-Ulrich *et al.*, 2010). Previous investigations have also found cases when overweight/over-fat was related to PA (Ward *et al.*, 2006). However, the relationship between SE for PA and PA in normal fat versus over-fat children, particularly in low income, minority populations, is unclear. The purpose of this study was to compare PA among four groups of children based on body fatness and SE for PA: 1) normal fat, low SE, 2) over-fat, low SE, 3) normal fat, high SE, and 4) over-fat, high SE.

24.2 METHODS

24.2.1 Participants

Participants were 154, 4th and 5th grade students (74 boys and 80 girls; mean age 10.6 ± 0.8 y; 62 % African American), from a convenience sample at four schools with populations that were predominantly minority (~60 % African American) and low income (~75 % eligible for free/reduced price lunch). Prior to beginning the project, participants provided assent and parents/guardians provided informed consent. The study was approved by the Michigan State University Biomedical Institutional Review Board.

24.2.2 Measures and procedures

PA was assessed using self-report (adopted from Youth Risk Behavior Surveillance System survey conducted by the U.S. Centers for Disease Control and Prevention). SE for PA was assessed using a 15-item, 5-point scale questionnaire (1-disagree a lot, 5-agree a lot) designed for children and adolescents (Saunders *et al.*, 1997). High and low SE were determined by median split. Body fatness was assessed by bioelectric impedance analysis (Tanita BC-534 Innerscan), and cut-points were used from the Fitnessgram standards for healthy fitness zone (over-fat: ≥25 % boys; ≥32 % girls). All measures were taken by trained staff.

24.2.3 Statistical analyses

Descriptive statistics were calculated for the entire sample. Gender, self-efficacy, and fatness group differences were examined using t-tests, and differences among fatness-SE groups were explored using ANOVA and Hochberg's post-hoc test.

24.3 RESULTS

On average, participants reported 4.8 ± 2.2 days of PA. There were no differences in reported days of PA between boys and girls or between normal and over-fat groups. The median value for SE was 3.8, with mean 3.7 ± 0.7. No difference in SE existed between genders. However, high SE children reported more days of PA than low SE children (5.3 ± 1.9 vs. 4.3 ± 2.3 days, respectively, $P<0.05$). Approximately 30 % of the sample was over-fat, with a mean fatness value for the entire sample of 24.4 ± 10.1 %. Gender differences in fatness did not exist. ANOVA revealed no PA difference across the four fatness-SE groups (see Table 24.1).

Table 24.1. Physical activity across the four self-efficacy-fatness groups.

Group	n	# of days of PA (mean SD)
Normal fat Low SE	50	4.3 ± 2.4
Over-fat Low SE	23	4.2 ± 1.9
Normal fat High SE	58	5.3 ± 2.0
Over-fat High SE	23	5.4 ± 1.8

24.4 CONCLUSION

No PA difference was found across fatness-SE groups, indicating lack of interaction between these factors. Previously, our research team found slightly different results for the same participants when using a different PA self-efficacy survey (unpublished data). In the previous investigation, the normal fat high SE and over-fat high SE groups reported more days of PA when compared to the normal fat low SE group. The previous SE for PA survey related to self-efficacy for meeting PA recommendations, while the current survey assessed overall SE for PA. Since the two surveys assessed slightly different aspects of SE, it is not surprising that results varied between the two studies. However, the fact that SE for PA was related to PA in both studies strengthens the case that SE is an influential variable and conceptually makes sense. Bandura (1977) noted that performance accomplishments are the most influential source of SE expectations, and these children likely based their answers on previous PA experiences.

The important message from both the previous and current investigations was that SE for PA was related to PA, independent of % fat classification. As previously noted, several investigations have found SE for PA to be an important correlate of PA in youth (Sallis *et al.,* 2000), including low income and minority youth (Kitzman-Ulrich *et al.,* 2010). SE for PA should be further addressed in future intervention studies, particularly among low income, minority youth, as it appears to be an effective method for identifying children at greatest risk for low PA.

24.5 REFERENCES

Bandura A., 1977, Self-efficacy: Toward a unifying theory of behavioural change. *Psychological Review*, **84**, pp. 191-215.
Butcher K., Sallis J.F., Mayer J.A. and Woodruff S., 2008, Correlates of physical activity guideline compliance for adolescents in 100 U.S. cities. *Journal of Adolescent Health*, **42**, pp. 360-368

Centers for Disease Control and Prevention. Youth Risk Behavior Surveillance – United States, 2007. Surveillance Summaries, June 6. Morbidity and Mortality Weekly Report 2008:57 (No.SS-4).

De Bourdeaudhuij I., Lefevre J., Deforche B., Wijndaele K., Matton L. And Philippaerts R., 2005, Physical activity and psychosocial correlates in normal weight and overweight 11 to 19 year olds. *Obesity Research*, **13**, pp. 1097-1105.

Flegal K.M., Ogden C.L., Yanovski J.A., Freedman D.S., Shepherd J.A. Graubard, B.I. and Borrud L.G., 2010, High adiposity and high body mass index-for-age in US children and adolescents overall and by race-ethnic group. *American Journal of Clinical Nutrition*, **91**, pp. 1020-1026.

Kitzman-Ulrich H., Wilson D.K., Van Horn M.L. and Lawman H.G., 2010, Relationship of body mass index and psychosocial factors on physical activity in underserved adolescent boys and girls. *Health Psychology*, **29**, pp. 506-513.

Ogden C.L., Carroll M.D., Curtin L.R., Lamb M.M. and Flegal K.M., 2010, Prevalenceof high body mass index in US children and adolescents, 2007-2008. *Journal of the American Medical Association*, **303**, pp. 242-249.

Sallis J.F., Prochaska J.J. and Taylor W.C., 2000, A review of correlates of physical activity of children and adolescents. *Medicine and Science in Sports and Exercise*, **32**, pp. 963-975.

Saunders R.P., Pate R.R., Felton G., Dowda M., Weinrich M.C., Ward D.S., Parsons M.A. and Baranowski T., 1997, Development of questionnaires to measure psychosocial influences on children's physical activity. *Preventive Medicine*, **26**, pp. 241-247.

Troiano R.P., Berrigan D., Dodd K.W., Masse L.C., Tilert T. and McDowell M., 2008, Physical activity in the United States measured by accelerometer. *Medicine and Science in Sports and Exercise*, **40**, pp. 181-188.

Trost S.G., Kerr L.M., Ward D.S. and Pate R.R., 2001, Physical activity and determinants of physical activity in obese and non-obese children. *International Journal of Obesity and Related Metabolic Disorders*, **25**, pp. 822-829.

Ward, D.S., Dowda, M., Trost, S.G., Felton, G.M., Dishman, R.K. and Pate, R.R., 2006, Physical activity correlates in adolescent girls who differ by weight status. *Obesity*, **14**, pp. 97-105.

PHYSICAL ACTIVITY IN CHILDREN: DOES IT VARY BY WHERE CHILDREN LIVE, LEARN AND PLAY? LESSONS FROM THE BUILT ENVIRONMENT AND ACTIVE TRANSPORT (BEAT) PROJECT

M.R. Stone, G. Faulkner, R. Buliung, and R. Mitra

University of Toronto, Canada

25.1 INTRODUCTION

The built environment consists of the neighbourhoods, roads, buildings, food sources, and recreational facilities in which people live, work, are educated, eat, and play. The physical layout of communities can promote or limit opportunities for physical activity. Using accelerometers to capture objective levels of physical activity, Frank and colleagues (2005) observed that community design was significantly associated with the accumulation of moderate-to-vigorous physical activity (MVPA) and the achievement of activity guidelines. However, these associations were explored in adults. While there is some evidence to support a link between the built environment and children's physical activity (Davison and Lawson, 2006; Rahman *et al.*, 2011), most studies have used self-reported measures of activity that show mixed results (Sandercock *et al.*, 2010), and, are known to have limited validity in children (Pate *et al.*, 2002). Thus, there is growing interest in understanding how neighbourhood design impacts children's objective (i.e., accelerometer-measured) habitual levels of physical activity.

The built environment is influenced by the needs of a society. Toronto is primarily a city with older, traditional neighbourhoods at its core (Buliung *et al.*, 2009), yet demands for affordable housing spurred a post-war suburban housing revolution, directing transportation options and patterns, and resulting in urban sprawl. The design of these sprawling communities typically makes it difficult to walk/cycle or perform the most basic errands, making car travel the fastest, most convenient, and sometimes only way to get around.

Multiculturalism has also diversified the city of Toronto and is central in community establishment and transformation. Socioeconomic status (SES) varies widely across urban and suburban settings. A resident's choices regarding opportunities for physical activity and the safety of engaging in physical activity are therefore affected.

To estimate the true effect of the built environment in influencing activity levels, a design must ensure sufficient representation in built-form characteristics, a type of geographical stratification typically absent in the literature. Therefore, the purpose of this study was to examine the relationship between neighbourhood/SES and physical activity using a sampling frame that purposefully locates schools in varying neighbourhoods to ensure variability in built environment characteristics.

25.2 METHOD

25.2.1 Experimental design

Project BEAT (Built Environment and Active Transport; www.beat.utoronto.ca) is a large scale, multidisciplinary and mixed method study examining how the BE influences school travel modes of elementary school children in Toronto. The results presented are based on data collected during the second of three interlinked studies.

In January 2010, all elementary/intermediate schools within the Toronto District School Board (TDSB) with Grade 5 and 6 students (n = 469) received an invitation to participate. A pool of interested schools was generated and 15 schools selected that varied with respect to built form (suburban: looping street layout versus urban: grid-based street layout) and socioeconomic status (SES; low and high income households based on medium household income reported in the Canada Census). Consent was obtained from participating school boards, individual schools, parents, and students. Student participation was voluntary.

A total of 881 parents/guardians completed a travel behaviour survey and gave consent for their children to participate. Children completed an assent form and a travel-behaviour questionnaire. Stature and body mass measurements were taken and BMI calculated (n=854).

25.2.2 Criteria for physical activity measurement and data analysis

Children's physical activity behaviour was objectively measured for 7 days using accelerometry (ActiGraph GT1M, Pensacola, FL). A 5 s epoch was used to capture rapid transitions in activity typical in children (Stone *et al.*, 2009). For inclusion in data analysis, each child required a minimum of 10 hours of wearing time for at least 3 weekdays and 1 weekend day. A string of 30 minutes of consecutive zeros was used to classify non-wear time. Biologically implausible data were assessed to determine whether files were included in final analyses. Time spent at various levels of movement intensity (sedentary, light, moderate, vigorous, hard) was classified according to published thresholds in children (Stone *et al.,* 2009).

25.2.3 Statistical analysis

One-way ANOVAs with post-hoc comparisons (Tukey) were used to examine gender-specific differences based on built form (street design and era of development) and SES (old BE, low-SES (OL); old BE, high-SES (OH); new BE, low-SES (NL); new BE, high-SES (NH)) in accelerometry summary measures (total activity (TPA) mean counts, light, and moderate-to-vigorous physical activity (MVPA)) for weekdays (WD) and across the week (WK). The alpha level was set at 0.05. These data are part of an ongoing study, with a final wave of data collection planned for the spring of 2011.

25.3 RESULTS

Valid accelerometer data were collected for 730 participants (11.0 ± 0.6 y; boys, $n=330$; girls, $n=400$). Boys in OH neighbourhoods accumulated significantly greater mean counts (WD, WK) than all other groups (Table 25.1). However, boys in OL neighbourhoods accumulated significantly more light activity on weekdays than boys in OH neighbourhoods. For boys, built form/SES did not impact TPA and MVPA. Girls in OH neighbourhoods accumulated more TPA (WK) and MVPA (WD, WK) than girls in NL neighbourhoods, and more achieved current physical activity guidelines (Table 25.2). The intensity of overall activity (mean counts) was greater in girls from high SES than low SES neighbourhoods (WD, WK). The combination of living in an older neighbourhood and low SES was associated with a greater accumulation of light activity across weekdays.

Table 25.1 Influence of built form and SES on characteristics of accelerometer-measured physical activity in boys ($n=330$).

Boys ($n=330$)	Total physical activity (counts·d⁻¹)		Mean counts per minute (counts·min⁻¹)		Light activity (min·d⁻¹)		Moderate-to-vigorous activity (MVPA; min·d⁻¹)	
	WD	WK	WD	WK	WD	WK	WD	WK
Old Built Environment, Low SES ($n=94$)	489297 (133430)	451168 (132491)	474.1 (139.7)[d]	441.0 (138.0)[d]	197.8 (36.4)[b]	187.4 (37.0)	37.2 (16.2)	33.1 (15.0)
Old Built Environment, High SES ($n=93$)	474654 (102570)	458581 (100692)	498.0 (134.9)[d]	489.9 (142.0)[d]	182.2 (31.4)[a]	179.0 (31.2)	37.4 (13.0)	35.4 (12.1)
New Built Environment, Low SES ($n=78$)	499750 (134368)	459260 (113750)	481.1 (149.2)[d]	444.6 (121.6)[d]	193.5 (37.3)	185.4 (35.1)	39.8 (17.2)	35.3 (14.3)
New Built Environment, High SES ($n=65$)	518239 (125721)	478735 (109852)	590.8 (161.5)[a,b,c]	554.1 (144.6)[a,b,c]	195.7 (25.3)	186.3 (22.6)	42.4 (17.3)	37.8 (14.6)

[a]Significantly different from old BE, low SES; [b]Significantly different from old BE, high SES; [c]Significantly different from new BE, low SES; [d]Significantly different from new BE, high SES. $P<0.05$.

Table 25.2 Influence of built form and SES on characteristics of accelerometer-measured physical activity in girls (n=400).

Girls (n=400)	Total physical activity (counts·d⁻¹)		Mean counts per minute (counts·min⁻¹)		Light activity (min·d⁻¹)		Moderate-to-vigorous activity (MVPA) (min·d⁻¹)	
	WD	WK	WD	WK	WD	WK	WD	WK
Old Built Environment Low SES (n=102)	401804 (112789)	371052 (106521)	391.3 (124.2)[b,d]	368.0 (120.2)[b,d]	180.3 (31.6)[b,d]	171.5 (29.3)[d]	25.8 (12.9)	23.0 (12.0)[b]
Old Built Environment High SES (n=126)	402514 (107433)	390546 (109908)[c]	437.8 (133.8)[a,c]	431.1 (139.9)[a,c]	166.0 (30.6)[a]	162.3 (29.5)	28.9 (12.9)[c]	27.5 (12.6)[a,c]
New Built Environment Low SES (n=91)	371894 (96442)	350283 (85398)[b]	359.9 (106.9)[b,d]	343.9 (101.2)[b,d]	172.2 (28.6)	166.4 (26.8)	23.5 (10.5)[b]	21.5 (9.1)[b]
New Built Environment High SES (n=81)	399599 (108435)	370405 (109709)	458.7 (132.7)[a,c]	431.7 (125.3)[a,c]	167.8 (30.0)[a]	157.8 (28.5)[a]	26.8 (10.0)	24.1 (9.0)

[a]Significantly different from old BE, low SES; [b]Significantly different from old BE, high SES;
[c]Significantly different from new BE, low SES; [d]Significantly different from new BE, high SES. P<0.05.

25.4 DISCUSSION

The type of physical activity accumulated varies according to neighbourhood design and SES, and is gender-specific. Older neighbourhoods with greater street connectivity encourage walking for transportation/activity. Children in these neighbourhoods are more likely to have a daily activity profile dominated by light activity, yet SES moderates this relationship. Families in newer neighbourhoods with economic means may encourage structured, localized, higher-intensity activities to avoid barriers posed by less connected, looping-streets. Greater street connectivity and economic means appears especially important for girls to accumulate MVPA and achieve guidelines.

Our findings highlight the value of geographical stratification in cross-sectional analyses of accelerometry data and the importance of investigating the PA profile of children as built form/SES impacts discrete characteristics of PA differently. Our preliminary findings confirm that characteristics of accelerometer-measured physical activity in children vary by where children live, learn and play, and, differences appear to be gender-specific. Investigations into how geographical stratifications, specific characteristics of BE (i.e., land-use mix, traffic volume) and parental/child attitudes (i.e., safety) influence segmented patterns of activity (hour-by-hour, school travel) and daily accumulation of MVPA are ongoing.

25.5 REFERENCES

Buliung, R.N., Mitra, R. and Faulkner, G., 2009, Active school transportation in the Greater Toronto Area, Canada: An exploration of trends in space and time (1986-2006). *Preventive Medicine*, **48**, pp. 507-512.

Davison, K. and Lawson, C.T., 2006, Do attributes in the physical environment influence children's physical activity? A review of the literature. *International Journal of Behavioural Nutrition and Physical Activity*, **3**, pp. 19, doi:10.1186/1479-5868-3-19.

Frank, L.D., Schmidt, T.L., Sallis, J.F. and Chapman, J., 2005, Linking objectively measured physical activity with objectively measured urban form: Findings from SMARTRAQ. *American Journal of Preventive Medicine*, **28**, pp. 117-125.

Pate, R.R., Freedson, P.S., Sallis, J.F., Taylor, W.C., Sirard, J., Trost, S.G. and Dowda, M., 2002, Compliance with physical activity guidelines: Prevalence in a population of children and youth. *Annals of Epidemiology*, **12**, pp. 303-308.

Rahman, T., Cushing, R. and Jackson, R.J., 2011, Contributions of built environment to childhood obesity. *Mount Sinai Journal of Medicine*, **78**, pp. 49-57.

Sandercock, G., Angus, C. and Barton, J., 2010, Physical activity levels of children living in different built environments. *Preventive Medicine*, **50**, pp. 193-198.

Stone, M.R., Rowlands, A.V., Middlebrooke, A.R., Jawis, M.N. and Eston, R.G., 2009, The pattern of physical activity in relation to health outcomes in children. *International Journal of Pediatric Obesity*, **4**, pp. 306-315.

FEASIBILITY OF PHYSICAL EDUCATION HOMEWORK ASSIGNMENTS IN HIGH-SCHOOL

M. Pantanowitz[1], R. Lidor[2], D. Nemet[1], and A. Eliakim[1]

[1]Pediatric Department, Child Health and Sport Center, Meir Medical Center, Sackler School of Medicine, Tel-Aviv University, Tel-Aviv, Israel. [2]Zinman College of Physical Education and Sport Sciences at the Wingate Institute, Netanya, Israel

26.1 INTRODUCTION

In most school classes, the in-school time for learning and practical work is enhanced by homework assignments. Homework assignments develop the ability of self-study and self-discipline, enhance the ability to organize and manage time, improve the attitude towards school and improve academic achievements (Cooper *et al.*, 2006). It is suggested, therefore, that homework in physical education (PE) may increase learning time, improve exercise performance and encourage a healthy life style. Consistent with this hypothesis, medical and educational organizations have recommended homework assignments in PE classes. For example, the Center for Disease Control and Prevention (CDC) recommended in 1997 giving practical PE homework, by PE assignments that the student can implement on his own and together with his family (Smith and Claxton, 2003). Despite this, there is no tradition for the use of homework in PE, compared to other subjects. The aim of the present study was to investigate the attitude and compliance of high school students in Israel to physical and theoretical PE homework assignments. We hypothesized that high school students understand the importance of homework in PE, and thus, will complete the PE homework assignments.

26.2 METHODS

26.2.1 Participants and protocol

Ninety-five 11th and 12th graders (in 5 classes) at a regional high school in southern Israel participated in the study. The study was approved by the Israeli Ministry of Education, and by the Meir Medical Center Institutional review board. Participants were divided randomly to four groups: (1) Physical homework (n=23), (2) Theoretical homework (n=25), (3) Integrated group (physical and theoretical) (n=24), and (4), Control group (n=23), that was not assigned any homework. The research hypothesis and goals were not revealed to the students.

Over the 3 month study period, homework assignments were given to the different study groups at the end of each PE class (24 assignments in total). *Physical* homework topics included physical activities that are usually performed in PE classes in Israeli high schools (long distance running, short distance interval sessions, general strength for upper/lower extremities and abdominal muscles, rope skipping, and ball games). The length of each physical homework assignment was 20-45 minutes. *Theoretical* homework assignment included reading materials, writing brief reports on the beneficial health effects of activities that were performed in PE classes, and self-selected writing reports on important historical sports events. The *integrated* homework group received both the *physical* and *theoretical* assignments.

26.2.2 Anthropometric measurements and fitness assessment

Standard, calibrated scales and stadiometers were used to determine stature and body mass. BMI percentiles were calculated at the beginning of the study. Body fat was determined by sum skinfolds at the triceps and sub-scapula.

26.2.3 Physical fitness assessment

Physical fitness was assessed at the beginning of the study and included a 2 km run for boys and 1.5 km run for girls, 2 minutes rope skipping (number of skips), abdomen strength (maximal continuous sit-ups number), and arm strength (number of pull-ups for boys, and seconds of static pull ups for girls). These tests reflect basic fitness components, practiced regularly at school and used by the Israeli Ministry of Education as the national fitness assessment test.

26.2.4 Students and parents questionnaires

Participants filled in a habitual physical activity questionnaire to determine after school involvement in light, moderate and intense physical activity, before and at the end of the study. Participants and their parents were asked to express their attitude towards PE homework. Students reported their compliance to the assignments.

26.2.5 Statistical analysis

Unpaired t-tests were used to compare anthropometric and fitness parameters between participants who did or did not comply with the homework assignments. Data presented as mean (SD). Statistical significance was set at P value ≤ 0.05.

26.3 RESULTS

More than half of the students supported the use of PE homework assignments. The reasons for the support included mainly increased knowledge and awareness of healthy lifestyles, fitness development and enjoyment. Approximately one third did not support giving homework assignments. Reasons for this included lack of time, the homework load in other topics, the feeling that this could affect perception of the unique status of PE class as fun, unburdened period, and the lack of ability to monitor homework in this field. Some of the students felt that PE homework assignments should be practiced only in elementary schools. The majority of parents supported the idea of assigning PE homework. The reasons for their support were the wish that their children will acquire healthier lifestyles, develop PA as a habit, and increase the general knowledge of the importance of PA. More than half the parents were not satisfied by the PA level of their children (Table 26.1).

Very few students did all homework assignments (4 %), and a third to half completed some of the assignments (29-48 %). The percentage of students that completed homework in the groups assigned for either theoretical or physical homework was higher than in the integrated group (48-52 % compared to 33 %). Due to the relatively small number of students who completed homework, and for comparison purposes, we combined all groups who did the homework into one group and those who did not into a separate group. There were no differences in baseline anthropometric measures and fitness characteristics between the homework and the non-completing homework groups.

Table 26.1. Attitude of students and their parents toward homework in PE, and self-report of the students on actual PE homework assignments completion (percentage)

	Physical	Theoretical	Integrated	Control	Average
Need for PE homework					
Students	47.8	60.0	60.0	47.8	53.9
Parents	100	80	100	100	95
Completion PE homework					
All	4.3	4.0	4.2		4.2
Some	47.8	44.0	29.2		40.3
All + some	52.1	48.0	33.3		44.5
Not done	47.8	52.0	58.3		52.7

Table 26.2. Anthropometrics and fitness characteristics of the study participants

		Homework	No homework
Stature (m):	boys	1.72±0.07	1.75±0.07
	girls	1.62±0.07	1.59±0.06
Body mass (kg):	boys	67.6±19.0	68.4±8.5
	girls	58.3±10.4	55.3±10.6
BMI (percentile):	boys	45.3±31.4	52.0±26.5
	girls	56.3±23.8	48.3±28.0
SSF (mm):	boys	20.4±8.7	21.0±6.3
	girls	25.4±7.3	26.4±7.5
Distance run (s):	boys	520.1±64.0	537.0±94.1
	girls	567.2±115.7	532.4±89.7
Abdominal strength:	boys	67.7±13.9	59.6±12.6
	girls	50.6±11.5	51.2±13.5
Arms strength:	boys	10.7±7.7	8.4±5.9
	girls	29.4±28.1	33.3±23.2
Rope skipping:	boys	192.9±48.9	195.8±82.2
	girls	144.1±68.4	122.9±44.4

26.4 DISCUSSION

PE homework assignments have the potential of increasing habitual physical activity, improving fitness and promoting healthier life style in high-school pupils. However, despite support of the majority of both students and parents, very few students completed all, and less than half completed at least some of the homework assignments. Reasons for not doing PE homework included lack of time, mainly due to heavy homework load in other topics and to the approaching matriculation examinations. Moreover, homework assignments were prepared mainly by groups assigned to physical *or* theoretical homework, but not by the group assigned to both. This suggests that increasing homework load (complexity and preparation time length) above a certain threshold results in non-compliance, pointing to the need for brief, short and doable homework assignments. We were unable to characterize pupils that comply with PE homework assignments. There was a trend of leaner and fitter boys, and fatter and less fit girls in the homework group compared to the no-homework group, however, this difference was not statistically significant. Finally, it is possible that introducing the idea of PE homework at earlier stages (e.g. elementary school) may lead to greater student adherence.

26.5 REFERENCES

Cooper H., Robinson J.C. and Patall E.A. 2006, Does homework improve academic achievement? A synthesis of research, 1987-2003. *Education Research*, **76**, pp. 1-62.

Smith M.A. and Claxton D.B. 2003, Using active homework in physical education. *Journal of Physical Education, Recreation and Dance*, **74**, pp. 28-32.

Part V

Exercise and Medicine

LONGITUDINAL ORAL CONTRACEPTIVE USE ON BONE PARAMETERS

A.J. McLardy[1], C.D. Rodgers[1], M.C. Erlandson[1],
S.A. Kontulainen[1], R.A. Pierson[2], and A.D.G. Baxter-Jones[1]
[1]College of Kinesiology, [2] Department of Obstetric, Gynecology and
Reproductive Science, University of Saskatchewan, Canada

27.1 INTRODUCTION

Osteoporosis is a disease typically affecting the elderly but onset can occur at any age. The prevalence of osteoporosis is growing in Canada, with a current two million Canadians diagnosed (Osteoporosis Canada, 2010). This disease is characterized by low bone density and increased fracture risk and has its antecedents in childhood; although the two major factors affecting bone accrual in childhood are exercise and diet, recently there has been increased interest in the effects of oral contraception (OC) usage. Bone accrues during adolescence by the action of continuous resorption and formation of bone cells. While 25 % of adult bone mass is accrued during the adolescent growth spurt (Bailey, 1999), up to 50 % increase in total bone mass occurs between the ages of 12-18 years (Cromer et al., 2008). This is of interest since bone mass peaks at approximately 18 years of age in females and starts to decline after the third decade of life (Frost, 1997; Busen, 2004), with the largest loss of bone occurring at the time of menopause. Therefore, with the age-related reductions in bone mass, women are at high risk for osteoporosis if they do not lay down enough bone during the growing years to survive the impact of bone loss in later life. As such, it is important for girls to accrue as much bone as possible in their youth, in order to ward off osteoporotic bone levels later in life (Busen, 2004).

While genetics account for 80 % of bone mass accrual, environmental and lifestyle account for 20-40 % (Ruffing et al., 2007). Major influencing factors on bone growth and bone maintenance are physical activity, diet and the hormonal milieu. Hormones such as oestrogen play a key role in bone accrual (Cromer et al., 2008). Oestrogen levels increase during puberty (Busen et al., 2004) due to the onset of the menstrual cycle. High levels of oestrogen lead to optimal peak levels of bone maintenance, since oestrogen suppresses cell apoptosis of osteoblasts cells, which are essential in bone remodeling. With a deficiency of oestrogen, bone resorption increases, without an equivocal rise in bone formation (ESHRE Capri Workshop Group, 2009). Hormones are affected by a number of factors, and pharmacology agents such as Hormonal Contraceptive Therapy (HCT) which affect the level of circulating estrogen in the body. Progesterone in HCT suppresses the levels of oestrogen; therefore, reducing the peak amounts of oestrogen during the menstrual cycle and ultimately decreasing circulating oestrogen (Reed et al., 2003). Liu and Lebrun (2006) found that there were positive effects of oral contraceptives (OC) on populations of peri-menopausal and oligio-amenorhhea women. However, since OC usage is often initiated in adolescence, long-term effects of OC in childhood on bone accrual are unknown. In the 1996/1997 Statistics Canada Health Report, a total of 18 % of the population was using OC; 27 % of whom were 15-19 year olds (Wilkins et al., 2000). A 2 year study by Scholes et al., (2010) assessed over 600 adolescent and adult female OCT users, aged 14 to 18 and 19 to 30 years respectively. In this study, mean duration of use was 9 months for adolescent users and 1 year for young adult users. While there was no impact on BMD noted at the adolescent age between users and non-users, the adult females indicated reduced BMD in the users group. Further analysis showed as duration of use increased, BMD decreased.

Considering skeletal maturation is assessed at the time point of peak height velocity (PHV); it is important to note that bone growth varies for each individual, and that PHV (time of maturation), occurs between the years of 10-12 y in females. Participants should be aligned by Biological Age (BA), which is deemed at the time of skeletal maturation, rather than chronological age in order to account for differences in individual growth. Thus, researchers must assess bone growth in the time before and after PHV (Malina, 1978). This time of accelerated bone growth is a period when influential factors such as OC may have a significant impact on this bone accrual.

Age of onset of OC use is gradually decreasing. While the primary medical use of HCTs is to prevent unplanned pregnancies, other medical conditions often use similar hormone therapy as part of the ongoing treatment. For example, OCT is the first prescribed method of controlling irregular menstrual function (Hartard et al., 2004), including persons diagnosed with oligomenorrhea and polycystic ovarian syndrome. HCT is also often prescribed as an acne medication. It is not unusual therefore to see OC use beginning as young as 12 years of age (Rome et al., 2004), the age coinciding with the average age of PHV. Considering the 6-year timeline of 50 % skeletal growth from 12-18 years (Cromer et al., 2008) and the delicate lifestyle influences, such as pharmalogical agents, the timing of initiation of HCT use with respect to maturation needs to be examined. Berenson et al. (2008) performed a 3-year study using 16 to 33 year old participants and showed an increase in the spine BMD in the first 12 months, then a gradual decrease. In contrast, Cromer et al.

(2008) found a decrease in spine BMD during the first year in a group of 12-18 year olds. Given these contradictory results more investigations are required in this area.

27.2 PURPOSE

The purpose of this study was to examine the interrelationship of OC use on bone mineral accrual. This study analyzed the effects of prior OC usage on young adults' aerial bone mineral density (aBMD) and bone mineral content (BMC). This research had three main objectives: Objective 1: To assess the longitudinal changes in BMC between OC users and non-users at the total body (TB), lumbar spine (LS) and femoral neck (FN). Objective 2: To assess the differences in aBMD and BMC at the TB, LS and FN in regards to duration of use between non users, users 1-5 years, users 6-10 years, and users 10 plus years. Objective 3: To 1) assess the differences in BMC at the TB, LS and FN between non-users and OC users who started in adolescence, approximately within 6 years of Post Peak Height Velocity (PPHV) (12-18 years of age), and young adulthood, 6 plus years PPHV, (19 years plus).

Hypothesis 1: Individuals that use OC will have less BMC at the TB, LS and FN than those who have never used OCT. Hypothesis 2: Increased OC usage will be related to lower aBMD and BMC at all sites tested. Hypothesis 3: Those using OC within 6 years of PPHV will have lower amounts of BMC in comparison to the other 2 subgroups

27.3 METHODS

27.3.1 Experiment design

Female participants (n=110), were drawn from the Pediatric Bone Mineral Accrual Study (PBMAS) at the University of Saskatchewan (U of S). PBMAS uses a mixed-longitudinal cohort design study and was initiated in 1991; a cohort of 251 males and females were recruited between the ages of 8 and 15 years. In 2011 the study entered the 20th year of data collection and as the cohort clusters remained the same, data was available from 8 to 35 years of age. Ethics were obtained through the U of S Biomedical Research Ethics Board. Prior to testing the subjects were informed of the testing protocols and consent was obtained using a consent form.

Dual-Energy X-Ray Absorpitometry (DXA) was utilized to assess BMC and aBMD. BMC and aBMD measurements were taken at the total body (TB), lumbar spine (LS) and femoral neck (FN) sites. Stature, sitting height, and body mass data were collected at each sequence of the study. Participants filled out a selection of questionnaires to assess diet, physical activity and hormonal contraceptive use.

27.3.2 Inclusion/ exclusion criteria

Participants, who had used depot medroxyprogesterone acetate injections (n=8), were excluded from the present analysis as it has been shown to negatively affect bone parameters (Cromer *et al.,* 2008). Women using the oral contraceptive pill, or contraceptive patches were included in this study.

27.3.3 Data analysis

Data were aligned against a biological age (BA; years from peak height velocity (PHV)). PHV was determined from serial height measures by fitting a cubic spline to annual velocity measures.

Subjects were group into OC users and non-users. Users were defined as those that used OCs for one or more years. The OC users group was sub grouped by years of OC use; Group a: 1-5 years, Group b: 5-10 years, Group c: 10 plus years and in relation to duration of use. Group i: non-users, Group ii: 1-6 years PPHV, and Group iii: 6 plus years PPHV relative to PHV.

Analysis of covariance ANCOVA was then used to analyze group difference among the HCT models (covariates: height, lean mass, physical activity, vitamin D and calcium) for BMC at each site. Level of significance was $P < 0.05$.

27.4 RESULTS

Objective 1: At 30 years plus, non-users had significantly greater TB BMC than OC users ($P<0.05$). There was no significant difference at any of the other sites between groups ($P>0.05$) of users and non-users. Objective 2: Duration of OC use indicated no significant difference between any groups at any site for aBMD or BMC. Table 27.1 indicates results from Objective 3: The initiation of OC use 7 years after attainment of PHV showed a significantly lower TB BMC at 30 years, than those who initiated OC use 1 to 6 years after attainment of PHV. At 19 years of age, those that had initiated OC use between 1-6 years post PHV had significantly more LS BMC accrual compared to non-users.

Table 27.1 Results of timing initiation of oral contraception (OC) use.

Time from PHV		Approximate Chronological Age	Total Body BMC	Lumbar Spine BMC	Femoral Neck BMC
Non User	PHV 0.00	12	1296.9	32.2	3.3
	PPHV 7.00	19	2095.8	56.4	4.4
	PPHV 20.00	32	2599.60*	59.591	5.116
User 1-7 y PPHV	PHV 0.00	12	1319.2	33.8	3.2
	PPHV 7.00	19	2206.1	63.3	4.4
	PPHV 20.00	32	2178.83	67.321	3.472
User 7+ y PPHV	PHV 0.00	12	1354.1	35.5	3.2
	PPHV 7.00	19	2073.5	53.7	4
	PPHV 20.00	32	2235.76*	57.459	4.452

Data expressed as Mean ± SEM; *Significant Difference $P < 0.05$

27.5 CONCLUSION

At the age of 30 years, the non-users of OC had more TB BMC than the users, suggesting that use of OCs may have a detrimental effect later on in life. Further analysis for duration of use did not show a significant difference at any of the sites. This could be due to the small number of participants in this particular analysis. At 32 years of age, non-users had greater mean TB BMC than those that initiated use after 18 years; however an interesting finding at 19 years is those who initiated OC use between 12-18 years had more LS BMC; however, this difference was no longer evident by the age of 30. Although these findings indicated OC usage in adolescence may not be harmful, long-term usage may be problematic. This finding indicates the need for further study to investigate the timing of initiation of use and OC use in the mid 30-40s in relation to bone maintenance, in order to seek preventative strategies for low BMC at the hip and spine, and possibly the prevention of osteoporotic bone mineral levels later in life.

27.6 REFERENCES

Bailey, D.A., McKay, H.A., Mirwald, R.L., Crocker, P.R.E. and Faulkner, R.A., 1999, A six-year longitudinal study of the relationship of physical activity to bone mineral accrual in growing children: The university of Saskatchewan bone mineral accrual study. *Journal of Bone and Mineral Research*, **14**, pp. 1672-1679.

Berenson, A.B., Rahman, M., Breitkopf, C.R. and Bi, L.X., 2008, Effects of depot medroxyprogesterone acetate and 20-microgram oral contraceptives on bone mineral density. *American College of Obstetricians and Gynecologists*, **112**, pp. 788-799.

Busen, N.H., 2004, Bone mineral density in adolescent women using depot medroxyprogesterone acetate. *Journal of the American Academy of Nurse Practitioners*, **16**, pp. 57-63.

ESHRE Capri Workshop Group, 2009, Bone fractures after menopause. *Human Reproduction Update*, **16**, pp. 1-13.

Cromer, B.A., Bonny, A.E., Stager, M., Lazebnik, R., Rome, E., Zielger, J., Camlin Shingler, K. and Scenic, M., 2008, Bone mineral density in adolescent females using injectable or oral contraceptives: A 24-month prospective study. *Fertility and Sterility*, **90**, pp. 2060-2067.

Frost, H.M., 1997. On our age-related bone loss: Insights from a new paradigm. *Journal of Bone and Mineral Research*, **12**, pp. 1539-1546.

Hartard, M., Kleinmond, C., Kirchbichler, A., Jeschke, D., Wiseman, M., Wissenbacher, E.R., Felsenberg, D. and Erben, R.G., 2004. Age at first oral contraceptive use as a major determinant of vertebral bone mass in female endurance athletes. *Bone*, **35**, pp. 836-841.

Liu, S.L. and Lebrun, C.M., 2005, Effect of oral contraceptives and hormone replacement therapy on bone mineral density in premenopausal and perimenopausal women: A systematic review. *British Journal of Sports Medicine*, **40**, pp. 11-24.

Malina, R.M., 1978, Adolescent Growth Maturation: Selected Aspects of Current Research. *Yearbook of Physical Anthropology*, **21**, pp. 63-94.

Osteoporosis Canada, 2010, Osteoporosis at-a-glance. Retrieved from http://www.osteoporosis.ca/index.php/ci_id/5526/la_id/1.htm

Reed, S.D., Scholes, D., LaCroix, A.Z., Ichikawa, L.E., Barlow, W.E. and Ott, S.M., 2003, Longitudinal changes in bone density in relation to oral contraceptive use. *Contraception*, **68**, pp. 177-182.

Rome, E., Ziegler, J., Secic, M., Bonny, A., Stager, M., Lazebnik, R. and Cromer, B.A., 2004. Bone biochemical markers in adolescent girls using either depot medroxyprogesterone acetate or an oral contraceptive. *North American Society for Pediatric and Adolescent Gynecology*, **9**, 13.

Ruffing, J.A., Nieves, J.W., Zion, M., Tendy, S., Garrett, P., Lindsay, R. and Cosman, F., 2007, The influence of lifestyle, menstrual function and oral contraceptive use on bone mass and size in female military cadets. *Nutrition and Metabolism*, **4**, pp. 17.

Scholes, D., Ichikawa, L., LaCroix, A.Z., Spangler, L., Beasley, J.M., Reed, S. and Ott, S.M., 2010, Oral contraceptive use and bone density in adolescent and young adult women. *Contraception*, **81**, pp. 35-40.

Wilkins, K., Johansen, H., Beaudet, M.P., and Neutel, C.I., 2000, Oral contraceptive use. *Statistics Canada Catalogue*, **11**, pp. 25-37.

THE TIMING OF BONE DENSITY AND ESTIMATED BONE GEOMETRY AT THE PROXIMAL FEMUR: A LONGITUDINAL HIP STRUCTURAL ANALYSIS STUDY

A.D.G. Baxter-Jones[1], S.A. Jackowski[1], D.M.L. Cooper[2], J.L. Lanovaz[1], and S.A. Kontulainen[1]

[1]College of Kinesiology, University of Saskatchewan, [2]Department of Anatomy and Cell Biology, University of Saskatchewan, Saskatoon, SK, Canada

28.1 INTRODUCTION

Bone is constantly renovated through the dynamic process of bone formation and resorption. Disequilibrium between periosteal bone formation and endosteal bone resorption is proposed to be the underlying mechanism for osteoporosis (Seeman, 2007). Recently it has been observed that the decrease in areal bone mineral density (aBMD) in adulthood is compensated by adaptations in bone geometry to maintain structural integrity and strength. Beck *et al.* (2000) using hip structural analysis (HSA), observed an age-related decline in aBMD at the proximal femur with a reduced age-related loss in section modulus (Z) due to a linear compensation in subperiosteal expansion. This suggests that although bone mass is lost, mechanical strength may be maintained through geometric adaptation. Although hip bone fragility and related fractures are largely experienced during adulthood, this disease has paediatric antecedents (Faulkner and Bailey, 2007). Thus it is important to understand potential childhood and adolescent mechanisms that may influence osteoporosis development.

28.1.1 Study purpose

The purpose of this study was to describe the development of bone density and estimated bone strength at the proximal femur and identify the ages at which peak values of areal bone mineral density (aBMD), cross sectional area (CSA) and section modulus (Z) occur.

28.2 PROCEDURES AND METHODS

28.2.1 Participants

Participants consisted of individuals from the University of Saskatchewan's Pediatric Bone Mineral Accrual Study (PBMAS) (Bailey *et al.,* 1999). 73 males and 92 females covering the age span of approximately 8-30 years of age were included. Ninety-eight percent of the participants were of Caucasian descent. Written consent was obtained from all participants. All procedures were approved by the University of Saskatchewan's biomedical review committee.

28.2.2 Maturation

Stature was assessed annually to the nearest 0.1 cm using a wall-mounted stadiometer (Holtain Limited, Crymych, UK). To determine the age at peak height velocity (PHV), whole year height velocities were calculated and a cubic spline fitting procedure was applied to each to identify the age at peak (GraphPad Prism 5, GraphPad Software, San Diego, CA, USA). Biological age (years from PHV) was then calculated by subtracting the age at PHV from the chronological age at time of measurement.

28.2.3 Bone measures

Bone measures were derived using the hip structural analysis (HSA) program (Beck *et al.,* 2000). In brief, the HSA program estimates the structural geometry at three locations (narrow neck, NN; intertrochanter, IT; femoral shaft, S) of the proximal femur using DXA derived images of the hip. From each location, the HSA program produces ten output variables, of which three were assessed for this study: *Areal bone mineral density* (aBMD) – the estimated amount of bone mineral within the program selected defined bone area; *Cross Sectional Area* (CSA) – the estimated amount of bone surface area in the cross section after excluding all the trabecular and soft tissue space; and, *Section Modulus* (Z) – an indicator of bending strength calculated as the CSMI/ the maximum distance from the center of mass to outer cortex.

28.2.4 Peak bone strength assessment

To determine the age at peak proximal femur aBMD, CSA and Z for each participant the annual absolute values for aBMD, CSA and Z were independently plotted against chronological age (years from birth) and the absolute highest values of aBMD (aBMDp), CSA (CSAp) and (Zp) were chosen as the peak at each of the three locations of the proximal femur. Once the peak values were identified, the chronological ages at which these peaks occurred was determined. These ages were then converted to a biological age (years away from PHV) as outlined above.

28.2.5 Statistical analyses

A 2x3 (sex by site) factorial MANOVA with repeated measures (bone strengths) was used to test for differences between the ages at aBMDp, CSAp and Zp in males and females at each site of the proximal femur. If significant sex by site by bone strength interactions were observed, subsequent analyses were sex segregated, and a single factor (site) MANOVA with repeated measure was conducted. If a significant multivariate main effect was found, a univariate ANOVA was conducted for each site. Site specific differences between the ages at peak bone strength measure were evaluated with post hoc paired t-test comparisons with Bonferroni adjustments. An alpha of $P<0.05$ was considered significant. All analyses were performed using SPSS 18.0 for Windows (SPSS, Chicago, IL, USA).

28.3 RESULTS

28.3.1 Bone strength timing at each site

There was a significant sex by site by bone strength interaction ($P<0.05$). There was also significant site by bone strength interactions ($P<0.05$) with differences in the age at peak bone strength at NN, IT, and S sites ($P<0.05$). There were significant sex differences in the chronological ages at which peak measurement occurred ($P<0.05$) (Table 28.1). When aligned by biological age only the biological age at ITZp continued to be significantly different between sexes ($P<0.05$), with females age at ITZp occurring 1.3 years earlier than males (Table 28.1).

Table 28.1. The chronological and maturation ages for peak bone strength and height measurements in males and females (Means SD).

Variable	Chronological age	Biological age	Chronological age	Biological age
PHV	13.4 ± 1.1*	0	11.9 ± 0.9	0
NN CSAp	21.6 ± 3.3	8.1 ± 3.2	20.6 ± 3.6	8.8 ± 3.6
NN BMDp	19.4 ± 2.7 *	6.0 ± 2.7	17.9 ± 2.9	6.0 ± 2.7
NN Zp	22.0 ± 3.2 *	8.7 ± 3.2	20.7 ± 3.4	8.8 ± 3.5
IT CSAp	21.1 ± 3.4 *	7.7 ± 3.4	19.4 ± 3.9	7.5 ± 3.5
IT BMDp	20.0 ± 3.4 *	6.6 ± 3.4	18.7 ± 3.5	6.8 ± 3.5
IT Zp	21.3 ± 3.4 *	7.9 ± 3.4 **	18.5 ± 3.9	6.6 ± 4.0
S CSAp	22.3 ± 2.9 *	8.9 ± 3.1	21.0 ± 3.3	9.2 ± 3.3
S BMDp	21.8 ± 2.8 *	8.4 ± 2.8	19.7 ± 3.3	7.8 ± 3.3
S Zp	21.2 ± 2.8	7.8 ± 2.8	20.6 ± 3.5	8.7 ± 3.5

PHV = Peak height velocity; NN = Narrow neck site; IT = Intertrochanter site; S = Femoral shaft site; CSAp = peak cross sectional area, BMDp = peak bone mineral density; Zp = Peak section modulus
* indicates a significant difference in chronological age between sexes
** indicates a significant difference in biological age between sexes

At all sites of the proximal femur, males' age at aBMDp (NN, 6.0 ± 2.7 y; IT, 6.6 ± 3.4 y; S, 8.4 ± 2.8 y) occurred significantly earlier than CSAp (NN, 8.1 ± 3.2 y; IT, 7.7 ± 3.4 y; S, 8.9 ± 3.1 y) and earlier than Zp at only the NN (8.7 ± 3.2 y) and IT (7.9 ± 3.4 y) sites. Additionally, the age of Zp occurred significantly earlier than the age of CSAp only at the S site ($P<0.05$). In females, the age at aBMDp (NN, 6.0 ± 2.7 y; IT, 6.8 ± 3.5 y; S, 7.8 ± 3.3 y) also occurred significantly earlier than CSAp at all sites (NN, 8.8 ± 3.6 y; IT, 7.5 ± 3.5 y; S, 9.2 ± 3.3 y) and earlier than Zp at only the NN (8.8 ± 3.5 y) and S (8.7 ± 3.5 y). Unlike males, the age of Zp occurred significantly earlier than the age of CSAp only at the IT site in females ($P<0.05$).

28.4 DISCUSSION

Following both males and females from childhood, through adolescence and into early adulthood it was observed that there were significant sex differences in the developmental timing of peak geometric bone measures. Despite these sex differences, males and females followed a similar pattern in the timing of BMDp and CSAp at all sites of the proximal femur. The age at BMDp occurred approximately one year prior to the occurrence of CSAp. These observations suggest that during development, optimization of bone strength continues after the attainment of peak bone density. This pattern parallels that proposed for later changes in architecture associated with aging (Beck *et al.*, 2000; Seeman, 2007). The peak in aBMD and geometric properties observed in the current study coincides with previous literature suggesting that bone strength peaks between

20-40 years of age (Bonjour *et al.,* 1994) and geometric properties plateau around 20 years of age (Zhang *et al.,* 2010).

In conclusion, there were observed sex differences in the developmental timing of geometric bone measures at the proximal femur, but despite these differences, in both males and females, the peak in BMD occurred significantly earlier than CSA at all assessment sites using HSA. These findings suggest that changes in bone mass precede geometric adaptations and are integral for the development and maintenance of bone strength. However, further research on geometric adaptations using three dimensional imagining is necessary.

28.5 REFERENCES

Bailey D.A., McKay, H.A., Mirwald, R.L., Crocker, P.R. and Faulkner, R.A., 1999, A six-year longitudinal study of the relationship of physical activity to bone mineral accrual in growing children: The University of Saskatchewan bone mineral accrual study. *Journal of Bone and Mineral Research,* **14**, pp. 1672-1679.

Beck, T.J., Looker, A.C., Ruff, C.B., Sievanen, H. and Wahner, H.W., 2000, Structural trends in the aging femoral neck and proximal shaft: Analysis of the Third National Health and Nutrition Examination Survey dual-energy X-ray absorptiometry data. *Journal of Bone and Mineral Research,* **15**, pp. 2297-2304.

Bonjour, J.P., Theintz, G., Law, F., Slosman, D. and Rizzoli, R., 1994, Peak bone mass. *Osteoporosis International,* **4**, pp. 7-13.

Faulkner, R.A. and Bailey, D.A., 2007, Osteoporosis: A pediatric concern? *Medicine and Sport Science,* **51**, pp. 1-12.

Seeman, E., 2007, The periosteum: A surface for all seasons. *Osteoporosis International,* **18**, pp 123-128.

Zhang, F., Tan, L.J., Lei, S.F. and Deng, H.W., 2010, The differences of femoral neck geometric parameters: Effects of age, gender and race. *Osteoporosis International,* **21**, pp. 1205-1214.

HEART RATE VARIABILITY AND AEROBIC FITNESS IN ADOLESCENTS BORN PREMATURELY WITH VERY LOW BIRTH WEIGHT

P.A. Nixon[1, 2], L.K. Washburn[2], and T.M. O'Shea[2]

[1]Department of Health and Exercise Science and [2]Department of Pediatrics, Wake Forest University, Winston-Salem, NC, USA

29.1 INTRODUCTION

Approximately 60,000 or 1.5 % of infants are born each year with very low birth weight (VLBW $\leq$ 1500 grams), and nearly all of these infants are born prematurely. Improved survival rates due to better prenatal care and medical advances are associated with both short- and long-term morbidities, and growing evidence indicates that these infants have increased risk for cardiovascular (CV) disease in adulthood (Saigal and Doyle, 2008). The increased risk may be partly explained by alterations in developing systems in response to environmental stressors as suggested by the concept of "fetal programming" (Barker, 2002). Although beneficial in the short-term, these alterations persist and may be maladaptive in later life.

Alterations in the developing autonomic nervous system may lead to autonomic dysfunction and sympathovagal imbalance in CV regulation (Young, 2002). Noninvasive assessment of autonomic function is commonly made via the measurement of heart rate variability (HRV), and reduced HRV has been associated with increased risk for CV morbidity and mortality (Liao *et al.,* 1997). Reduced HRV has also been reported in preterm infants compared to their term-born peers (Longin *et al.,* 2006). Furthermore, HRV has been shown to be directly associated with aerobic fitness (Gutin *et al.,* 2005), and several studies indicate reduced fitness levels in persons born prematurely (Hebestreit and Bar-Or, 2001). The purpose of this study was therefore to examine the correlation between aerobic fitness and HRV in prematurely-born VLBW adolescents. It was hypothesized that lower fitness would be associated with reduced HRV.

29.2 METHODS

29.2.1 Participants

Participants with the following inclusion criteria were identified from our computerized neonatal database and invited to participate: 1) birth occurred between 01/01/92 to 06/30/96; 2) birth weight $\leq$ 1500 g; 3) hospital of birth was Forsyth Medical Center; 4) singleton birth; 5) no major congenital anomaly; 6) follow up visit at one year adjusted-age; and 7) 15th year of life for all study visits.

29.2.2 Measurements and procedures

Prior to participation, the study was explained and written informed consent was obtained from the parent/guardian and assent from the adolescent.

Measurements of aerobic fitness and HRV were taken at the 2nd visit (as part of a larger 3-visit study). At this visit, the participant's weight and height were measured, and BMI was calculated (kg·m^{-2}) and BMI percentile was determined from age- and gender-specific reference data (CDC 2000). Aerobic fitness was determined from peak oxygen uptake (peak VO$_2$) obtained from progressive maximal exercise testing. Prior to exercise testing, a resting ECG was recorded for 10 min using a Biopac MP36 system with the participant lying supine in a quiet room.

Nevrokard software was used to analyze the ECG, and HRV was determined in both the time and frequency domains from the second 5 min of the 10 min recording. The square root of the mean of the sum of the squares of the differences in successive R-R intervals (RMSSD) was chosen to reflect the time domain. Low (LF) and high (HF) frequency powers (in normalized units) were used to reflect HRV in the frequency domain, with the ratio of LF to HF (LF-HF ratio) providing an indication of sympathovagal balance.

Descriptive analyses were performed (SPSS 18.0) to examine measures of central tendency and dispersion. Group comparisons for continuous variables were made using Mann-Whitney U tests, and Chi-square analysis was used to compare proportions. Relationships were examined using Spearman correlational analysis.

29.3 RESULTS

Participants were 151 14 y old adolescents (43 % male, 57 % female; 58 % Caucasian, 37 % Africa American, 5 % other) who completed all three visits and had valid fitness and HRV data. Neonatal and current characteristics are presented in Table 29.1. Current height and birth weight z-values were significantly higher in males than females. Twenty-nine % of males and 36 % of females were overweight or obese as indicated by a BMI $\geq 85^{th}$ percentile.

Table 29.1. Participant neonatal and current characteristics expressed as median (5th, 95th percentile)

	Male	Female
Neonatal		
Gestational age, wk	28 (24, 33)	28 (23, 33)
Birth weight, g	1090 (690, 1477)	1040 (592, 1460)
Birth weight, z-value	-0.22 (-1.88, 2.20)*	-0.43 (-1.96, 0.56)
Current		
Age, y	14.6 (14.1, 15.0)	14.6 (14.1, 14.9)
Weight, z-value	0.51 (-1.43, 2.72)	0.40 (-1.81, 2.16)
Height, z-value	0.23 (-2.24, 1.44)*	-0.51 (-2.51, 1.07)
BMI percentile	67 (9, 99)	66 (7, 99)

* $P<0.05$, Male>Female

Aerobic fitness and HRV results are presented in Table 29.2. Male adolescents had significantly higher peak VO_2 when expressed in $ml \cdot kg^{-1} \cdot min^{-1}$. Thirty-six % of males and 42 % of females had a peak $VO_2 < 80$ % of predicted, with no group differences. Males also had higher LF and LF-HF ratio compared to females, but RMSSD did not differ between genders.

Table 29.2. Aerobic fitness and HRV parameters expressed as median (5th, 95th percentile)

	Male	Female
Peak VO_2		
$mL \cdot kg^{-1} \cdot min^{-1}$	44.7 (28.3, 60.2)*	32.9 (20.2, 45.4)
Peak VO_2 % predicted	89 (56, 120)	82 (51, 113)
RMSSD, ms	64.4 (21.7, 211.8)	75.0 (24.0, 204.9)
LF, nu	31.0 (9.5, 55.5)*	25.9 (14.4, 53.4)
HF, nu	52.8 (27.9, 85.4)	55.1 (35.0, 75.0)
LF-HF ratio	0.63 (0.11, 1.67)*	0.48 (0.24, 1.58)

*$P<0.05$, Male>Female

Spearman correlational analyses revealed a significant inverse correlation between fitness and RMSSD ($r=-0.29$, $p=0.008$), and a direct correlation with LF ($r=0.22$, $P=0.04$) and LF-HF ratio ($r=0.19$, $P=0.09$) in females, indicating that lower fitness was associated with greater HRV and less sympathetic dominance. No significant correlations between fitness and HRV were observed in male adolescents.

29.4 CONCLUSIONS

The results of our study are consistent with previous studies in that a large number of our participants had reduced fitness, and males exhibited lower HRV than females (Faulkner *et al.,* 2003). However, our results do not support our hypothesis and are inconsistent with other studies (Gutin *et al.,* 2005), in that lower fitness was not associated with HRV in adolescent males, and females with lower fitness exhibited greater HRV in both the time and frequency domains. Failure to find positive associations between fitness and HRV might be due to confounding effects of factors such as obesity and parental history of CV disease. It is also possible that complications and treatments associated with preterm birth may have altered other developing systems involved with CV regulation and fitness, consequently disrupting the relationship of fitness and HRV in our sample of prematurely-born, VLBW adolescents.

29.5 REFERENCES

Barker, D.J., 2002, Fetal programming of coronary heart disease. *Trends in Endocrinology and Metabolism*, **13**, pp. 364-368.

Faulkner, M.S., Hathaway, D. and Tolley, B., 2003, Cardiovascular autonomic function in healthy adolescents. *Heart Lung*, **32**, pp. 10-22.

Gutin, B., Howe, C., Johnson, M.H., Humphries, M.C., Snieder, H. and Barbeau, P., 2005, Heart rate variability in adolescents: Relations to physical activity, fitness, and adiposity. *Medicine and Science in Sports and Exercise*, **37**, pp. 1856-1863.

Hebestreit, H. and Bar-Or, O., 2001, Exercise and the child born prematurely. *Sports Medicine*, 31, 591-599.

Liao, D., Cai, J., Rosamond, W.D., Barnes, R.W., Hutchinson, R.G., Whitsel, E.A., Rautaharju, P. and Heiss, G., 1997, Cardiac autonomic function and incident coronary heart disease: A population-based case-cohort study. The ARIC Study. Atherosclerosis Risk in Communities Study. *American Journal of Epidemiology*, **145**, pp. 696-706.

Longin, E., Gerstner, T., Schaible, T., Lenz, T. and Konig, S., 2006, Maturation of the autonomic nervous system: Differences in heart rate variability in premature vs. term infants. *Journal of Perinatal Medicine*, **34**, pp. 303-308.

Saigal, S. and Doyle, L.W., 2008, An overview of mortality and sequelae of preterm birth from infancy to adulthood. *Lancet*, **19**, 371, pp. 261-269.

Young, J.B., 2002, Programming of Sympathoadrenal Function. *Trends in Endocrinology and Metabolism*, **13**, pp. 381-385.

CARDIOPULMONARY OUTCOMES IN YOUNG ADULTS BORN PREMATURELY WITH VARYING BIRTH WEIGHTS

M.C. Sullivan[1,2], P.A. Mitchell[3], R.J. Miller[2], S.B. Winchester[2], and J.W. Ziegler[3]

[1]University of Rhode Island, Kingston, RI, USA; [2]Women and Infants Hospital, Brown Center for the Study of Children at Risk, Providence, RI, USA; [3]Rhode Island Hospital/Hasbro Children's Hospital, Pediatric Heart Center, Providence, RI, USA

30.1 INTRODUCTION

Cardiopulmonary problems dominate the first days of life for prematurely born infants especially those with lower birth weight. Despite improved ventilation, exogenous surfactant and postnatal corticosteroids, bronchopulmonary dysplasia rates remain high. Yet, the extent to which birth weight and neonatal cardiopulmonary morbidity affects adult cardiac and pulmonary function has not been examined. The Developmental Origins Theory proposes that prenatal stress provokes adaptive changes in endocrine and metabolic processes that become permanently programmed (Barker, 2007). The purpose of this study is to examine cardiac and pulmonary function at age 23 years in a prospectively followed sample of prematurely born infants and a term born comparison group. Secondly, we aimed to examine the relative effects of birth weight, neonatal acuity, gender and current fitness on cardiac and pulmonary outcomes at age 23 years.

Cardiovascular and metabolic disorders have been found worldwide in retrospective studies of adults born preterm (Barker, 2002; Ward et al., 2004). Findings in support of Developmental Origins Theory, include animal studies of permanent physiological and behavioral alterations due to neonatal stress (Welberg and Seckl, 2001) now found in human studies raising concern for later health. The major hormonal system that mediates the stress response involves glucocorticoids and catecholamines which have potent effects on metabolic and vascular systems. Cortisol, argued as the most powerful human glucocorticoid, is essential for regulation and support of metabolism, immune response, vascular tone, and general homeostasis. These systems are plastic and become re-programmed due to fetal or neonatal events which have been repeatedly demonstrated by higher cortisol levels in adults born preterm (Phillips *et al.*, 2000; Reynolds *et al.*, 2001). When prolonged stress reactions occur during sensitive developmental periods there is a marked effect on neural organization which may result in permanent changes in structure and physiology. Robust correlations have been found between cortisol concentrations, birth weight, and the development of hypertension and type 2 diabetes mellitus (Matthews, 2002). Specifically, it has been shown that low birth weight predicts increased cortisol concentrations in adults; additionally, high cortisol concentrations correlate positively with higher blood pressure and coronary artery calcification in adulthood (Phillips *et al.*, 2000; Whitworth *et al.*, 2005).

For the current NICU survivors, there is limited information about cardiopulmonary function as young adults. Frequent invasive, painful NICU procedures (e.g., skin breaks, endotracheal suctioning, and clustered nursing care) induce chronic stress in high-risk preterm infants (Grunau *et al.*, 2001). We know that respiration in preterm infants is compromised by immaturity of the lungs, insufficient clearing of lung secretions, and possible mechanical ventilation and/or oxygen supplementation (Vrijlandt *et al.*, 2007). Even though there is a tendency for normalization of lung function in adolescence, "they persist with reduced flows, lower exercise tolerance, and bronchial hyperresponsiveness" (Friedrich *et al*, 2005, p. 79). More recently, airway obstruction and lower level of fitness in adolescents and young adults has been reported (Anand *et al.*, 2003; Vrijlandt *et al.*, 2006). Preterm infants with VLBW and BPD have poorer and more rapid deterioration of lung function than those preterm infants with VLBW without BPD at late adolescence (Doyle *et al*, 2006). Most researchers have found that maximum aerobic capacity of children born preterm is similar to that of control children. However, children born preterm and with BPD experience exertional desaturation.

30.2 METHODS

30.2.1 Sample

The infants were born in the US at Women and Infants Hospital, the major regional source of care for high-risk infants in Rhode Island and Southern New England. This study reports on a subsample of 69 preterm infants grouped by birth weight and 19 full term infants recruited at birth. There are four groups defined by birth weight as Extremely Low Birth Weight (ELBW, <1000 g), Very Low Birth Weight (VLBW, 1000-1499 g), Low Birth Weight (LBW, 1500-2499 g), and Normal Birth Weight (NBW, ≥2500 g). Neonatal acuity of cardiac and respiratory risk were calculated using the Hobel Risk Score (Hobel *et al.*, 1973). Neonatal characteristics are displayed in Table 30.1.

Table 30.1. Mean (SD) neonatal characteristics by birth weight groups

	ELBW n=21	VLBW n=28	LBW n=19	NBW n=19
Birth weight**	826.7±94.8	1224.0±146.5	1618.4±83.8	3494.5±488.5
Gestational age**	27.6±1.9	30.1±1.8	31.9±1.6	39.7±0.6
Length of NICU stay**	82.4±20.8	48.5±17.1	31.5±11.2	3±0.5
O$_2$ duration (hours)**	819.8±858.9	297.1±468.5	36.1±50.4	0
Mechanical ventilation (hours)**	457.1±560.5	113.8±201.5	26.8±6.3	0
Hobel cardiac risk*	4.8±5.1	3.6±4.5	2.4±3.5	0.5±1.6
Hobel respiratory risk**	20.9±7.6	15.0±8.8	9.5±7.0	0.0±0.0
Male/female	5/16	12/16	10/9	6/13
BPD (n/total)**	8/21	3/28	0	0

*P = 0.009; ** P < 0.0001

30.2.2 Measures and procedure

Evaluation of cardiopulmonary response to exercise and pulmonary function testing were performed at the Rhode Island Hospital Pediatric Heart Center, Providence, RI, US, by a master's prepared cardiopulmonary exercise physiologist with a licensed, board-certified physician present. Prior to testing, a cursory cardiac examination was performed by the physician. In addition, a baseline HR, BP, oxygen saturation, and ECG were obtained. Height and weight was used to compute body surface area. Health history was reviewed with particular attention to cardiovascular, respiratory, and medication history. If any abnormalities were detected on baseline assessment, the stress test was deferred until the patient was cleared by his/her primary physician or an adult cardiologist.

Pulmonary function testing (PFTs) were conducted per the American Thoracic Society's standard protocol (ATS, 2007). The exercise physiologist explained each manoeuver and expectation before connecting the subject to the system. Spirometry was performed to assess baseline pulmonary function and repeated until there were 3 consistent flow/volume loops recorded. Subjects were standing with a nose clip during testing and asked to take a slow, deep inhalation, followed by a forced, long, sharp exhalation.

To determine cardiopulmonary response to exercise, subjects underwent full metabolic exercise testing using a ramp protocol on a cycle ergometer to maximal exertion. Electrodes were applied in a modified 12 lead configuration for exercise testing. Once the leads were attached, excess wire was tucked in, pulse oximetry was attached and subject data was entered into the CPX Ultima system (MedGraphics, 2007). VO_2 L·min^{-1} was determined by subject's stature, body mass, age, sex, and exercise level. Subjects were seated on the bicycle ergometer at a seat height adjusted to have the knees slightly bent on full extension of bicycle pedals. Feet were secured to pedals using toe straps. Resting blood pressure was obtained. Subjects were asked to maintain a pedal rate between 70-80 revolutions per minute. The appropriate starting watt level was determined by the exercise physiologist using the formula (VO_2 L·min^{-1} − 0.5) x 10 = starting watts. Spirometry was performed before, 6 and 10 minutes after exercise and then again after administration of albuterol if needed. In addition to ECG readings, breath-by-breath analysis and rapid response O_2 and CO_2 were analyzed; there was automated detection of anaerobic threshold, respiratory compensation and peak VO_2 and additional monitoring of pulse-oximetry, HR, BP, and outputs from the cycle. ECG monitoring continued for 5 minutes after maximum exercise. BP was obtained 2 and 4 minutes after maximum exercise until subject returned to baseline values (usually within 5 minutes). Key variables reported to differ in preterm groups including VE, V/Q, FEV_1, and Peak VO_2 were used in the primary analysis (Doyle *et al.*, 2006; Doyle, 2008).

30.2.3 Analysis

To answer the first aim, ANOVA was used to test the effect of birth weight on pulmonary and cardiac outcomes. Chi-square analyses were used for categorical variables to test the effect of birth weight on blood pressure (BP) risk, decreased fitness (as indicated by peak VO_2 <80 % predicted value), and PFT results. To answer the second aim, multiple regression models were built to test the effect of neonatal variables of birth weight, respiratory and cardiac neonatal acuity, gender, and current fitness on pulmonary and cardiac outcomes at age 23 years.

30.3 RESULTS

Premature infants with birth weight < 1000 g (ELBW) had poorer power output

(W), peak VO_2 , FVC, and FEV_1 at age 23 years (Table 30.2). Resting systolic and diastolic BP was higher for ELBW and VLBW groups. Forty percent of adults born preterm had decreased fitness indicated by peak VO_2 <80 % predicted value. PFTs did not differ across birth weight groups (χ=4.7, P=0.192).

Table 30.2. Mean (SD) exercise testing outcomes at age 23 years by birth weight groups

	ELBW n=21	VLBW n=28	LBW n=19	NBW n=19	ANOVA
BP systolic (resting)	115.2±21.0	111.8±14.5	114.2±15.7	106.4±16.9	F (3,86) =1.04, P=0.37
BP diastolic (resting)	72.6±11.4	71.6±8.2	68.8±9.0	70.2±9.5	F (3,86) =0.60, P=0.61
RPE	6.5±1.9	7.7±1.8	6.7±1.1	6.6±.1.5	F (3,84) =2.7, P=0.04
Power output (W)	128.8±36.5	169.8±57.7	187.1±60.5	159.7±58.3	F (3,86) =4.18, P=0.008
Peak VO_2 ($mL \cdot kg^{-1} \cdot m^{-1}$)	26.1±6.3	31.1±8.2	33.5±6.6	28.0±7.4	F (3,86) =4.2, P=0.008
FVC (L)	3.3±0.7	4.1±0.7	4.3±0.8	4.0±0.9	F (3,86) =6.07, P=0.001
FEV_1 (L)	2.8±0.46	3.4±0.61	3.6±0.77	3.5±0.74	F (3, 86) =26.2, P=0.001
FEV_1/FVC	85.5±5.7	83.1±5.2	84.2±8.6	88.3±7.9	F (3, 86) =2.3, P=0.08
$PETCO_2$mmHg	37.9±3.5	38.0±4.8	42.8±13.2	39.4±7.2	F (3,86) =2.05, P=0.113
$PETO_2$mmHg	113.8±4.6	115.4±4.7	113.2±4.6	113.1±3.9	F (3, 86) =1.38, P=0.254

In regression models, when neonatal acuity, gender, and current fitness were included, the effect of birth weight was diminished. Gender and fitness predicted power output (W) [F(5,84)=27.8, P=0.000; r^2-0.64). Birth weight and gender predicted FEV_1 [F(4,84)=15.88, P=0.000; r^2-0.50) and peak VO_2

[F(4,86)=24.5, P=0.000; r^2-0.54]. Models with measures of ventilatory efficiency (VE/VO$_2$, PETO$_2$, PETCO$_2$) approached statistical significance.

30.4 CONCLUSION

Male gender and birth weight impact early adult pulmonary function, however, respiratory and cardiac neonatal acuity did not. Fitness level and higher resting BP suggests cardiac risk for those born prematurely with lowest birth weight. Similar to Doyle (2008), the poorest pulmonary outcomes and higher resting BP were for those born ELBW. Additional health data for age 23 years has not been analyzed yet, but our data from age 17 revealed that physical health, growth, and subtle neurological outcomes were poorer in the preterm groups. For infants with medical and neurological acuity there was a 24-32 % increase in acute and chronic health conditions. Clearly continued monitoring of adults born prematurely is warranted, not only at young adulthood but as they reach middle age. One approach that we plan to take is to create a Pathobiological Determinants of Atherosclerosis in Youth (PDAY) Risk Score at age 23 because it is strongly associated with coronary artery disease 10-15 years later (Loria *et al.*, 2007). Continued monitoring of preterm survivors will enhance our understanding of the relative impact of prematurity and neonatal intensive care on later adult cardiopulmonary disease. This aligns with a recent Institute of Medicine report that recommends long term studies into young adulthood to determine extent of recovery, if any, and to monitor individuals who were born preterm for the onset of disease during adulthood as a result of being born preterm (Behrman and Stith Butler, 2006).

Acknowledgement

Research support by National Institutes of Health, National Institute of Child Health and Development # 19195, and National Institute of Nursing Research # 003695.

30.5 REFERENCES

American Thoracic Society. 2007, Pulmonary Function and Exercise Testing. *ATS Documents, Statements, Guidelines and Reports*.
[http://www.thoracic.org/sections/publications/statements/index.html]
Accessed June 1, 2007.

Anand D., Stevenson, C.J., West, C.R. and Pharoah, P.O.D. 2003, Lung function and respiratory health in adolescents of very low birth weight. *Archives of Disease in Childhood*, **88**, pp. 135-138.

Barker D.J. 2002, Fetal programming of coronary heart disease. *Trends in Endocrinology and Metabolism,* **13**, pp. 364-368.

Barker D.J. 2007, The origins of the Developmental Origins Theory. *Journal of Internal Medicine*, **261**, pp. 412-417.

Behrman R. and Stith Butler, A. 2006, Preterm birth: Causes, consequences, and prevention 2006, *National Academy of Sciences*. Washington, DC: The National Academies Press.

Doyle, L.W., Faber, B., Callanan, C., Freezer, N., Ford, G.W. and Davis, N.M. 2006, Bronchopulmonary dysplasia in very low birth weight subjects and lung function in late adolescence. *Pediatrics*, **118**, pp. 108-113.

Doyle, L. W. 2008, Cardiopulmonary outcomes of extreme prematurity. *Seminars in Perinatology*, **32**, pp. 28-34.

Friedrich, L., Corso, A.L. and Jones, M.H. 2005, Pulmonary prognosis in preterm infants. *Journal of Pediatrics*, **81**, pp. 79-88.

Grunau R.E., Oberlander T.F., Whitfield M.F., Fitzgerald C. and Lee S.K. 2001, Demographic and therapeutic determinants of pain reactivity in very low birth weight neonates at 32 weeks' postconceptional age. *Pediatrics*, **107**, pp. 105-112.

Hobel, C.J., Hyvarien, M., Okada, D. and Oh, W. 1973, Prenatal and intrapartum high risk screening. *American Journal of Obstetrics and Gynecology*, **117**, pp. 1-9.

Loria, C.M., Liu, K., Lewis, C.E., Hully, S.B., Sidney, S., Schreiner, P.J., Williams, O.D., Bild, D.E. and Debrano, R., 2007, Early adult risk factor levels and subsequent coronary artery calcification. *Journal of the American College of Cardiology*, **49**, pp. 2013-2020.

Matthews, S.G., 2002, Early programming of the hypothalamo-pituitary-adrenal axis. *Trends in Endocrinology and Metabolism*, **13**, pp. 373-380.

MedGraphics. 2007, Cardiopulmonary Exercise and Nutritional Assessment Systems. *CPX Ultima System*.

Phillips, D.I., Walker, B.R., Reynolds, R.M., Flanagan, D.E.H., Wood, P.J., Osmond, C., Barker, D.J.P and Whorwood, C.B., 2000, Low birth weight predicts elevated plasma cortisol concentrations in adults from 3 populations. *Hypertension*, **35**, pp. 1301-1306.

Reynolds, R.M., Walker, B.R., Syddall, H.E., Wood, P.J., Phillips, D.I.W. and Whorwood, C.B. 2001, Altered control of cortisol secretion in adult men with low birthweight and cardiovascular risk factors. *Journal of Clinical Endocrinology and Metabolism*, **86**, pp. 245-250.

Vrijlandt, E.J., Gerritsen, J., Boezen, H.M., Grevink, R.G. and Duiverman, E.J. 2006, Lung function and exercise capacity in young adults born prematurely. *American Journal of Respiratory and Critical Care Medicine*, **173**, pp. 890-896.

Vrijlandt, E.J., Boezen, H.M., Gerritsen, J., Stremmelaar, E.F. and Duiverman, E.J. 2007, Respiratory health in prematurely born preschool children with and without bronchopulmonary dysplasia. *Journal of Pediatrics*, **150**, pp. 256-261.

Ward, A.M.V., Syddall, H.E., Wood, P.J., Chrousos, G.P. and Phillips, D.I.W. 2004, Fetal programming of the hypothalamic-pituitary-adrenal (HPA) axis: Low birth weight and central HPA regulation. *Journal of Clinical Endocrinology and Metabolism*, **89**, pp.1227-1233.

Welberg L.A.M. and Seckl J.R. 2001, Prenatal stress, glucocorticoids and the programming of the brain. *Journal of Endocrinology*, **13**, pp. 113-128.

Whitworth, J.A., Williamson, P.M., Mangos, G. and Kelly, J.J., 2005, Cardiovascular consequences of cortisol excess. *Vascular Health Risk Management*, **1**, pp. 291-299.

PHYSICAL ACTIVITY AND MUSCLE HYPOFUNCTION IN CHILDREN WITH CROHN'S DISEASE: IMPLICATIONS FOR BONE HEALTH

J. Hay[1], D.R. Mack[2], F. Rauch[3], E. Benchimol[2], M. Matzinger[4], N. Shenouda[4] and L.M. Ward[2]

[1] Brock University, Ontario, Canada; [2] University of Ottawa, Ottawa, Ontario, Canada; [3] Shriners Hospital for Children, McGill University, Montréal, Québec, Canada; [4] University of Ottawa, Ottawa, Ontario, Canada

31.1 INTRODUCTION

Inflammatory bowel disease (IBD) is an idiopathic, destructive chronic inflammatory condition of the gastrointestinal tract. The prevalence of IBD in children below 15 years of age is 20/100,000 (Kim and Ferry, 2004). About 80 % of pediatric IBD patients have Crohn's Disease (CD); the remainder have ulcerative colitis. Apart from the gastrointestinal tract, IBD affects many organ systems, including the skeleton. The aetiology of the bone mass deficit in CD remains incompletely understood (Burnham et al., 2004). The effect on the skeleton is often difficult to distinguish from the effect of osteotoxic medications that are used to control the inflammatory process, such as glucocorticoids. The development of bone is a complex process in healthy children and that complexity is heightened further in children with CD both by the disease itself, treatment, and its effects on diet and exercise. It is clear that IBD by itself has an effect on the skeleton even prior to treatment as ilial histomorphometric analyses indicate a disturbance in skeletal architecture (thinning of the cortices), and in skeletal metabolism (Ward et al., 2010). The serum of children with IBD contains factors that inhibit osteoblasts (Sylvester et al., 2002). Mechanical stress exerted by skeletal muscle increases bone mass (Schoneau et al., 2002) and strength (Rittweger et al., 2000) which suggest that the osteopenia seen at diagnosis may have partly resulted from a lack of muscle development (sarcopenia). Sarcopenia may in turn result from systemic inflammatory cachexia (Burnham et al., 2005). At this juncture the potential role of physical activity/inactivity on muscle/bone development in children with CD has not been explored and is therefore the focus of this report.

31.2 METHODS

31.2.1   Patients and study design

This cross-sectional study was conducted through the IBD clinic at the Children's Hospital of Eastern Ontario (Ottawa, Canada), a tertiary care children's hospital. The study protocol was approved by the hospital's Institutional Review Board. Informed consent (and assent, where appropriate) was obtained from all participants prior to enrollment in the study. Between April 2008 and 31 December, 2010 children suspected of having CD and with confirmatory diagnostic were invited to participate in this study. The other study procedures were performed within two weeks of diagnosis. Histologic evaluation of mucosal biopsies confirmed the diagnosis of CD in each of the study participants. Forty children, 24 boys and 16 girls with a mean age of 12.2 ($\pm$ 2.6) and 13.9 ($\pm$ 2.7) y respectively are reported in this study. Boys had a mean BMI of 17.41 ($\pm$ 2.9) and girls 17.42 ($\pm$ 3.7) kg·m^{-2}. There were 26 children at Tanner Stage 3 or lower, 19 boys - (mean age 11.7 $\pm$ 2.2) y, with a mean of BMI 16.8 ($\pm$ 2.1) kg·m^{-2} and 7 girls mean age 11.6 ($\pm$ 2.4) y, with a mean BMI of 14.9 ($\pm$ 2.1) kg·m^{-2}.

Disease severity ratings were determined according to the Pediatric Crohn's Disease Activity Index (Hyams *et al.,* 2005). Pubertal development was assessed by physical examination according to Tanner staging, using published photographs as a normal reference. Height was determined on a Harpenden stadiometer. Weight was measured using a digital weight scale. Physical activity and inactivity were assessed using the Habitual Activity Estimation Scale (HAES) for both a typical weekday and a typical Saturday in the previous 2 weeks (Hay and Cairney, 2006; Wells *et al.,* 2008). The two inactive, non-weight-bearing categories (inactive – lying down and somewhat inactive – sitting) and the two active weight-bearing categories (somewhat active – walking and very active – running) were combined for each day and again to provide an overall assessment of overall inactivity and activity expressed in hours/waking day. Children underwent a bone health evaluation within 2 weeks of diagnosis including lateral spine radiograph for vertebral fracture assessment according to Genant semi-quantitative (GSQ) and Algorithm-Based Qualitative (ABQ) methods. The radiographs were assessed independently by two pediatric radiologists. Discrepancies between readers were resolved by consensus.

Muscle function was measured by peak jump power on a single, two-legged jump using a mechanography force plate (Leonardo™). Bone and muscle structural indices were measured by peripheral quantitative computed tomography (pQCT) at the 4 %, 38 % and 66 % tibia sites. Peak jump power and pQCT results were compared to age- and gender-matched healthy controls.

31.2.2 Clinical findings

Ninety-two percent of children had a paediatric Crohn's Disease activity score (PCDAI) that was severe, the rest were moderate. Peak jump power ($W \cdot kg^{-1}$) was significantly reduced in CD (33 ± 9 compared to 43 ± 8 in controls, $P<0.001$). Children with CD had low diaphyseal muscle cross-sectional area (CSA) 4174 ($\pm$ 1092) vs. controls 5066 ($\pm$ 125) mm^2 ($P<0.01$). Complete HAES results were available for 40 of the 43 eligible children (96 %) and are reported here. Subjects were significantly less active than healthy peers with 50 % reporting no very active time on one of either the school-day or the Saturday. Three children reported no very active and somewhat active time on either day.

31.2.3 Statistical analysis

Pearson correlations were determined controlling for age, gender, BMI and Tanner stage between the variable of interest. There were almost no significant relationships between activity/inactivity and unadjusted muscle CSA, muscle power with only total week activity significantly related to muscle power (Table 31.1). As associations with these unadjusted variables may have masked differences due to the muscle size (length) differences between children, we then repeated the correlations adjusting for tibial length with area and power expressed in terms of tibial length (Table 31.1). The relationship between muscle function (power relative to tibial length) was significantly positive with activity and significantly negative for inactivity for both weekdays and weekend days. There were no corresponding relationships with muscle area (area relative to tibial length) suggesting that physical activity affected muscle function but not muscle size. Inactivity and activity on weekend days produced higher correlations than on weekdays demonstrating that children, more active on those days where children have more opportunity for activity, demonstrated greater power. Weekday free-choice activity is attenuated by the large portion of the waking day spent in school which by default is largely somewhat inactive. When examining the results of those children in Tanner stages 1-3 alone to remove the confounding effects of muscle and bone growth and maturation during and after peak height velocity (Tanner and Whitehouse, 1976) the results are more striking, demonstrating stronger correlations with power for both activity and inactivity (Table 31.2). In this sub-group there are also significant correlations with muscle area corrected for tibial length in the same directions as with power. The three girls who reported 0 total very active hours had significantly lower mean power scores (19.2 vs. 32.2; $P<0.03$, F=5.76).

Table 31.1. Correlations between physical activity/inactivity, muscle and bone – full sample (controlled for age, gender, BMI, and Tanner Stage)

N=40 24m, 16f	Muscle Area mm^2	Max Power W·kg^{-1}	Area/Size*	Power/Size*
Inactive Weekday	0.0481	-0.1635	-0.1195	-0.2505
Inactive Saturday	0.0267	-0.2598	-0.2904	-0.4323***
Active Weekday	-0.0141	0.2968	0.1202	0.3450**
Active Weekend Day	-0.00003	0.2749	0.2590	0.4245***
Total Inactive	0.0409	-0.2342	-0.2276	-0.3780**
Total Active	-0.0078	0.31376**	0.2097	0.4288***

*corrected by tibial length; **P<0.05; ***P<0.01

Table 31.2. Correlations between physical activity/inactivity muscle and bone - Tanner stages 1-3 (controlled for age, gender, BMI, and Tanner Stage)

N=26 19m,7f	Muscle Area mm^2	Max Power W·kg^{-1}	Area/Size*	Power/Size*
Inactive Weekday	-0.2334	-0.3488	-0.3107	-0.3949**
Inactive Saturday	-0.2363	-0.3368	-0.5067***	-0.5035***
Active Weekday	0.1927	0.4043**	0.2904	0.4525**
Active Weekend Day	0.2313	0.3026	0.4881***	0.4626**
Total Inactive	-0.2537	-0.3701**	-0.4452**	-0.4873***
Total Active	0.2288	0.3747**	0.4256**	0.4925***

* corrected by tibial length; ** P<0.05; ***P<0.01

31.3 CONCLUSIONS AND LIMITATIONS

Children with CD had significantly less muscle CSA and peak power than healthy controls. The muscle function of more active children was superior to that of inactive children. This difference was not due to size so it appears that the more active children may have been able to develop and employ more functional muscle. Hypothetically this could have positive long-term implications for bone development.

Cross-sectional designs cannot determine the direction of the relationships reported. This research was limited by a relatively small sample size and a subjective, if well validated, clinical measure of physical activity. These would tend to work against finding a true difference or to mask relationships. That the results are sufficiently strong to reach statistical significance is evidence that physical activity/inactivity may play an integral role in the development of muscle function. The sample size precludes more sophisticated modelling analyses that would allow consideration of the multiple variables involved. The timing and contribution of PA to the muscle-bone axis cannot be determined from this data. However, these findings are sufficiently promising to stimulate further work to determine the duration and intensity of physical activity required to promote healthy muscle and bone development in children during treatment for CD. The potential role of physical activity, in remediating the sarcopenia seen in children with CD, in an attempt to promote healthy bone development warrants full investigation.

31.4 REFERENCES

Burnham, J.M., Shults, J., Semeao, E., Foster, B., Zemel, B.S., Stallings, V.A. and Leonard, B., 2004, Whole body BMC in pediatric Crohn Disease: Independent effects of altered growth, maturation, and body composition. *Journal of Bone and Mineral Research*, **19**, pp. 1961–1968.

Burnham, J.M., Shults, J., Semeao, E., Foster, B., Zemel, B.S, Stallings, V.A. and Leonard, B., 2005, Body-composition alterations consistent with cachexia in children and young adults with Crohn disease. *American Journal of Clinical Nutrition*, **82**, pp. 413–420.

Hay, J. and Cairney, J., 2006, Development of the habitual activity estimation scale for clinical research: A systematic approach. *Pediatric Exercise Science*, **18**, pp. 193-206.

Hyams, J., Markowitz, J., Otley, A., Rosh, J., Mack, D., Bousvaros, A., Kugathasan, S., Pfefferkorn, M., Tolia, V., Evans, J., Treem, W., Wyllie, R. and Rothbaum, R., 2005, Evaluation of the pediatric Crohn disease activity index: A prospective multicenter experience. *Journal of Pediatric Gastroenterology and Nutrition*, **41**, pp. 416–421.

Kim, S.C. and Ferry, G.D., 2004, Inflammatory bowel diseases in pediatric and adolescent patients: Clinical, therapeutic, and psychosocial considerations. *Gastroenterology*, **126**, pp. 1550-1560.

Rittweger, J., Beller, G., Ehrig, J., Jung, C., Koch, U., Ramolla, J., Schmidt, F., Newitt, D., Majumdar, S., Schiessl, H. and Felsenberg, D., 2000, Bone-muscle strength indices for the human lower leg. *Bone*, **27**, pp. 319–326.

Schoenau, E., Neu, C.M., Beck, B., Manz, F. and Rauch, F., 2002, Bone mineral content per muscle cross-sectional area as an index of the functional muscle-bone unit. *Journal of Bone Mineral Research*, **17**, pp. 1095-1101.

Sylvester, F.A., Wyzga, N., Hyams, J.S. and Gronowicz, G.A., 2002, Effect of Crohn's disease on bone metabolism in vitro: A role for interleukin-6. *Journal of Bone Mineral Research*, **17**, pp. 695-702.

Tanner, J.M. and Whitehouse, R., 1976, Clinical standards for height, weight, height velocity, and stages of puberty. *Archives of Diseases in Childhood*, **51**, pp. 170-179.

Ward, L.M., Rauch, F., Matzinger, M., Boland, M. and Mack D., 2010, Iliac bone histomorphometry in children with newly diagnosed inflammatory bowel disease. *Osteoporosis International*, **21,** pp. 331-337.

Wells, G.D., Wilkes, D.L., Schneiderman-Walker, J., Elmi, M., Tullis, E., Lands, L.C., Ratjen, F. and Coates, A.L., 2008, Reliability and validity of the habitual activity estimation scale (HAES) in patients with cystic fibrosis. *Pediatric Pulmonology*, **43**, pp. 345-353.

REDUCED FAT OXIDATION RATES DURING SUBMAXIMAL EXERCISE IN ADOLESCENTS WITH A CHRONIC INFLAMMATORY DISEASE

T. Nguyen[1], J. Obeid[1], H.E. Ploeger[1,2], T. Takken[1,3], L. Pedder[4], R.M. Issenman[4], and B.W. Timmons[1]

[1]McMaster University, Canada. [2]University of Groningen, The Netherlands. [3]University Medical Center Utrecht, The Netherlands. [4]McMaster Children's Hospital, Canada.

32.1 INTRODUCTION

Adolescents with cystic fibrosis (CF) and Crohn's disease (CD) tend to experience chronic inflammation and suffer from impaired growth. Poor growth may be a result of malnutrition (Thomas *et al.,* 1993; Burdge *et al.,* 1994). While exercise is known to improve clinical outcomes for patients with CF (Wilkes *et al.,* 2009) and CD (Narula and Fedorak, 2008), promoting exercise as a therapy would be of greater value if it does not compromise adequate nutritional intake, and consequently growth.

Carbohydrate (CHO) utilization during submaximal exercise in patients with chronic inflammation is comparable to healthy individuals (Ward *et al.,* 1999; Wideman *et al.,* 2009), however, the use of fat as fuel during exercise has not yet been investigated in adolescents with CF or adolescents with CD. High-fat diets are promoted in patients with CF (Burdge *et al.,* 1994), which emphasizes its role in malnutrition and its importance as a fuel. In contrast, low-fat diets are associated with good clinical outcomes in the CD population, and may reduce inflammation (Fernández-Bañares *et al.,* 1994). Therefore, determining substrate utilization during exercise would provide valuable information to guide patients in which energy fuel may be required to support an active lifestyle. This study set out to determine whether substrate utilization, in particular the use of fat as fuel, during submaximal exercise is altered in adolescents with CF and CD, compared to adolescents without a chronic disease.

32.2 METHODS

32.2.1 Participants

Four clinically stable males with CF (mean age: 16.1 y, FEV_1: 73-123 % predicted), four males with CD in remission (15.7 y), and four healthy active males (15.0 y) participated in the study. Chronological age does not necessarily indicate biological maturity (Mirwald *et al.,* 2002), and since biological maturity has a strong influence on substrate utilization during exercise (Timmons *et al.,* 2007) we selected to match our participants according to their biological rather than chronological age. Therefore, the estimated years to age of peak height velocity (Mirwald *et al.,* 2002) was used to match our participants.

32.2.2 Experimental design

Participants completed two visits. Peak mechanical power (PMP) was assessed at Visit one using the *McMaster All-Out Progressive Continuous Cycling Test* on a mechanically braked cycle ergometer (Fleisch-Metabo, Geneva, Switzerland). Visit two occurred at least 2 days after Visit one to avoid residual effects from the previous exercise session. Participants were asked to refrain from any food or liquid consumption 3 hours prior to Visit two. Submaximal exercise consisted of 2×30 min bouts of cycling with 6 min of rest between bouts. The participant cycled at a constant pace of 60 revolutions per min with the intensity set at 50 % PMP. Breath-by-breath gas exchange (O_2 and CO_2) was assessed (Vmax29, SensorMedics, Palm Springs, California, USA) for 6 min at the mid-way (at 12-18 min) and at the end (at 23-29 min) of each 30 min bout. The last 3 min of each gas collection period were averaged and used for analysis. Therefore, a total of four time points were analyzed (EX-1, EX-2, EX-3, and EX-4).

32.2.3 Substrate calculations

Whole body oxidation rates of total fat and total CHO were calculated using the following equations (Peronnet and Massicotte, 1991):

$$FAT_{total} \ (\text{g·min}^{-1}) = -1.70 \cdot \dot{V}CO_2 \ (\text{L·min}^{-1}) + 1.69 \cdot \dot{V}O_2 \ (\text{L·min}^{-1})$$
$$CHO_{total} \ (\text{g·min}^{-1}) = 4.59 \cdot \dot{V}CO_2 \ (\text{L·min}^{-1}) - 3.23 \cdot \dot{V}O_2 \ (\text{L·min}^{-1})$$

The energy potentials of fat (9.75 kcal·g^{-1}) and CHO (3.87 kcal·g^{-1}) were used to calculate the energy provided, and expressed as a percent of total energy expenditure (EE).

32.2.4 Statistical analysis

Date was determined to be normally distributed using Shapiro-Wilk ($P<0.05$) (PASW version 18.0, SPSS, Inc., Chicago, IL). Therefore, two-way repeated measures ANOVA (Statistica version 5.0, Statsoft, Inc., Tulsa, OK) was performed on total fat oxidation rate, total CHO oxidation rate, % fat of total EE, and % CHO of total EE. The two factors examined were group (three levels: CF, CD, Healthy) × time (four levels: EX-1, EX-2, EX-3, EX-4). If a main effect for group and/or a group × time interaction was present, Tukey's HSD post hoc analyses were performed to test for specific mean differences. Significance was set at $P<0.05$.

32.3 RESULTS

32.3.1 Oxidation rates

Compared to healthy adolescents, fat oxidation rates (expressed in mean mg·kg body mass^{-1}·min^{-1} ± SD) in adolescents with CF were significantly lower at EX-2 (CF: 5.8 ± 2.2, Healthy: 10.0 ± 2.6, $P<0.001$), EX-3 (CF: 6.9 ± 2.4, Healthy: 9.9 ± 3.2, $P<0.05$), and EX-4 (CF: 6.7 ± 2.2, Healthy: 11.3 ± 1.6, $P<0.001$), while adolescents with CD were significantly lower at EX-1 (CD: 2.5 ± 1.2, Healthy: 6.5 ± 1.8, $P<0.001$), EX-2 (CD: 4.4 ± 1.1, $P<0.001$), EX-3 (CD: 7.0 ± 1.4, $P<0.05$), and EX-4 (CD: 7.5 ± 1.3, $P<0.01$). CHO oxidation rates were similar between groups at all time points (Figure 32.1).

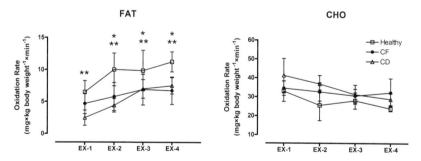

Figure 32.1. Oxidation rates of fat and CHO during exercise.
*Significantly different between CF and Healthy.
** Significantly different between CD and Healthy.

32.3.2 Energy expenditure

Adolescents with CF and healthy adolescents utilized a similar proportion of fat (CF: 32 ± 9 %, healthy: 46 ± 8 %, P=0.06) and CHO (CF: 68 ± 9 %, healthy: 54 ± 9 %, P=0.06). Adolescents with CD relied significantly less on fat (CD: 28 ± 6 %, P<0.05) and more on CHO (CD: 72 ± 6 %, P<0.05) compared to healthy adolescents (Figure 32.2). There were no differences between adolescents with CF and CD.

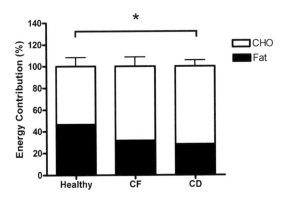

Figure 32.2. Percent of fat and CHO of total EE.
* Significantly different between CD and Healthy.

32.4 CONCLUSION

Adolescents with a chronic disease associated with impaired growth displayed suppressed whole body fat oxidation rates during submaximal exercise, but normal CHO oxidation rates compared to healthy adolescents. Differences in substrate utilization were more apparent between adolescents with CD and healthy adolescents. Collectively, these results indicate altered fat metabolism in adolescents with chronic inflammation, and that adolescents with CD rely more on CHO to meet energy demand required for submaximal exercise. Future work is required to decipher whether a lack of available lipids or altered lipid metabolism machinery is responsible for the suppressed fat oxidation rates observed.

32.5 REFERENCES

Burdge, G.C., Goodale, A.J., Hill, C.M., Halford, P.J., Lambert, E.J., Postle, A.D. and Rolles, C.J., 1994, Plasma lipid concentrations in children with cystic fibrosis: The value of a high-fat diet and pancreatic supplementation. *British Journal of Nutrition*, **71**, pp. 959-964.

Fernández-Bañares, F., Cabré, E., González-Huix, F. and Gassull, M.A., 1994, Enteral nutrition as primary therapy in Crohn's disease. *Gut*, **35**, pp. S55-59.

Mirwald, R.L., Baxter-Jones, A.D., Bailey, D.A. and Beunen, G.P., 2002, An assessment of maturity from anthropometric measurements. *Medicine and Science in Sports and Exercise*, **34**, pp. 689-694.

Narula, N. and Fedorak, R.N., 2008, Exercise and inflammatory bowel disease. *Canadian Journal of Gastroenterology*, **22**, pp. 497-504.

Peronnet, F. and Massicotte, D., 1991, Table of nonprotein respiratory quotient: An update. *Canadian Journal of Sport Sciences*, **16**, pp. 23-29.

Thomas, A.G., Taylor, F. and Miller, V., 1993, Dietary intake and nutritional treatment in childhood Crohn's disease. *Journal of Pediatric Gastroenterology and Nutrition*, **17**, pp. 75-81.

Timmons, B.W., Bar-Or, O. and Riddell, M.C., 2007, Influence of age and pubertal status on substrate utilization during exercise with and without carbohydrate intake in healthy boys. *Applied Physiology, Nutrition and Metabolism*, **32**, pp. 416-425.

Ward, S.A., Tomezsko, J.L., Holsclaw, D.S. and Paolone, A.M., 1999, Energy expenditure and substrate utilization in adults with cystic fibrosis and diabetes mellitus. *The American Journal of Clinical Nutrition*, **69**, pp. 913-919.

Wideman, L., Baker, C.F., Brown, P.K., Consitt, L.A., Ambrosius, W.T. and Schechter, M.S., 2009, Substrate utilization during and after exercise in mild cystic fibrosis. *Medicine and Science in Sports and Exercise*, **41**, pp. 270-278.

Wilkes, D.L., Schneiderman, J.E., Nguyen, T., Heale, L., Moola, F., Ratjen, F., Coates, A.L. and Wells, G.D., 2009, Exercise and physical activity in children with cystic fibrosis. *Paediatric Respiratory Reviews*, **10**, pp. 105-109.

SEDENTARY BEHAVIOUR IN YOUTH WITH CEREBRAL PALSY AND AGE-, GENDER- AND SEASON-MATCHED CONTROLS

J. Obeid, S. Noorduyn, J.W. Gorter, and B.W. Timmons
on behalf of the Stat-FIT Study Group
Child Health and Exercise Medicine Program, McMaster University, Canada

33.1 INTRODUCTION

Cerebral palsy (CP) refers to a group of non-progressive neurologic conditions affecting approximately 2-3 in 1,000 children worldwide (Claassen *et al.*, 2011). The condition, caused by disturbances to the developing brain, is characterized by poor voluntary muscle control, muscle paresis, and spasticity resulting in abnormal movement and posture. From a functional perspective, these impairments in motor abilities are known to affect the child's capacity to perform activities of daily living, and will also limit engagement in physical activity (van Brussel *et al.*, 2011). In fact, children and adolescents with CP are known to be less physically active than their typically developing peers, a finding that may have significant implications for the development of secondary health complications (Stevens *et al.*, 2010; Claassen *et al.*, 2011).

While much of the focus to date has been on the relationship between physical activity and health outcomes, sedentary behaviour has recently emerged as a significant contributor to the development of chronic disease in both children and adults (Tremblay and Willms, 2003; Tremblay *et al.*, 2010; Healy *et al.*, 2011). Interestingly, increased sedentary time, independent of physical activity, has been linked with overweight and obesity, as well as cardiovascular and metabolic risk factors (Tremblay *et al.*, 2010). Not only is it important to consider the amount or volume of sedentary time, but also the manner in which it is accumulated. Findings in the adult population suggest that more interruptions in sedentary time (i.e., shorter sedentary "bouts") were beneficially associated with metabolic risk factors (Healy *et al.*, 2008). Given the breadth of evidence supporting the relationship between sedentary behaviour (time, frequency, duration, and breaks) and health outcomes, it seems likely that sedentary behaviour in CP may play an important role in mediating risk for chronic disease; however, this variable has not yet been objectively quantified in youth with CP. As such, the primary objective of this study was to examine sedentary behaviour in a sample of children with CP compared with healthy, age-, gender-, and season-of-wear-matched controls.

33.2 METHODS

Sixteen youth with CP (mean ± SD, age: 13.1 ± 2.3 y) participated in this study, among these were eight children with the Gross Motor Function Classification System level I, five were level II, and three were level III. Sixteen healthy children were matched with the CP sample based on gender, chronological age (± 0.5 y), and season the device was worn (± 1.5 months).

Sedentary behaviour and physical activity were measured via accelerometry (ActiGraph GT1M; Fort Walton Beach, FL), an objective and valid method of quantifying free-living activity in children and adolescents. Activity counts were recorded in 3 s epochs to provide the resolution required to capture the intermittent and spontaneous physical activity patterns previously observed in children (Baquet et al., 2007).

Participants were outfitted with an accelerometer securely fastened to an elastic belt around their waist and instructed to wear the device over the right hip during all waking hours for 7 consecutive days, except when engaging in water activities. They were also asked to record the times the accelerometer was worn or removed over the course of the week. Actual monitoring days varied from 4 to 7 days (mean SD, 6.2 ± 0.9 days). Monitoring time for each day ranged from 0.4 to 16.8 hours. Only participants who wore the accelerometer for ≥ 5 hours on ≥ 4 days were included in the analyses.

Accelerometer data were visually inspected to ensure the time recorded in the activity log book matched the accelerometer output. Any activity counts recorded by the accelerometer during non-wear time, as reported in the log book, were excluded from analysis. All remaining zero counts were treated as inactive time. The data were then uploaded to a Microsoft Excel-based Visual Basic data reduction program to determine total monitoring time, total active and sedentary time, as well as frequency and duration of continuous bouts of sedentary bouts and breaks in sedentary time. Breaks were defined as any interruption in sedentary time in which the activity count was ≥ 6 counts/3 s. To categorize activity and sedentary time, we used cut-points previously developed using the ActiGraph accelerometer (Evenson et al., 2008). Sedentary was defined as 0-5 counts/3 s, and physical activity (light, moderate and vigorous activity) as ≥ 6 counts/3 s.

Independent sample t-tests were used to compare activity and sedentary time, as well as frequency and duration of sedentary bouts and breaks between children with CP and controls. Statistical significance was set at $P \leq 0.05$.

33.3 RESULTS

No differences were seen in monitoring and total sedentary time between children with CP and matched controls (sedentary: 569.5 ± 89.0 vs. 568.9 ± 81.3 min·d^{-1}, P=0.98). Conversely, total physical activity was lower in CP (152.4 ± 61.2 vs. 203.0 ± 45.8 min·d^{-1}, P=0.01). Despite the lack of difference in daily sedentary minutes, children with CP spent a larger proportion of monitoring time being sedentary (78.9 ± 8.3 vs. 73.4 ± 6.3 %, P=0.042).

When it came to the manner in which sedentary time was accumulated, fewer (1466 ± 489 vs. 1881 ± 524 bouts·day^{-1}, P=0.03) but longer (253.5 ± 39.3 vs. 39.7 ± 10.7 s·bout^{-1}, P=0.03) sedentary bouts were seen in children with CP compared with healthy controls. Moreover, the frequency of breaks in sedentary time was lower in CP (1649 ± 481 vs. 2126 ± 406 breaks·day^{-1}, P<0.01), while the mean duration of breaks was similar between groups (CP: 13.0 ± 2.1 vs. healthy: 12.2 ± 3.7 s·break^{-1}, P=0.47) (Figure 33.1).

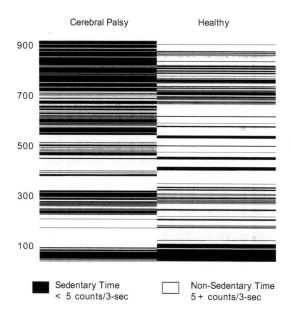

Figure 33.1. Bouts of sedentary activity with intermittent breaks in a child with cerebral palsy and age-, gender-, and season-matched control over the course of 1 monitoring day. Total monitoring and sedentary times were matched between participants.

33.4 CONCLUSION

The results suggest that while total sedentary time is similar in CP and healthy controls, differences exist in the manner in which it is accumulated. More specifically, sedentary behaviour in youths with CP is characterized by longer bouts of sedentary time with less frequent breaks when compared with their healthy peers.

There is emerging evidence that sedentary time, the frequency and duration of sedentary bouts, and breaks in sedentary bouts are related to risk of chronic disease (Healy *et al.*, 2008, 2011; Tremblay *et al.*, 2010). Given that children with CP are at an increased risk of developing a number of secondary health complications including obesity, type II diabetes and cardiovascular disease (Claassen *et al.*, 2011; van Brussel *et al.*, 2011), future work should aim to examine the relationship between sedentary behaviour and health outcomes in this population.

33.5 NOTE

This study was funded by the McMaster Children's Hospital Foundation.

33.6 REFERENCES

Baquet, G., Stratton, G., Van Praagh, E. and Berthoin, S., 2007, Improving physical activity assessment in prepubertal children with high-frequency accelerometry monitoring: A methodological issue. *Preventive Medicine*, **44**, pp. 143-147.

Claassen, A., Gorter, J., Stewart, D., Verschuren, O., Galuppi, B. and Shimmell, L., 2011, Becoming and staying physically active in adolescents with cerebral palsy: Protocol of a qualitative study of facilitators and barriers to physical activity. *BMC Pediatrics*, **11**, pp. 1-10.

Evenson, K., Catellier, D., Gill, K., Ondrak, K. and McMurray, R., 2008, Calibration of two objective measures of physical activity for children. *Journal of Sports Sciences*, **26**, pp. 1557-1565.

Healy, G., Dunstan, D., Salmon, J., Cerin, E., Shaw, J., Zimmet, P. and Owen, N., 2008, Breaks in sedentary time: Beneficial associations with metabolic risk. *Diabetes Care*, **31**, pp. 661-666.

Healy, G., Matthews, C., Dunstan, D., Winkler, E.A.H. and Owen, N., 2011, Sedentary time and cardio-metabolic biomarkers in US adults: NHANES 2003-06. *European Heart Journal*, **32**, pp. 590-597.

Stevens, S., Holbrook, E., Fuller, D. and Morgan, D., 2010, Influence of age on step activity patterns in children with cerebral palsy and typically developing children. *Archives of Physical Medicine and Rehabilitation*, **91**, pp. 1891-1896.

Tremblay, M.S. and Willms, J.D., 2003, Is the Canadian childhood obesity epidemic related to physical inactivity? *International Journal of Obesity*, **27**, pp. 1100-1105.

Tremblay, M., Colley, R., Saunders, T., Healy, G. and Owen, N., 2010. Physiological and health implications of a sedentary lifestyle. *Applied Physiology, Nutrition, and Metabolism*, **35**, pp. 725-740.

van Brussel, M., van der Net, J., Hulzebos, E., Helders, P. J. M. and Takken, T., 2011, The Utrecht approach to exercise in chronic childhood conditions: The decade in review. *Pediatric Physical Therapy*, **23**, pp. 2-14.

AN ADAPTATION OF CENTRAL AND PERIPHERAL CARDIOVASCULAR EXERCISE RESPONSES IN CHILDREN AS A DETERMINANT OF MICROVASCULAR FUNCTION

M.N. Jawis[1], A.R. Middlebrooke[2], A.V. Rowlands[2], and N. Armstrong[2]

[1] Sports Science Unit, School of Medical Sciences, University Sains Malaysia, Malaysia, [2] Children's Health and Exercise Research Centre, University of Exeter, UK

34.1 INTRODUCTION

The vascular endothelium has an influence on the progression of atherosclerosis via anticoagulant, anti-inflammatory, and vascular remodelling properties (Ross, 1999). Studies have indicated that subjects with cardiovascular disease or risk factors for cardiovascular disease may exhibit impaired endothelium-dependent vasomotor responses (Al Suwaidi *et al.*, 2001) and attenuated vascular nitric oxide (NO) activity. The relevance of endothelial dysfunction has been highlighted by many studies indicating that endothelial dysfunction is an independent predictor of cardiac events (Vita and Keaney, 2002). Regular physical exercise is believed to improve endothelium-dependent vasodilation in a number of populations (Walsh *et al.*, 2003) including those of heart failure (Maiorana *et al.*, 2000), type 2 diabetes (Middlebrooke *et al.*, 2005) and hypertension (Higashi *et al.*, 1999).

The cardiovascular system plays a major role in the body's ability to respond to the increased demands of physical activity and exercise. Cardiac variables may be important determinants of microvascular function in the adult population. Studies have demonstrated that the level of aerobic fitness might relate to the maximal performance of the skin microcirculation (Colberg *et al.*, 2005; Middlebrooke *et al.*, 2005). To date, there are no published data on the adaptation of both central and peripheral cardiovascular responses to exercise in children as a determinant of microvascular function or whether aerobic fitness is reflected in the skin microvascular function. Therefore, the aim of this study was to investigate the adaptations of the cardiovascular system in relation to skin blood flow of the microvascular function.

34.2 METHODS

34.2.1   Experimental design

Sixteen boys, aged 9-10 years, were recruited from a local school at Exeter. No participant had a personal history of any cardiovascular disease risk factors such as hypertension, diabetes, high blood pressure and atherosclerosis. Each participant was requested to attend the testing on two occasions. Skin blood flow responses were tested using a combination of two methods, iontophoresis and Laser Doppler Perfusion Imaging (LDPI) (PeriScan, PIM II Laser Doppler, Perimed AB, Sweden) in both occasions. On the second visit, the children completed an incremental cycle ergometer protocol for the determination of maximum peak VO_2 followed by 30 minutes post-maximal exercise microvascular function test. All exercise testing took place in the morning at approximately the same time for each child.

34.2.2   Determination of cardiac output (Q), stroke volume (SV) and peak oxygen uptake (peak VO_2)

Cardiac output (Q) was estimated using a thoracic electrical bioimpedance method (Physioflow, Manatec Biomedical, France) following the procedures described by Welsman *et al.* (2005). Physioflow is a non-invasive Q measurement system that can be used on subjects at rest and during exercise. Changes in thoracic impedance during cardiac ejection were used to calculate stroke volume (SV). A high frequency current was used to eliminate the risk of interference with the heart and brain bioelectrical activity. Maximal exercise testing on a cycle ergometer was performed by measuring the peak oxygen uptake (peak VO_2) achieved during a graded maximal exercise test to exhaustion. The test was performed on an electronically braked cycle ergometer (Lode, Gronigen, the Netherlands).

34.2.3   Determination of microvascular function of iontophoresis and LDPI

Following the termination of the maximal exercise, the participant was taken immediately into the microvascular laboratory for post–maximal microvascular function test. The participant was required to rest down in supine position for about 30 minutes to get acclimatized to the temperature-controlled room (21.5 ± 0.5°C) to ensure the blood pressure and heart rate return to resting values. Skin microvascular perfusion was measured at the drug delivery site using LDPI (PeriScan, PIM II Laser Doppler, Perimed AB, Sweden). LDPI was used to map skin perfusion. A 1-mW Helium Neon laser beam (wavelength 633 nm) sequentially scanned an area of tissue.

34.2.4 Statistical analysis

The paired Student's t-test was used to compare HR, peak VO_2, Q, SV and skin blood flow of the microvascular function before and after acute maximal exercise. A P-value of ≤ 0.05 was considered as statistically significant. Data were expressed as mean (SD).

34.3 RESULTS

There was a significant difference on the peak sodium nitroprusside (SNP) response between pre- and post-maximal exercise (P = 0.04). Similarly, the peak percentage change of SNP response was greater at post-maximal exercise relative to baseline ($P = 0.03$). Heart rate increased significantly with exercise intensity from rest to maximal (74 ± 7 vs 194 ± 18 b·min^{-1}). On the other hand, SV rose significantly at the onset of exercise (45.6 ± 6.9 vs 55.5 ± 7.6 mL). Peak SNP was significantly correlated with maximum Q ($P = 0.02$) at post-maximal exercise.

34.4 CONCLUSION

The main findings from the current study are: 1) acute exercise is reflected in the skin microvascular function; 2) the iontophoresis of acetylcholine (ACh) could not last longer when compared to SNP at post-peak VO_2 test; and 3) when Q and SV were related to the ACh, microvascular function, no significant difference was obtained either at rest or post-maximal exercise. Overall, the iontophoresis of ACh and SNP caused vasodilation of the microvascular blood vessels and smooth muscle cells at the forearm location at both pre- and post-maximal exercise. However, the perfusion of SNP causes greater vasodilation of the blood vessel in the system, than the perfusion of ACh. An explanation for this finding may relate to the importance of the endothelium, which the ACh binds to endothelial cells in producing nitric oxide (Vallance and Collier, 1994). This mechanism delays the relaxation of smooth muscle cell, resulting in the lethargic behaviour of the vasodilation of blood vessels (Higashi and Yoshizumi, 2004).

34.5 REFERENCES

Al Suwaidi, J., Higano, S.T., Hamasaki, S., Holmes, D.R., and Lerman, A., 2001, Association between obesity and coronary atherosclerosis and vascular remodeling. *American Journal of Cardiology*, **88**, pp. 1300-1303.

Colberg, S. R., Parson, H.K., Nunnold, T., Holton, D.R., Swain, D.P. and Vinik, A.I., 2005, Change in cutaneous perfusion following 10 weeks of aerobic training in Type 2 diabetes. *Journal of Diabetes Complications*, **19**, pp. 276-283.

Higashi, Y., Sasaki, S., Kurisu, S., Yoshimizu, A., Sasaki, N., Matsuura, H., Kajiyama, G. and Oshima, T., 1999, Regular aerobic exercise augments endothelium-dependent vascular relaxation in normotensive as well as hypertensive subjects: Role of endothelium-derived nitric oxide. *Circulation*, **100**, pp. 1194-2202.

Higashi, Y. and Yoshizumi, M., 2004, Exercise and endothelial function: Role of endothelium-derived nitric oxide and oxidative stress in healthy subjects and hypertensive patients. *Pharmacology and Therapeutics*, **102**, pp. 87-96.

Maiorana, A., O'Driscoll, G., Dembo, L., Cheetham, C., Goodman, C., Taylor, R. and Green D., 2000, Effect of aerobic and resistance exercise training on vascular function in heart failure. *American Journal of Physiology. Heart and Circulatory Physiology*, **279**, pp. H1999-2005.

Middlebrooke, A.R., Armstrong, N., Welsman, J.R., Shore, A.C., Clark, P. and MacLeod, K.M., 2005, Does aerobic fitness influence microvascular function in healthy adults at risk of developing Type 2 diabetes? *Diabetic Medicine*, **22**, pp. 483-489.

Ross, R., 1999, Atherosclerosis is an inflammatory disease. *American Heart Journal*, **138**, pp. S419-420.

Vallance, P. and Collier, J., 1994, Biology and clinical relevance of nitric oxide. *British Medical Journal*, **309**, pp. 453-457.

Vita, J.A. and Keaney, J.F. Jr., 2002, Endothelial function: A barometer for cardiovascular risk? *Circulation*, **106**, pp. 640-642.

Walsh, J.H., Bilsborough, W., Maiorama, A., Best, M., O'Driscoll, G.J., Taylor, R.R., and Green, D.J., 2003, Exercise training improves conduit vessel function in patients with coronary artery disease. *Journal of Applied Physiology*, **95**, pp. 20-25.

Welsman, J., Bywater, K., Farr, C., Welford, D. and Armstrong, N., 2005, Reliability of peak VO_2 and maximal cardiac output assessed using thoracic bioimpedance in children. *European Journal of Applied Physiology*, **94**, pp. 228-234.

THE EFFECTIVENESS OF A SHORT-TERM LOW-INTENSITY WALKING INTERVENTION ON LIPID PROFILE IN OBESE ADOLESCENTS

A.M. McManus[1], R.R. Mellecker[1], C. Yu[1], and P.T. Cheung[2]

[1]Institute of Human Performance, [2]Department of Paediatric and Adolescent Medicine, University of Hong Kong

35.1 INTRODUCTION

There is considerable support for shifting the focus away from moderate-to-vigorous exercise toward increasing low-to-moderate intensity physical activity. Experimental work has shown that low-intensity incidental activity rather than moderate- or vigorous-intensity activity distinguishes the lean from the obese (Levine *et al.,* 2008a,b). Convincing evidence in animals verifies this proposition, showing benefit in lipid metabolic pathways from increasing low-intensity activity, as opposed to vigorous-intensity exercise (Hamilton *et al.,* 2007*)*. Serum cholesterol and triglyceride have been found to decrease after only 1 week of increased moderate intensity physical activity, combined with the consumption of a low fat and high fibre diet (Schmidt *et al.,* 2011). With the current interest in the use of low-to-moderate intensity activity-enhanced video games as an alternative form of physical activity, it is necessary to establish if similar metabolic benefit is conferred by this lower intensity activity. The purpose of this study was to determine whether a short-term low-intensity interactive video-game treadmill walking programme, without dietary manipulation, was effective in altering the lipid profile of obese adolescents.

35.2 METHODS

35.2.1 Participants

Thirty consecutive obese adolescents (11-16 years) attending a hospital obesity clinic were identified as fulfilling the entry criteria of primary obesity, with BMI

>95th percentile using a local reference (So *et al.*, 2008). After excluding those with underlying congenital abnormalities, type II diabetics, active smokers, pre-term birth (< 37 weeks) and delayed puberty, 22 youngsters were assigned either to an intervention group (n=12) or a control group (n=10). Written informed consent was obtained from all parents and the experimental procedures were approved by the Institutional Review Board for Human Ethics.

35.2.2 Procedures

All participants visited the laboratory in the early morning prior to and within 4 days of completion of the intervention. Assessment of anthropometric measures and body composition was completed and participants provided a venous blood sample. Those in the intervention group underwent assessment of semi-supine and interactive video-game treadmill walking energy expenditure using indirect calorimetry. Dietary and physical activity habits were assessed prior to and in the fourth week of the intervention.

35.2.3 Measures

Stature and body mass were assessed to the nearest 0.1 cm and 0.1 kg respectively. Body composition was measured from a dual x-ray absorptiometer whole-body scan (Hologic Explorer, USA). A venous blood sample was drawn by a trained phlebotomist and assayed for total cholesterol, triglycerides, HDL- and LDL-cholesterol using standard procedures. Energy expenditure was measured using a Medgraphics (Ultima, CPX) indirect calorimeter. Daily physical activity was monitored using a triaxial accelerometer (RT3, StayHealthy Inc, USA). Dietary habits were assessed using a short food frequency questionnaire designed for Chinese adolescents (Ho *et al.*, 2010).

35.2.4 Intervention

The intervention consisted of interactive video-game treadmill walking without any dietary intervention. Participants were asked to complete sixteen 45-minute sessions on an adapted treadmill, with a minimum attendance criteria of 12 sessions. The sessions were completed within 4 weeks. Participants played XBOX360 games while walking at 1.4 km·h[-1]. The speed was chosen on the basis of previous findings which showed that this was the speed at which youngsters could play XBOX360 games normally without having to divert attention to the walking (Mellecker *et al.*, 2009).

35.3 RESULTS

We were unable to collect venous blood from one intervention group participant at baseline and three declined the post-test blood sample (one intervention group and two control group participants). The food frequency questionnaire showed diet remained constant and body mass and composition remained stable over the 4 week period. Descriptive statistics for the participants by group are shown in Table 35.1.

Table 35.1. Descriptive characteristics of the participants. Values are means (SD)

	Control Group (n=10)	Intervention Group (n=12)
Age (y)	13.9 (1.8)	14.2 (1.2)
Height (cm)	165.0 (11.2)	163.4 (7.1)
Body Mass (kg)	83.6 (15.9)	79.9 (15.7)
BMI (mass·h^{-2})	31.7 (4.0)	29.6 (5.0)
Percent Body Fat (%)	39.6 (5.0)	37.4 (5.5)

No time or group significant main effects, nor time by group interactions were noted for any of the blood lipid parameters ($P>0.05$; see Table 35.2).

The average energy cost above rest of a 45 minute interactive video game walking session was 81.2 ($\pm$ 26.9) kcal. This resulted in a mean weekly energy expenditure from the programme of 408 ($\pm$ 128) kcal or 1.71 ($\pm$ 0.53) MJ. Despite this increase in energy expenditure daily physical activity expressed as total vector magnitude did not increase in the intervention group (P>0.05).

Table 35.2. Blood lipid profile pre- and post-intervention by group. Values are means (SD)

	Control (n=8)		Intervention (n=10)	
	Pre	Post	Pre	Post
Triglycerides	1.0 (0.7)	1.0 (0.9)	1.3 (0.9)	1.2 (0.8)
Total Cholesterol	3.9 (0.5)	3.8 (0.6)	4.4 (0.9)	4.2 (0.7)
HDL-Cholesterol	1.0 (0.2)	1.0 (0.3)	1.1 (0.3)	1.1 (0.3)
LDL-Cholesterol	2.4 (0.4)	2.4 (0.5)	2.8 (0.6)	2.7 (0.5)

35.4 DISCUSSION

Compliance was high with 8 of the 12 intervention group participants completing all 16 sessions and all participants completing 12 sessions. Regardless, the 4 weeks of low-intensity walking did not affect blood lipids in this group of obese adolescents. Although changes in lipid profile have been shown after as little as 1 week of increased exercise (Schimdt *et al.*, 2011), the volume of physical activity that is required for clinically significant effects on the blood lipid profile has been disputed. Some suggest that a threshold of approximately 4.2 MJ·wk^{-1} is necessary prior to any beneficial blood lipid effects (Lee and Skerrett, 2001; Durstine *et al.*, 2002). Significant effects on LDL-cholesterol have been shown in overweight Chinese adolescents with a low-to-moderate intensity activity programme (Sun *et al.*, 2011); however, the positive change in the blood lipid profile in Sun *et al.*'s study was accompanied by a reduction in BMI and central adiposity, most likely a result of the longer duration of the programme (10 weeks). Most probably the intensity of activity in the present programme was insufficient to elicit metabolic benefit within the 4 week period, but it is important to note that no change in daily physical activity was apparent in the intervention group participants. This signals that compensatory behaviour occurred, which would render the intervention inert even if the volume of activity of the programme was increased. Finding ways to over-come compensatory behaviour will be key to designing effective long-term activity-enhanced interactive video game interventions in obese adolescents.

35.5 REFERENCES

Durstine, J.L., Grandjean, P.W., Cox, C.A., and Thompson, P.D. 2002, Lipids, lipoproteins, and exercise. *Journal of Cardiopulmonary Rehabilitation*, **6**, pp. 385-398.

Hamilton, M.T., Hamilton, D.G., and Zderic, T.W. 2007, Role of low energy expenditure and sitting in obesity, metabolic syndrome, type 2 diabetes, and cardiovascular disease. *Diabetes*, **56**, pp. 2655-2667.

Ho, S.Y., Wong, B.Y.M., Lo, W.S., Mak, K.K., Thomas G.N. and Lam, T.H. 2010, Neighbourhood food environment and dietary intakes in adolescents: Sex and perceived family affluence as moderators. *International Journal of Pediatric Obesity*, **5**, pp. 420-427.

Lee, I.M. and Skerrett, P.J. 2001, Physical activity and all-cause mortality: What is the dose-response relation? *Medicine and Science in Sports and Exercise*, **6**, pp. S459–S471.

Levine, J.A., Lanningham-Foster, L.M., McCrady, S.K., Krizan, A.C., Olson, L.R., Kane, P.H., Jensen, M.D. and Clark, M.M. 2008a, Interindividual variation in posture allocation: Possible role in human obesity. *Science*, **307**, pp. 584-586.

Levine, J.A., McCrady, S.K., Lanningham-Foster, L.M., Kane, P.H., Foster, R.C., and Manohar, C.U. 2008b, The role of free-living daily walking in human weight gain and obesity. *Diabetes*, **57**, pp. 548-554.

Mellecker, R.R., McManus, A.M., Lanningham-Foster, L. and Levine, J.A. 2009, Development of a motion-enhancing gaming unit for children. *International Journal of Pediatric Obesity*, **4**, pp. 106-111.

Schmidt, S.L., Hickey, M.S., Koblenz, K.M., Klamer, H., Botero, M.F., Pfaffenbach, K.T., Pagliassotti, M.J. and Melby, C.L. 2011, Cardiometabolic plasticity in response to a short-term diet and exercise intervention in young hispanic and non-hispanic white adults. *PLoS ONE,* **6**, pp. e16987.

So, H.K., Nelson, E.A.S., Li, A.M., Wong, E.M.C., Lau, J.T.F., Guldan, G.S., Mak, K.H., Wang, Y., Fok, T.F. and Sung, R.Y.T. 2008, Secular changes in height, weight and body mass index in Hong Kong Children. *BMC Public Health,* **8**, pp. 320.

Sun, M.X., Huang, X.Q., Yan, Y., Li, B.W., Zhong, W.J., Chen, J.F. and Zhang, Y.M. 2011, One-hour after-school exercise ameliorates central adiposity and lipids in overweight Chinese adolescents: A randomized controlled trial. *Chinese Medical Journal,* **124**, pp. 323-329.

Part VI

Testing and Performance

REPRODUCIBILITY OF FUNCTIONAL AND PHYSIOLOGICAL OUTCOMES OF EXERCISE TESTING IN AMBULATORY CHILDREN WITH SPINA BIFIDA

J.F. De Groot, T. Takken, M.A.C.G. Schoenmakers, R. Gooskens, S. Goossens, S. den Haak, L. Vanhees, and P.J.M. Helders

Wilhelmina Children's Hospital, University Medical Center Utrecht, in cooperation with the HU University of Applied Sciences Utrecht, The Netherlands

36.1 INTRODUCTION

Due to advances in the medical approach, mortality rates have decreased in recent years and more children with neuromotor disability can now be expected to live to be adults (Roebroeck *et al.*, 2009). This requires a different approach in medical management of these patients from childhood through adolescence into adulthood, with attention not only to the pathological aspects, but also to the (preventable) medical, functional and social consequences of neuromotor disability. Spina Bifida (SB) is the most frequently seen congenital deformity of the neural tube, with an incidence ranging from 2–8 per 10000 live births worldwide (Kondo *et al.*, 2009). As a result of the neural tube deformity, patients experience a variety of deficits in cognition, motor function, sensory function and bowel and bladder function (Ryan *et al.*, 1991). Several studies have shown children and adolescents and young adults with SB to be less active, resulting in obesity, reduced health-related quality of life and significantly reduced levels of physical fitness when compared with healthy peers (van den Berg-Emons *et al.*, 2003; Buffart *et al.*, 2008; Schoenmakers *et al.*, 2008). Ambulatory children with SB do not only perform poorer compared to their healthy peers, but also compared to children with other chronic conditions (Hassan *et al.*, 2010). Besides, a relationship was found between aerobic capacity and energy expenditure during ambulation (De Groot *et al.*, 2008).

The emerging interest in physical fitness, physical activity and implementation of lifestyle and exercise programmes in children, adolescents and young adults with neuromotor disability, emphasizes the need to develop appropriate protocols to monitor change in these areas. For evaluation of intervention programmes, information is needed regarding validity and reliability of exercise testing in children with SB. The purpose of this study was to analyse reproducibility of both maximal and submaximal outcomes of exercise testing in ambulatory children with SB. Since research labs and clinical settings differ in both equipment and experience in exercise testing, both physiologic and performance parameters were analysed in this study.

36.2 METHODS

36.2.1 Study design

The study was a reproducibility study of maximal and submaximal exercise measures, with retesting taking place 2 weeks later, at the same time of day by the same tester.

36.2.2 Subjects

The study group consisted of 23 ambulatory children with SB, type myelomeningocele (MMC), known at the SB outpatient clinic of Wilhelmina Children's Hospital in Utrecht, The Netherlands. Study procedures took place at the Child Development and Exercise Center. All study procedures were approved by the University Medical Ethics Committee. Children were included when they were (1) at least community ambulatory, (2) able to follow instructions regarding testing and (3) between 6 and 18 years of age. Parents and children signed informed-consent forms prior to testing. Exclusion criteria were medical events that might interfere with the outcomes of the testing and/or medical status that did not allow maximum exercise testing.

36.2.3 Measurements

Maximal measures
In this study, maximal exercise testing was measured using a graded treadmill test (EnMill, Enraf, Delft, The Netherlands). In previous studies, treadmill protocols have been used to test peak VO_2 in children with disability (Hoofwijk *et al.*, 1995; Verschuren *et al.*, 2006), including children with SB (De Groot *et al.*, 2009). In order to accommodate children with different ambulatory abilities, two progressive exercise test protocols were used. Children ambulating < 400 metres during a 6 minute walking test (6MWT) were tested with a starting speed of 2 km·h^{-1}, which was gradually increased by 0.25 km·h^{-1} every minute, with a set grade of 2 %. Children ambulating > 400 metres during the 6MWT were

started at a speed of 3 km·h^{-1}, with the speed being increased 0.5 km·h^{-1} every minute, with a set grade of 2 %. The protocols were continued until the patient stopped due to exhaustion, despite verbal encouragement from the test leader. During the incremental exercise test, physiologic responses, including breath-by-breath gas analysis, were measured using a heart rate (HR) monitor (Polar Accurex, Polar-Nederland BV, Almere, The Netherlands) and calibrated mobile gas analysis system (Cortex Metamax B^3, Cortex Medical GmbH, Leipzig, Germany). Heart rate response (HRR) not to be confused with heart rate reserve and oxygen pulse (O$_2$ pulse) were derived from VO$_2$ and HR measures. HRR was chosen because it assumes a linear relationship between increase in VO$_2$ and the increase in HR during exercise, independent of the patient's motivation or ending the test prematurely, e.g. when a test is considered "symptom-limited". HRR was calculated as (HR$_{peak}$-HR$_{rest}$)/(peak VO$_2$-VO$_{2rest}$) (Eschenbacher and Mannina, 1990). O$_2$-pulse, used as an index of stroke volume, was calculated as peak VO$_2$/HR$_{peak}$ (Wasserman et al., 1999). Besides physiologic responses, maximal walking or running speed was recorded.

Submaximal measures
Measures at the ventilatory threshold (VT)
VO$_2$ and HR were determined at the VT. The VT was determined using the criteria of an increase in the ventilatory equivalent of oxygen (VE/VO$_2$) with no increase in the ventilatory equivalent of carbon dioxide (VE/VCO$_2$), while respiratory exchange ratio (RER), defined as VCO$_2$ / VO$_2$ remained below 1.0 (Whipp et al., 1981).

Oxygen uptake efficiency slopes (OUES)
The OUES is considered a submaximal measure, introduced by Baba et al., (1996) as an alternative to the VT, when VT cannot be determined and because of the questionable reliability of the VT when using different examiners. The OUES reflects efficiency of ventilation in relation to oxygen uptake. The OUES is calculated by making use of the following regression equation: VO$_2$ = a·log(V$_E$) + b, in which the constant 'a' represents the rate of increase in VO$_2$ in response to an increase in V$_E$, called the OUES.

Energy expenditure during the 6 minute walk test (6MWT)
The test was performed on a 20 m track in a straight corridor. Patients were instructed to cover the largest possible distance in 6 minutes at a self-selected walking speed. The test and encouragements during the test were performed in accordance with the American Thoracic Society guidelines (2002). Steady state (SS) normalized oxygen uptake (VO$_2$·kg^{-1}·min^{-1}) was calculated as the average value over the period during which oxygen consumption changed 5 % or less. Respiratory exchange ratio (RER) was calculated as VCO$_2$/VO$_2$ during steady state. Speed (m·min^{-1}) was calculated as distance (m)/6 (min). Subsequently the

following parameters were derived: Gross energy consumption (ECS_{gross}) and gross energy cost (EC_{gross}). ECS was expressed in $J \cdot kg^{-1} \cdot min^{-1}$, using SS VO_2 and RER in the following equation: $J \cdot kg^{-1} \cdot min^{-1} = (4.960 \times RER + 16.040) \times VO_2 \cdot kg^{-1}$ (Garby and Astrup, 1987). Furthermore gross energy cost (EC_{gross}) expressed in $J \cdot kg^{-1} \cdot m^{-1}$ was calculated, dividing ECS_{gross} by speed. For net energy expenditure, resting values were deducted from gross measures.

36.2.4 Data analysis

For initial analyses, data were checked for normality and heteroscedasticity, the latter being defined as a correlation coefficient between the differences of test–retest and the mean of the observations greater than 0.3 (Atkinson and Nevill, 1998). Reproducibility encompasses both reliability and agreement (De Vet *et al.*, 2005). Subsequently, for reliability, the intra-class correlation$_{consistency}$ (ICC) was calculated using the following formula: $variance_{patient}^2/variance_{patient}^2 + variance_{residual}^2$ (De Vet *et al.*, 2005). An ICC of 0.8 or higher was considered good.

For clinicians, agreement of the measurements is more of interest, because they look to determine meaningful improvements in a single patient. For agreement in normal distributed differences, the Standard Error of Measurement (SEM) and the Smallest Detectable Difference (SDD) were calculated, using the following equations: $SEM = SD * \sqrt{1 - ICC_{consistency}}$ and $SDD = 1.96 * \sqrt{2} * SEM$. (Portney and Watkins 2008). For heteroscedastic data, the coefficient of variance (CV) was calculated as a measure for stability within individual results. When dealing with heteroscedastic data, log transformation is recommended (Atkinson and Nevill, 1998). To examine the 95 % confidence interval of the CV %, data was antilogged and expressed to the power of 1.96, using the available spreadsheet calculations by Hopkins (1996). Statistical analyses were performed using SPSS for Windows (version 15.0, SPSS Inc., Chicago, IL.) or MS Excel, (Microsoft, Amsterdam, The Netherlands).

36.3 RESULTS

Reproducibility measures can be found in Table 36.1. ICC is high and agreement shows a SEM of 3 % and 3.2 % for respectively maximum speed during the treadmill test and the 6MWT. ICC's for peak VO_2, HRR and O_2-pulse maximum speed were > 0.8 (0.97-0.99) and moderate for HR_{peak}. CV for maximal measures ranged from 5.0 % for HR_{peak} to 17.3 % for HRR. ICCs varied from 0.53 for HR_{VT} to 0.94 for HR_{6MWT}. CV ranged from 4.6 for HR_{VT} up to 13.2 for VO_{2VT} and 24.3 % for the OEUS. ICCs for energy expenditure measures vary from 0.86 and 0.88 for net EC and ECS to 0.96 for resting ECS. ICC for speed is 0.97. The SDD expressed as a percentage of the mean was 18-24 % for gross energy expenditure, and up to over 30 % for net energy expenditure.

Table 36.1. Reproducibility data for exercise testing in children with SB

	ICC	SEM	SDD	CV %	95 % interval of CV %
Performance measures					
$Speed_{max}$ $(km \cdot h^{-1})$	0.99	0.2	0.5		
6MWD	0.98	13.1	36.3		
Maximal measures					
Peak VO_2 $(L \cdot min^{-1})$	0.97			8.2	6.1 – 12.5
HR_{peak}	0.78			5.0	3.6 – 7.8
HRR	0.87			17.3	12.3 – 29.4
O_2-pulse	0.95			9.7	7.2 – 14.9
Submaximal measures					
VO_{2VT} $(L \cdot min^{-1})$	0.89			13.2	9.6 – 21.1
HR_{VT}	0.53			4.6	3.3 – 7.3
OUES	0.8			24.3	17.9 – 38.9
HR_{6MWT}	0.94			5.4	3.2 – 7.5
ECS_{gross} $(J \cdot kg^{-1} \cdot min^{-1})$	0.91	31.0	86.1		
EC_{gross} $(J \cdot kg^{-1} \cdot m^{-1})$	0.91	0.6	1.7		
ECS_{net} $(J \cdot kg^{-1} \cdot min^{-1})$	0.88	32.3	89.4		
EC_{net} $(J \cdot kg^{-1} \cdot m^{-1})$	0.86	0.6	1.5		

ICC =Intraclass correlation; SEM=Standard error of measurement; SDD=Smallest detectable difference

36.4 CONCLUSION

The aim of this study was to assess both the reliability and agreement of maximal and submaximal exercise parameters in ambulatory children with SB. While exercise testing is advised and feasible in children with disability, it is important to determine reproducibility of testing for the populations at stake as the psychometric measures differ from each other and from the healthy paediatric population. Examples include agreement for the 6 MWT varying from 43 meters in children with Cerebral Palsy (Maher *et al.*, 2008), up to 139 metres in children with Cystic Fibrosis (Cunha *et al.*, 2006), compared to the 36 metres for children with SB. CV or ICC for HR_{peak} are less commonly reported, but generally CV remains below 2.2 % (Johnston *et al.*, 2009), which is lower than the 5% in this population. In this study, CV for HRR, OUES and O_2 pulse were > 10 %, therefore not recommended for use in the individual evaluation and interpretation of exercise testing. As far as energy expenditure measures are concerned, Thomas *et al.* (2009) have demonstrated the CV % for gross ECS and EC in healthy children to be around 9-10 %, while variability in net measures increased to 14-15 %, which is much lower than in this study.

36.5 REFERENCES

Atkinson, G. and Nevill, A.M., 1998, Statistical methods for assessing measurement error (reliability) in variables relevant to sports medicine. *Sports Medicine*, **26**, pp. 217-238.

ATS, 2002, ATS statement: Guidelines for the six-minute walking test. *American Journal for Respiratory Critical Care Medicine*, **166**, pp. 111-117.

Baba, R., Nagashima, M., Goto, M., Nagano, Y., Yokota, M., Tauchi, N. and Nishibata, K., 1996, Oxygen uptake efficiency slope: A new index of cardiorespiratory functional reserve derived from the relation between oxygen uptake and minute ventilation during incremental exercise. *Journal for American College of Cardiology*, **28**, pp. 1567-1572.

Buffart, L.M., Roebroeck, M.E., Rol, M, Stam, H.J. and van den Berg-Emons, H.J., 2008, Transition Research Group South-West Netherlands. Triad of physical activity, aerobic fitness and obesity in adolescents and young adults with myelomeningocele. *Journal of Rehabilitation Medicine*, **40**, pp. 672-677.

Cunha, M.T, Rozov, T., de Oliveira, R.C. and Jardim, J.R., 2006, Six-minute walk test in children and adolescents with cystic fibrosis. *Pediatric Pulmonology*, **41**, pp. 618-622.

De Groot, J.F., Takken, T., Schoenmakers M.A.C.G., Vanhees, L. and Helders, P.J.M., 2008, Interpretation of maximal exercise testing and the relationship with ambulation parameters in ambulation children with Spina Bifida. *European Journal of Applied Physiology*, **104**, 657-665.

De Groot, J.F., Takken, T., de Graaff, S., Gooskens, R.H., Helders, P.J.M, and Vanhees L., 2009, Treadmill testing of children who have spina bifida and are ambulatory: Does peak oxygen uptake reflect maximum oxygen uptake? *Physical Therapy*, **89**, pp. 679-687.

De Vet, H.C.W., Terwee, C.B., Knol, D.L. and Bouter L.M., 2005, When to use agreement versus reliability measures? *Journal of Clinical Epidemiology*, **59**, pp. 1033-1039.

Eschenbacher, W.L. and Mannina, A., 1990, An algoritm for the interpretation of cardiopulmonary exercise tests. *Chest*, **97**, pp. 263-267.

Garby, L, and Astrup, A., 1987, The relationship between the respiratory quotient and the energy equivalent of oxygen during simultaneous glucose and lipid oxidation and lipogenesis. *Acta Physiologica Scandinavica*, **129**, pp. 443-444.

Hassan, J., van der Net, J., Helders, P.J., Prakken, B.J. and Takken, T., 2010, Six-minute walk test in children with chronic conditions. *British Journal of Sports Medicine*, **44**, pp. 270-274.

Hoofwijk, M., Unnithan, V.B. and Bar-Or, O., 1995, Maximal treadmill performance of children with cerebral palsy. *Pediatric Exercise Science*, **7**, pp. 305-313.

Hopkins, W.G. 2000, http://www.sportsci.org/resource/stats/xrely.xls.

Johnston, K.N., Jenkins, S.C.and Stick, S.M., 2009, Repeatibility of peak oxygen uptake in children who are healthy. *Pediatric Physical Therapy*, **17**, pp. 11-17.

Kondo, A., Kamihira, O. and Ozawa, H., 2009, Neural tube deficits: Prevalence, etiology and prevention. *International Journal of Urology*, **16**, pp. 49-57.

Maher, C.A., Williams, M.T. and Olds, T.S., 2008, The six-minute walk test for children with cerebral palsy. *International Journal of Rehabilitation Residence*, **31**, pp. 185-188.

Portney, L.G. and Watkins, M.P., 2008, Foundations of Clinical Research: Applications to practice. Third edition. Upper Saddle River, NJ, USA: Pearson Prentice Hall.

Roebroeck, M.E., Jahnsen, R., Carona, C., Kent, R.M. and Chamberlain, M.A., 2009, Adult outcomes and lifespan issues for people with childhood-onset physical disability. *Devopmental Medicine Child Neurology*, **51**, pp. 670-678.

Ryan, D.K., Ploski, C. and Emans, J.B., 1991, Myelodysplasia-the musculoskeletal problem: Habilitation from infancy to adulthood. *Physical Therapy*, **71**, pp. 67-78.

Schoenmakers, M.A.G.C., De Groot, J.F., Gorter, J.W., Hilleart, J.L.M., Helders, P.J.M. and Takken, T., 2008, Muscle strength, aerobic capacity and physical activity in independent ambulating children with lumbosacral spina bifida. *Disability and Rehabilitation*, **31**, pp. 259-266.

Thomas, S.S., Buckon, C.E., Schwartz, M.H., Sussman, M.D. and Aiona, M.D., 2009, Walking energy expenditure in able-bodied individuals: A comparison of common measures of energy efficiency. *Gait and Posture*, **29**, pp. 592-596.

van den Berg-Emons, H.J., Bussmann, J.B., Meyerink, H.J., Roebroeck, M.E. and Stam, H.J., 2003, Body fat, fitness and level of everyday physical activity in adolescents and young adults with meningomyelocele. *Journal of Rehabilitation Medicine*, **35**, pp. 271-275.

Verschuren, O., Takken, T., Ketelaar, M., Gorter, J.W. and Helders, P.J., 2006, Reliability and validity of data for 2 newly developed shuttle run tests in children with cerebral palsy. *Physical Therapy*, **86**, pp. 1107-1117.

Wasserman, K., Hansen, J.E., Sue, D.L.Y., Casaburi, R. and Whipp, B.J., 1999, *Principles of Exercise Testing and Interpretation*. Third edition. Philadelphia, PA, USA. Lippincott Williams and Wilkins.

Whipp, B.J., Davis, J.A., Torres, F. and Wasserman, K., 1981, A test to determine parameters of aerobic function during exercise. *Journal of Applied Physiology*, **50**, pp. 217-221.

VALIDITY OF THE OXYGEN UPTAKE EFFICIENCY SLOPE IN CHILDREN WITH CYSTIC FIBROSIS

B.C. Bongers, H.J. Hulzebos, H.G.M. Arets, and T. Takken

University Medical Center Utrecht, the Netherlands

37.1 INTRODUCTION

Maximal oxygen uptake (VO_{2max}) is generally considered the most reliable single measure of an individual's maximal cardiopulmonary exercise capacity. Although many healthy children as well as paediatric patients do not show a plateau in oxygen uptake (VO_2) during exercise, several authors (Rowland 1993; Armstrong et al., 1996) showed that this levelling-off of VO_2 is not essential for defining the highest VO_2 in children. Therefore, VO_{2max} is often replaced by peak VO_2 (peak VO_2), the highest VO_2 measured during incremental exercise testing (IET).

Questions can be raised about the validity of peak VO_2 in children with Cystic Fibrosis (CF) during maximal exercise. Some authors have reported a reduced exercise capacity during IET in children with CF compared with healthy peers (Keochkerian et al., 2008; Wideman et al., 2009), however, the observed peak heart rates (HR_{peak}) in these studies were significantly lower compared to values observed in healthy children. Therefore, this lower peak VO_2 might be due to a really lower peak VO_2 or to an incapability of the patient to reach a 'true' peak VO_2. Moreover, peak VO_2 can be strongly influenced by motivation, the exercise protocol, and the experience of the tester (Andreacci et al., 2002).

The oxygen uptake efficiency slope (OUES) might be an alternative measurement for peak VO_2. The OUES describes the linear relation between the VO_2 and the common logarithm of the minute ventilation (VE) throughout IET. Theoretically, due to its linearity throughout IET, the OUES should be resistant to disruption by early termination during IET (Davies et al., 2006). Since the original rationale of the OUES was to provide a sub-maximal measure of cardiopulmonary exercise capacity, which could be used as a possible alternative for the peak VO_2 in populations unable to perform maximal exercise, the aim of the present study was to investigate whether the OUES could be used as a valid, sub-maximal measure of maximal cardiopulmonary exercise capacity in children with CF.

37.2 MATERIALS AND METHODS

37.2.1 Experimental design

Twenty-two children with mild to moderate CF (mean FEV_1 of 81.5 % [± 15.6]) and 22 healthy children, 11-18 years of age, 13 boys and 9 girls in each group, performed IET with respiratory gas analysis (Jaeger Oxycon Pro, Care Fusion, Houten, the Netherlands) using an electronically braked cycle ergometer (Lode Corrival, Lode, Groningen, the Netherlands). The work rate was increased by a constant increment of 15 or 20 $W \cdot min^{-1}$ until voluntary exhaustion. Output from the gas analyzers and airflow meter were averaged at 10 second intervals.

37.2.2 Measurements

The OUES was calculated at three different exercise intensities by making use of the following equation: $VO_2 = a \cdot Log(VE) + b$, in which the constant 'a' represents the rate of increase in VO_2 in response to an increase in VE, called the OUES (Baba *et al.,* 1996). To reduce the variability between subjects due to growth and maturation, OUES values were normalized for body surface area (BSA) (OUES/BSA). The OUES 50/BSA, OUES 75/BSA, and OUES 100/BSA were determined using respectively the first 50 %, the first 75 %, and 100 % of the exercise data. The efficiency of ventilation was also assessed with the VE/VO_2 ratio and the ventilatory threshold (VT) was determined using the V-slope method.

37.2.3 Statistical analysis

Independent samples t-tests were performed in order to test for significant between group differences. Repeated measures ANOVA, with Bonferroni adjustment for multiple testing, was used to evaluate within group differences in OUES/BSA values calculated at three different exercise intensities. Pearson correlation coefficients were calculated to examine the relationship between exercise variables and the OUES/BSA. Significance was a priori set at the 0.05 level.

37.3 RESULTS

Only the OUES 50/BSA appeared to be significantly different between the two groups (Figure 37.1), with lower values achieved in the children with CF (1378.1 [± 294.6] vs. 1616.3 [± 333.0], *P*=0.016). Figure 37.1 also shows the effect of exercise duration on the OUES/BSA, thereby showing its linearity characteristics within the two groups.

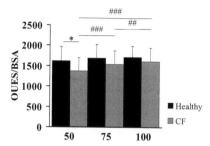

Figure 37.1. The OUES values normalized for BSA at the three different relative exercise intensities (% of total exercise duration); mean ± SD.*: between group difference; #: differences within the group with patients with CF. * *P*<0.05; ## *P*<0.01; ### *P*<0.001.

The OUES 50/BSA in children with CF (1378.1 [± 294.6]) appeared to be significantly lower than both the OUES 75/BSA (1542.4 [± 327.6], *P*<0.001) and the OUES 100/BSA (1610.0 [± 335.9], *P*<0.001). In addition, the OUES 75/BSA was significantly lower than the OUES 100/BSA (*P*=0.006). In contrast, no significant within group differences were found between the OUES 100/BSA (1714.2 [± 273.8]), OUES 75/BSA (1689.9 [± 339.3]), and OUES 50/BSA (1616.3 [± 333.0]) in the healthy children.

In children with CF, the OUES/BSA correlated moderately with the peak $VO_2 \cdot kg^{-1}$, peak $VO_2 \cdot kg^{-1}$ expressed as a percentage of predicted, and the VT (*r* ranging from 0.350 to 0.541), whereas moderate to strong correlations were found between the OUES/BSA and the peak $VO_2 \cdot kg^{-1}$, peak $VO_2 \cdot kg^{-1}$ expressed as a percentage of predicted, and VT (*r* ranging from 0.395 to 0.781) in the healthy children. Overall, associations weakened when a smaller amount of data points were used for the calculation of the OUES, with OUES 50/BSA having the lowest correlation coefficients. No significant associations were observed between the OUES/BSA and lung function parameters.

37.4 CONCLUSION

The main findings implicate that the OUES seems to be of limited value in children with CF and mild to moderate airflow obstruction as a measure of cardiopulmonary exercise capacity derived from sub-maximal exercise data.

This is attributable to its limited ability to distinguish between children with moderate CF and healthy peers together with its nonlinearity during the last part of IET and its moderate correlations with peak VO_2 and the VT.

In contrast to the construct of the OUES and our healthy children, the OUES appeared to be nonlinear in our patients with CF. Post-hoc analyses showed that children with moderate CF have a reduced efficiency of ventilation during sub-maximal exercise as specified by both the OUES/BSA (Figure 37.1) and the VE/VO_2 ratio calculated using exercise data up to 50 % of the total exercise duration.

When exercise progresses to 75 % and 100 % of the total exercise duration, children with CF show an improved efficiency of ventilation, as indicated by their OUES/BSA (Figure 37.1) and VE/VO_2 ratio values approaching the values attained by their healthy peers. This increasing efficiency of ventilation might be explained by slowed VO_2 kinetics or altered substrate utilization at lower exercise intensities.

A possible explanation for the limited distinguishing ability of the OUES is that although the included patients with CF had a significantly reduced peak VO_2, they were not ventilatory limited enough during IET to cause a significantly reduced OUES. Whether the OUES is a valid indicator of cardiopulmonary exercise capacity in patients with severe CF will need additional research.

37.5 REFERENCES

Andreacci, J.L., LeMura, L.M., Cohen, S.L., Urbansky, E.A., Chelland, S.A. and Von Duvillard, S.P., 2002, The effects of frequency of encouragement on performance during maximal exercise testing. *Journal of Sports Sciences*, **20**, pp. 345-352.

Armstrong, N., Welsman, J. and Winsley, R., 1996, Is peak VO_2 a maximal index of children's aerobic fitness? *International Journal of Sports Medicine*, **17**, pp. 356-359.

Baba, R., Nagashima, M., Goto, M., Nagano, Y., Yokota, M., Tauchi, N. and Nishibata, K., 1996, Oxygen uptake efficiency slope: A new index of cardiorespiratory functional reserve derived from the relation between oxygen uptake and minute ventilation during incremental exercise. *Journal of the American College of Cardiology*, **28**, pp. 1567-1572.

Davies, L.C., Wensel, R., Georgiadou, P., Cicoira, M., Coats, A.J.S., Piepoli, M.F. and Francis, D.P., 2006, Enhanced prognostic value from cardiopulmonary exercise testing in chronic heart failure by non-linear analysis: Oxygen uptake efficiency slope. *European Heart Journal*, **27**, pp. 684-690.

Keochkerian, D., Chlif, M., Delanaud, S., Gauthier, R., Maingourd, Y. and Ahmaidi, S., 2008, Breathing pattern adopted by children with cystic fibrosis with mild to moderate pulmonary impairment during exercise. *Respiration*, **75**, pp. 170-177.

Rowland, T.W., 1993, Does peak VO_2 reflect VO_{2max} in children? Evidence from supramaximal testing. *Medicine and Science in Sports and Exercise*, **25**, pp. 689-693.

Wideman, L., Baker, C.F., Brown, P.K., Consitt, L.A., Ambrosius, W.T. and Schechter, M.S., 2009, Substrate utilization during and after exercise in mild cystic fibrosis. *Medicine and Science in Sports and Exercise*, **41**, pp. 270-278.

THE VALIDITY OF THE STEEP RAMP PROTOCOL TO PREDICT PEAK OXYGEN UPTAKE IN ADOLESCENTS WITH CYSTIC FIBROSIS

H.J. Hulzebos[1], M.S. Werkman[1], P.B. van de Weert-van Leeuwen[2], H.G.M. Arets[2], T. Takken[1]

[1]Child Development and Exercise Center, University Medical Center Utrecht
[2]Pediatric Respiratory Medicine, University Medical Center Utrecht, The Netherlands

38.1 INTRODUCTION

Cardiopulmonary exercise testing (CPET) has an integral place in cystic fibrosis care and follows up because of its high yield of diagnostic, prognostic and functional information. The most important parameter of aerobic exercise capacity is the peak oxygen uptake (peak VO_2) (Ferraza *et al.*, 2009; Midgley and Carroll, 2009).

Traditionally, CPET is performed on a bicycle ergometer and ordinary, large work rate increments (10-20 $W \cdot min^{-1}$) are used to provide volitional exhaustion in a 10-12 minute period (Godfrey *et al.*, 1974; Ferraza *et al.*, 2009). Currently, ramp protocols (e.g. the Steep Ramp protocol (SR)) have gained popularity due to their short, intensive origin, and ability to predict peak VO_2 (Meyer *et al.*, 1996; de Backer *et al.*, 2007). For clinical purposes, there is a need for short, inexpensive and easy to administer exercise testing in children and adolescents. SR protocols have also gained popularity due to the anaerobic nature of children's physical activity behaviour. A SR protocol could possibly provide an alternative method for the more time consuming slower protocols, not only in cardiac patients, but also in chronic lung disease. A simple, short and feasible exercise test might help to increase the utilization of exercise testing in this patient group (Barker *et al.*, 2004).

The objectives of this investigation were to study: 1) the concurrent-validity of the SR protocol in measuring peak VO_2; and 2) to develop a model to estimate peak VO_2 from the W_{peak} obtained during the SR protocol in adolescents with CF.

38.2 MATERIALS AND METHODS

Design

Forty-six adolescents with CF (23 boys and 23 girls; 14.6 ± 1.7 y) of the Cystic Fibrosis Center of the University Children's Hospital and Medical Center Utrecht, The Netherlands, were measured for body mass, height, lung function and exercise capacity as part of their annual medical check-up. As all measurements were part of usual care, according to the policy of the medical ethical committee of the University Medical Center Utrecht, ethical approval and informed consent were not obliged. Individual data were collected in one test session. Lung function (Master Lab system, E. Jaeger, Würzburg, Germany) and anthropometric values, using an electronic scale (Seca, Birmingham, UK) and a stadiometer (Ulmer stadiometer, Prof. E. Heinze, Ulm, Germany), were determined before CPET. Adolescents were asked to avoid heavy meals and strenuous exercise from the evening before testing. To be able to study the concurrent-validity of the SR protocol, an ordinary, slower, Godfrey protocol was used as the criterion test (Godfrey, 1974). The sequence of the two test protocols was counterbalanced in group 1: SR-Godfrey and group 2: Godfrey-SR, and was allocated to the participants by randomization. Patients had 10 minutes passive recovery between both tests.

Exercise tests

The Godfrey protocol was performed on an electronically braked cycle ergometer (Ergoline, Cardinal Health, Houten, The Netherlands). Cycling started unloaded and was increased based on height (10 $W \cdot min^{-1}$ < 120 cm; 15 $W \cdot min^{-1}$ 120–150 cm; 20 $W \cdot min^{-1}$ > 150 cm), independent of gender, every minute until the patient stopped due to volitional exhaustion (Godfrey, 1974). The SR protocol was performed on the same electronically braked cycle ergometer. A modified SR protocol was used (Meyer *et al.,* 1996). The protocol was as follows: after 1 minute of resting measurement and 1 minute of unloaded cycling, the test started and work rate was increased every 10 seconds based on the subject's height as in the Godfrey protocol. The two tests ended when the pedal frequency fell below 60 $rev \cdot min^{-1}$ despite verbal encouragement.

Adolescents breathed through a mouthpiece, connected to a calibrated metabolic cart (Oxycon pro, Care Fusion, Houten, The Netherlands). Expired gas passed through a flow meter, oxygen analyzer, and a carbon dioxide analyzer. The flow meter and gas analyzer were connected to a computer, which calculated breath-by-breath minute ventilation (V_E), oxygen consumption (VO_2), carbon dioxide production (VCO_2), and respiratory exchange ratio (RER) from conventional equations. While testing, heart rate (HR) was monitored continuously by a 3-lead electrocardiogram (Hewlett-Packard, Amstelveen, The Netherlands), and transcutaneous oxygen saturation ($SpO_2\%$)

was measured by pulse oximetry on the index finger (Nellcor 200 E, Breda, The Netherlands).

38.2.1 Statistical analysis

Data were expressed as mean (SD). Data were analyzed using SPSS Statistics 17.0 for Windows (SPSS Inc., Chicago, IL, USA) and tested for normality with the Kolmogorov-Smirnov test. A P-value < 0.05 was considered statistically significant. Differences between the Godfrey and SR protocol within groups were analyzed and differences between groups were analyzed using ANOVA. Differences between protocols in the total sample were analyzed using paired sample t-tests. A linear regression model was used to predict the Godfrey peak VO_2 $(L \cdot min^{-1})$ from the SR W-peak values.

38.3 RESULTS

All 46 participants performed both exercise protocols without any complications or adverse events. All exercise variables were normally distributed. The mean exercise time of the Godfrey protocol was 11.0 ± 2.8 min and 4.1 ± 0.7 min for the SR protocol, both including 1 minute of resting measurements and 1 minute of reference cycling. The ventilatory and cardiovascular demand of the SR protocol was lower compared to the Godfrey protocol, as reflected by significant lower V_E (65 ± 26 vs. 72 ± 24 $L \cdot min^{-1}$; $P<0.001$) and HR (172 ± 14 vs. 180 ± 10 $b \cdot min^{-1}$; $P<0.001$). Resting HR and V_E ($P< 0.01$) were significantly higher before the SR protocol when it was preceded by the Godfrey protocol. In both groups, peak $VO2 \cdot kg^{-1}$ was lower in the SR protocol, and this difference decreased from 6.1 $mL \cdot min^{-1} \cdot kg^{-1}$ (SEM $= 2.3$ mL), when started with the SR protocol, to 1.5 $mL \cdot min^{-1} \cdot kg^{-1}$ (SEM $= 1.6$), when started with the Godfrey protocol. $W_{peak} \cdot kg^{-1}$ were significantly higher (~ 50 %) in the SR protocol within and between groups.

The linear regression model was influenced by test sequence:
Group 1: peak VO_2 $(L \cdot min^{-1})$ = $0.053 + 0.006$ x SR (W_{peak}) + 0.195 x FEV_1 $(L \cdot min^{-1})$; $r^2 = 0.66$ (SEE = 0.37).
Group 2: peak VO_2 $(L \cdot min^{-1})$ = $-0.008 + 0.23$ x FEV_1 $(L \cdot min^{-1})$ + 0.005 x SR (W_{peak}); $r^2 = 0.91$ (SEE = 0.20)).
The regression equation in the total group was peak VO_2 $(L \cdot min^{-1})$ = $0.014 + 0.005$ x SR (W_{peak}) + 0.226 x FEV_1 $(L \cdot min^{-1})$ with an $r^2 = 0.82$ (SEE= 0.27).

38.4 CONCLUSION

We found significant differences between peakVO$_2$ and peakVO$_2$·kg^{-1} obtained during the Godfrey protocol and SR protocol within groups, between groups and in the entire group. This overall finding is in contrast to previous literature, in which equal peak VO$_2$ values were found between traditional and short, supramaximal (work rate 105 % of work rate obtained during the traditional test) exercise protocols. Furthermore, as shown in previous studies, the ventilatory and cardiovascular demand of the SR protocol was lower compared to the slower Godfrey protocol, as reflected by significant lower VE$_{peak}$ and HR$_{peak}$ values in the SR protocol for the entire group (Meyer *et al.*, 1996).

We found a higher resting HR and V$_E$ before the SR protocol when it was preceded by the Godfrey protocol, pointing to incomplete recovery after the Godfrey protocol, which could possibly result in a faster onset of oxygen uptake kinetics at the start of the SR protocol. So, with an adequate warming-up, no statistically significant difference would be found between SR and Godfrey peak VO$_2$·kg^{-1}. The significant higher obtained W$_{peak}$ in the SR protocol compared to the Godfrey protocol can be explained by the possibility of a greater contribution of anaerobic energy metabolism during the SR protocol. However, although the linear regression model was influenced by test sequence peak VO$_2$ (L·min^{-1}) could still be predicted accurately from the SR W$_{peak}$ and FEV$_1$ (L·min^{-1}).

38.4.1 Implications for clinical practice

Although in adolescents with CF, the SR protocol does not seem to be valid in measuring peak VO$_2$ directly, the SR W$_{peak}$ in combination with the FEV$_1$ (L·min^{-1}) might still be used as a feasible, less time consuming, inexpensive and acceptable alternative for the traditional exercise protocols in estimating peak VO$_2$. The implementation of this test in clinical practice might help to increase the use of exercise testing in this patient group.

38.5 REFERENCES

Barker, M., Hebestreit, A., Gruber, W. and Hebestreit, H., 2004, Exercise testing and training in German CF centers. *Pediatric Pulmonology*, **37**, pp. 351-355.

de Backer, I.C., Schep, G., Hoogeveen, A., Vreugdenhil, G., Kester, A.D. and van Breda, E., 2007, Exercise testing and training in a cancer rehabilitation program: The advantage of the steep ramp test. *Archives of Physical Medicine and Rehabilitation*, **88**, pp. 610-616.

Ferrazza, A.M., Martolini, D., Valli, G. and Palange, P., 2009, Cardiopulmonary exercise testing in the functional and prognostic evaluation of patients with pulmonary diseases. *Respiration*, **77**, pp. 3–17.

Godfrey, S., 1974, *Exercise Testing in Children*. (London: W.B. Saunders Company Ltd), 1-168.

Meyer, K., Samek, L., Schwaibold, M., Westbrook, S., Hajric, R., Lehmann, M., Essfeld, D. and Roskamm, H., 1996, Physical responses to different modes of interval exercise in patients with chronic heart failure – application to exercise training. *European Heart Journal*, **17**, pp. 1040–1047.

Midgley, A.W. and Carroll, S., 2009, Emergence of the verification phase procedure for confirming true VO_{2max}. *Scandinavian Journal of Medicine and Science in Sport*, **19**, pp. 313-322.

A NEW TREADMILL PROTOCOL FOR THE CLINICAL EVALUATION OF CHILDREN WITH CARDIAC DISEASE

R.J. Sabath, K.M. Teson, J.E. Hulse, M. Gelatt

Children's Mercy Hospitals and Clinics, Section of Cardiology, Kansas City, Missouri, USA

39.1 INTRODUCTION

Exercise testing is frequently used for evaluation of exercise capacity and cardiopulmonary function in children with congenital cardiac defects or acquired cardiac disease. An often-used protocol for treadmill testing is the Bruce protocol (Bruce *et al.*, 1973), which was originally designed for adults (van der Cammen-van Zjip *et al.*, 2010). Although exercise testing is widely used in children, there is no agreement in specific practice guidelines for paediatric exercise testing (Chang *et al.*, 2006).

One of the main advantages of the Bruce protocol is that it may be used for all age groups (Washington *et al.*, 1994). However, several investigators have revealed practical difficulties with the Bruce protocol. The problems with the Bruce protocol that we and others have identified include: large work increments between successive stages, steep inclines, long stage duration which may lead to patient boredom in younger patients and in highly fit patients who must exercise for 12 minutes before reaching running speeds (Houlsby, 1986; Rowland, 1993; Washington *et al.*, 1994).

The purpose of this study was to compare the peak exercise responses of patients undergoing treadmill testing on the Bruce protocol to patients evaluated on the CMH Max treadmill protocol that was designed to alleviate or minimize the problems described above.

39.2 METHODS

39.2.1 Experimental design

A retrospective analysis was performed on the data from a total of 785 consecutive exercise tests on pediatric cardiology patients who had undergone

265

treadmill testing to volitional exhaustion or until test termination criteria were observed (i.e. ST segment changes, abnormal blood pressures responses, significant arrhythmias, etc.) on either the Bruce or CMH Max treadmill protocol (Table 39.1). All subjects received strong verbal encouragement during their test. There were no patients eliminated from the analysis. Therefore the data contain patients with heart block and those on medications designed to reduce myocardial work rate. Each cohort contained patients with repaired and unrepaired congenital heart defects as well as patients with acquired cardiac disease.

Heart rate and rhythm were monitored continuously by 12 lead ECG using a Quinton Q-Stress ECG System (version 3.0; Cardiac Science, Bothell, WA, USA). Blood pressure was measured by auscultation at rest, during exercise, and in recovery. Oxygen saturation was monitored at rest, periodically during exercise, and in recovery by pulse oximetry using a Nellcor Oximax N-595 monitor (Tyco Healthcare, Pleasanton, CA, USA).

Table 39.1. Bruce and CMH Max Protocols. Speed (miles per hour/kilometres per hour) and Grade (%).

Bruce Protocol (3 min stages)				CMH Max Protocol (1 min stages)			
Stage	Speed	Grade	METS	Stage	Speed	Grade	METS
1	1.7/2.7	10	4.6	1-3	3.0/4.8	0	3.3
2	2.5/4.0	12	7.0	4	4.0/6.4	0	4.8
3	3.4/5.4	14	10.1	5	4.0/6.4	2.5	6.0
4	4.2/6.7	16	12.8	6	4.0/6.4	5.0	7.2
5	5.0/8.0	18	14.8	7	5.0/8.0	5.0	10.3
6	5.5/8.8	20	16.9	8	5.5/8.8	5.0	11.3
7	6.0/9.6	22	19.2	9	6.5/10.5	5.0	13.1
				10	7.0/11.3	5.0	14.1
				11	7.0/11.3	7.5	15.3
				12	7.5/12.1	7.5	16.3
				13	8.0/12.9	7.5	17.3
				14	8.5/13.7	7.5	18.3
				15	8.5/13.7	10.0	19.8

39.2.2 Statistical analysis

Group data and descriptive statistics were analyzed using two-tailed t-test (SPSS Statistics Version 17.0). Alpha level was set at $P \leq 0.05$.

39.3 RESULTS

The patients in the CMH Max cohort were significantly taller, heavier and older than those in the Bruce cohort (Table 39.2). There were also more males and fewer females in the CMH Max group compared to Bruce. On the primary outcome variables, the CMH Max cohort had significantly higher peak heart rates (no difference in resting heart rate), higher peak systolic and diastolic blood pressure, greater peak METs and shorter total treadmill time (Table 39.3).

Table 39.2. Demographic Data (*$P \leq 0.05$)

	Bruce (n=404)	CMH Max (n=381)
Age (y)	12.9 ± 4.0	13.5 ± 3.0*
Stature (cm)	154.4 ± 18.2	161.3 ± 16.1*
Body mass (kg)	51.4 ± 20.9	54.0 ± 18.3*
Gender	Male=257 (64 %)	Male=277 (73 %)
	Female=147 (36 %)	Female=104 (27 %)

Table 39.3. Exercise Data (*$P \leq 0.05$)

	Bruce	CMH Max	95% CI
Resting Heart Rate (b·min^{-1})	77.5 ± 14.2	75.6 ± 13.5	-3.811 to 0.090
Peak Heart Rate (b·min^{-1})	179.2 ± 18.3	186.8 ± 14.6*	5.267 to 9.900
Resting SBP (mmHg)	108.8 ± 15.0	112.5 ± 17.1*	1.449 to 5.957
Peak SBP (mmHg)	149.5 ± 24.2	159.0 ± 25.7*	5.936 to 12.958
Resting DBP (mmHg)	58.8 ± 9.8	63.1 ±11.5*	2.825 to 5.823
Peak DBP (mmHg)	59.1 ± 9.4	64.5 ± 10.8*	3.944 to 6.796
Exercise time (min)	10.72 ± 2.6	9.75 ± 2.1*	-1.272 to -0.589
METS Achieved	12.4 ± 2.4	13.2 ± 2.5*	0.453 to 1.156

39.4 CONCLUSION

Subjects performing the CMH Max protocol achieved higher peak exercise values for heart rate and METs than the Bruce patients, even though resting heart rates were quite similar between the groups. The observed differences in these parameters may be due to the design of the CMH Max protocol. In the CMH Max protocol, grades are much lower, the stage times are markedly shorter, and the speeds more reflective of how children walk and run than the Bruce protocol. However, it is possible that the observed differences in peak exercise parameters may be secondary to differences in age, height, and weight between the two cohorts. The CMH Max protocol resulted in a more even distribution of METs compared to the Bruce protocol (Figure 39.1). The marked, uneven increases in work rate in Bruce often resulted in test termination mid-stage and we postulate at lower levels of maximal exertion.

The CMH Max protocol produces peak cardiorespiratory parameters that are equal to or greater than the values observed for the Bruce protocol. The CMH Max protocol is a viable alternative to the Bruce protocol in the clinical evaluation of patients with cardiac disease.

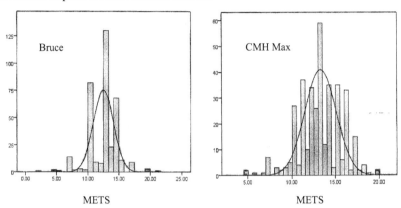

Figure 39.1. Peak METS achieved on Bruce and CMH Max

39.5 REFERENCES

Bruce, R.A., Kusumi, F. and Hosmer, D., 1973, Maximal oxygen intake and nomographic assessment of functional aerobic impairment in cardiovascular disease. *American Heart Journal*, **85**, pp. 546-562.

Chang, R., Gurvitz, M., Rodriguez, S., Hong, E. and Klitzner, T.S., 2006, Current practice of exercise stress testing among pediatric cardiology and pulmonology centers in the United States. *Pediatric Cardiology*, **27**, pp. 110-116.

Houlsby, W.T., 1986, Functional aerobic capacity and body size. *Archives of Disease in Childhood*, **61**, pp. 388-393.

Rowland, T.W., 1993, *Pediatric Laboratory Exercise Testing Clinical Guidelines*. (Champaign, IL: Human Kinetics), pp. 21-25.

van der Cammen-van Zijp, M.H.M., IJsselstijn, H., Takken, T., Willemsen, S.P., Tibboel, D., Stam, H.J., and van den Berg-Emons, R.J.G., 2010, Exercise testing of pre-school children using the Bruce treadmill protocol: New reference values. *European Journal of Applied Physiology*, **108**, pp. 393-399.

Washington, R.L., Bricker, J.T., Alpert, B.S., Daniels, S.R., Deckelbaum, R.J., Fisher, E.A., Gidding, S.S., Isabel-Jones, J., Kavey, R.E., and Marx, G.R., 1994, Guidelines for exercise testing in the pediatric age group. *Circulation Journal of the American Heart Association*, **90**, pp. 2166-2179.

INFLUENCE OF TWO SPRINT TRAINING PROGRAMMES ON FITNESS OF YOUNG SOCCER PLAYERS

Y. Meckel[1], Y. Gefen[1], D. Nemet[2], and A. Eliakim[1, 2]

[1]Zinman College of Physical Education and Sport Sciences, Wingate Institute, Israel; [2]Child Health and Sport Center, Meir Medical Center, Sackler School of Medicine, Tel-Aviv University, Israel

40.1 INTRODUCTION

During a soccer game, elite level players cover 8-13 km (Reilly and Thomas, 2003). The majority of the activity in the game is performed as low-intensity exercise such as walking, jogging or slow running. The sub-maximal nature of this activity predominantly uses aerobic energy sources. However, within this endurance context, numerous explosive bursts of activity are required, including sprinting, jumping, turning and tackling. Sprint-type activities account for about 8-12 % of the total distance covered in the game (Rampinini et al., 2007). The maximal nature of these activities stresses anaerobic energy sources of ATP-CP and glycolysis. Therefore, soccer training should enhance both aerobic and anaerobic abilities.

In modern soccer, the high frequency of matches during the competitive season limits the number of training sessions devoted to fitness development. Thus, it would be valuable to identify a single training method that could efficiently improve the player's aerobic and anaerobic abilities. Various studies have shown that sprint training consisting of high intensity short-term efforts of 5-30 s can improve anaerobic capabilities (Dawson et al., 1998; Burgomaster et al., 2005). Sprint training can also improve VO2max and aerobic enzyme activity (MacDougall et al., 1998; Rodas et al., 2000). Therefore, sprint or high-intensity interval training appears to be appropriate training to improve overall fitness requirements of soccer players. However, what is the most effective sprint training method for soccer players is still unclear. Thus, the aim of the present study was to determine the effect of all-out short sprint repetition training (SST) versus high-intensity long sprint repetition training (LST), matched for total distance, on aerobic and anaerobic fitness of young soccer players.

40.2 METHODS

40.2.1 Study design

Twenty-four 13-14 year old male soccer players completed two similar sets of fitness tests before and after 7 weeks of pre-season training. Following the pre-training tests, participants were matched for aerobic fitness and randomly assigned to one of two training groups (3 times·wk^{-1}): 1. all-out short sprint repetition training (SST); or 2. high-intensity long sprint repetition training (LST). Training for the SST group consisted of 4-6 sets of 4 x 50 m all-out sprints repetitions with 2 min rest between repetitions and 4 min rest between sets. Training for the LST group consisted of 4-6 x 200 m intervals at 85 % of max speed with 5 minutes rest between each run. Overall, the two groups performed similar training distances over the 7 weeks of training.

40.2.2 Testing procedures

Each set of tests, before and after training, consisted of the following: Standing long jump – Power test, 4 x 10 m run – Agility test, 30 m run – Speed test, 250 m run – Anaerobic endurance test, and 20 m shuttle run – Aerobic power test (Stolen *et al.,* 2005). Both set of tests were performed using the same procedures, at the same time of the day, under the same environmental conditions, and with the same technician, who was blinded to the training-group affiliation. Participants were familiar with the testing procedures since they had routinely performed them in previous years. Running times were recorded using a photoelectric cell timing system (Alge-Timing Electronic, Vienna, Austria).

40.2.3 Statistical analysis

A two-way repeated-measure ANOVA was used to compare fitness difference with time serving as the within group and training as the between group factor. Data are presented as mean ± SD. Significance level was set at $P<0.05$.

40.3 RESULTS

There were no baseline differences in predicted VO_2 max prior to training between the groups. Both training programmes led to a significant improvement in VO_2 max ($P<0.01$), with no between group difference ($P=0.14$; Table 40.1, Figure 40.1). There were no baseline anaerobic fitness differences, prior to training, between the groups. Both training programs led to a significant improvement in 30 m sprint time ($P<0.01$), 4 x 10 m shuttle running time ($P<0.01$) and 250 m running time ($P<0.01$), but had no significant effect on standing long jump ($P=0.21$).

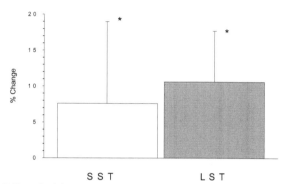

Figure 40.1. Effect of training programme on predicted VO_2 max percent changes (*$P<0.01$ for within group changes).

Table 40.1. The effect of different training programs on selected aerobic and anaerobic performances.

	Short Sprint Training (SST, n=11))		Long Sprint Training (LST, n=13)	
	Pre	Post	Pre	Post
VO_2max ($mL \cdot kg^{-1} \cdot min^{-1}$)	44.6±5.3	47.5±3.7*	44.9±5.2	49.5±5.4*
250 m run (s)	39.82±2.17	38.40±2.27*	38.58±2.48	37.51±2.52*
30 m run (s)	4.86±0.19	4.74±0.20*	4.82±0.23	4.74±0.22*
4x10 m run (s)	9.83±0.23	9.55±0.33*	9.69±0.34	9.59±0.36*
Standing long jump (m)	2.13±0.13	2.16±0.17	2.10±0.18	2.15±0.16

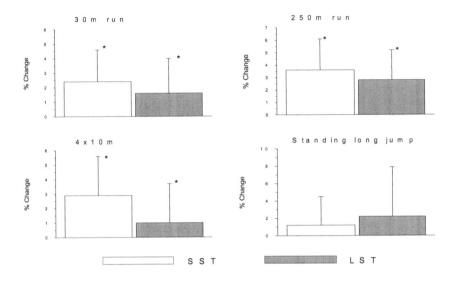

Figure 40.2. The effect of training programme on percent changes of selected anaerobic performance variables (*P<0.01 for within group changes).

40.4 DISCUSSION

The study showed that long, near maximal, sprints and short, all-out sprint training, matched for total distance, are equally effective in enhancing aerobic and anaerobic fitness characteristics of young soccer players. Moreover, both training programs used in the study did not negatively influence either aerobic or anaerobic performance. Therefore, although a combined aerobic/anaerobic training program may be recommended during the pre-season period, it is possible that during the competitive seasons, when frequency of matches and activity load is high, and the number of fitness sessions is limited, a short sprint training regimen may be an additional efficient training strategy to improve aerobic and anaerobic fitness characteristics of young soccer players.

40.5 REFERENCES

Burgomaster, K.A., Hughes, S.C., Heigenhauser, G.J., Bradwell, S.N. and Gibala, M.J., 2005, Six session of sprint interval training increases muscle oxidative potential and cycle endurance capacity in humans. *Journal of Applied Physiology*, **98**, pp. 1985-1990.

Dawson, B., Fitzsimons, M., Green, S., Goodman, C., Carey, M. and Cole, K., 1998, Changes in performance, muscle metabolites, enzyme and fiber types after short sprint training. *European Journal of Applied Physiology*, **78**, pp. 163-169.

MacDougall, J.D., Hicks, A.L., MacDonald, J.R., McKelvie, R.S., Green, H.J. and Smith K.M., 1998, Muscle performance and enzymatic adaptations to sprint interval training. *Journal of Applied Physiology*, **84**, pp. 2138-2142.

Rampinini, E., Coutts, A.J., Costagna, C., Sassi, R. and Impellizzeri, F.M., 2007, Variation in top level soccer match performance. *International Journal of Sports Medicine*, **28**, pp. 1018-1024.

Reilly, T. and Thomas, V., 2003, Motion analysis and physiological demands. In *Science and Soccer*, edited by Reilly, T. and Williams A.M., (Routledge, London), pp. 59-72.

Rodas, G., Ventura, J.L., Cadefau, J.A., Cusso, R. and Parra, J., 2000, A short training program for the rapid improvement of both aerobic and anaerobic metabolism. *European Journal of Applied Physiology*, **82**, pp. 480-486.

Stolen, T., Chamari, K., Castagna, C., and Wisloff, U., 2005, Physiology of soccer. *Sports Medicine*, **35**, pp. 501-536.

WEIGHT RESISTANCE FOR A CYCLE ERGOMETER WINGATE TEST PERFORMED BY DIFFERENT MATURATIONAL GROUPS OF MALE SWIMMERS

P. Duarte, R.J. Fernandes, and S. Soares

CIFI2D, Faculty of Sport, University of Porto, Portugal

41.1 INTRODUCTION

The athletes' performance evaluation and the training control are important tasks for coaches, allowing the accurate definition of the training loads and the reorganization of the training process (Bampouras and Marrin, 2009). Several performance components are evaluated on a training control programme, one of which refers to the expended energy that comes predominantly from the anaerobic system. Accordingly to Wilmore and Costill (1999), when the effort leads to exhaustion, the anaerobic system has a total time capacity of 90 s. Nevertheless, other authors suggest that this same total time capacity varies from 60 to 120 s (Gastin, 2001; Guyton and Hall, 2002).

In competitive swimming, the 50–200 m events are efforts that have an apparent anaerobic predominance (Bar-Or, 1987; Bar-Or *et al.*, 1994; Trappe, 1996; Troup, 1999). As those competitive distances are the majority of the World and Olympic events, the evaluation of anaerobic potential is crucial in swimming evaluation and training control. To assess this physical capacity the literature suggests several tests whose main purpose is to evaluate the capacity of a muscle or muscles to support a supramaximal effort. The time effort of these tests varies from 15 to 120 s: short durations are used to evaluate the power of the anaerobic system, and long durations intend to evaluate the system capacity. Within those tests, the most popular are the vertical jump (Sands *et al.*, 2004), the Margaria step test (Salonia *et al.*, 2004), the running tests (i.e. the yo-yo Intermittent Recovery Test, Atkins, 2006), and the Wingate Test (Bar-Or, 1987).

The Wingate Test is probably the most used in the diagnosis of anaerobic potential (Inbar and Bar-Or, 1986), gaining acceptance for its use comparatively with other tests, but is not a specific test for swimmers. When conducting a Wingate Test with a mechanically-breaked ergometer, it is important to precisely define the resistance applied to the ergometer (Dotan and Bar-Or, 1983; Dore *et al.,* 2001). Specifically, too high or too low a resistance will result in the underestimation of an athlete's anaerobic potential. The resistance that is usually applied in the literature is 0.075 $g \cdot kg^{-1}$ of body mass, and but this may not be optimal for trained subjects. Reference values for swimmers are currently unknown.

The present study aimed to verify the accuracy of an n x 10 s maximal Wingate cycle ergometer pedal test to determine the optimal load resistance (expressed as a percentage of body mass), to apply to different maturational groups of male swimmers.

41.2 METHODS

The study protocol consisted of a pre-test of n x 10 s maximal cycle ergometer test (*Monark*^{TM}, Sports Medicine Industries, Minnesota, USA), applied to 8 pre-pubertal, 10 pubertal and 7 post-pubertal male swimmers. The first 10 s bout was performed against a resistance load of 0.075 $g \cdot kg^{-1}$ of body mass. The following bouts were randomly added and subtracted in 0.005 $g \cdot kg^{-1}$ of body mass. A minimum rest interval of 15 min was completed between bouts. The tests stopped when the resistance able to produce the maximal value of power output was reached. This procedure allowed for the determination of the individual weight resistance theoretically able to induce the highest maximal power value in the 30 s Wingate Test (optimal load). After a minimum 24 h rest, a 30 s Wingate Test was performed using the optimal load determined in the pre-test. Two other 30 s Wingate Tests were then performed, adding and subtracting 0.005 $g \cdot kg^{-1}$ of body mass to the optimal load. A rest interval of 30 min was accomplished between bouts. The procedures relative to the Wingate Test followed the protocol usually described in literature (Bar-Or, 1987). Statistical procedures consisted in ANOVA test ($P \leq 0.05$).

41.3 RESULTS

In Figure 41.1 it is possible to observe that the prepubertal swimmers individual optimal load values determined in the n x 10 s maximal pedal rate to attain maximal power values varied between 0.095 and 0.105 $g \cdot kg^{-1}$ of body mass. Mean optimal load values were 10.39 ± 0.33 $g \cdot kg^{-1}$. Pubertal swimmers optimal values varied between 0.085 and 0.105 $g \cdot kg^{-1}$ of body mass, with a mean optimal load value of 8.79 ± 0.57 $g \cdot kg^{-1}$. Postpubertal swimmers minimum and maximum optimal load values were 0.085 and 0.10 $g \cdot kg^{-1}$ of body mass. Mean optimal load value was 9.67 ± 0.52 kg. Mean load values were higher for pre-pubertal swimmers. No differences were found between mean load values of pubertal and postpubertal swimmers.

a)

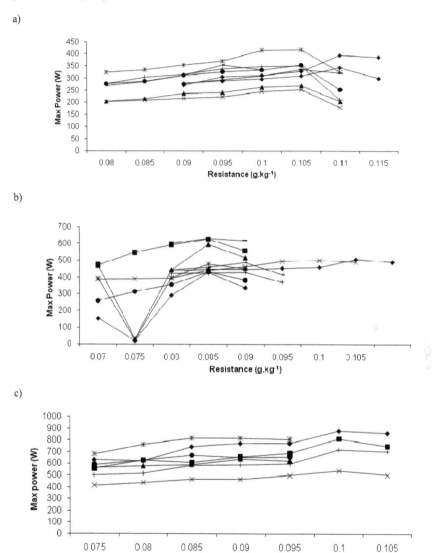

Figure 41.1. Maximal power values attained in n x 10s maximal pedal pre-test by a) pre-pubertal, b) pubertal, and c) postpubertal male swimmers.

Figure 41.2 is representative of maximal power (Pmax) values attained by pubertal and postpubertal swimmers in the Wingate Test, when the optimal load was applied as it was determined in the n x 10 s test and added and subtracted 0.005 g·kg^{-1}. As it can be observed, Pmax values showed a bell shape variation with the resistance load. When optimal load was added and subtracted 0.005 g·kg^{-1}, Pmax values were lower than those obtained with the pre-determined optimal load. Prepubertal swimmers values were not plotted once a large number (5 in 8) of swimmers did not reach the end of the Wingate Test when predetermined optimal load was used as it was calculated, and/or added an subtracted 0.005 g·kg^{-1}.

a)
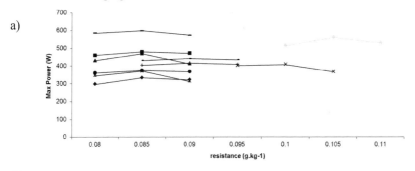

b)
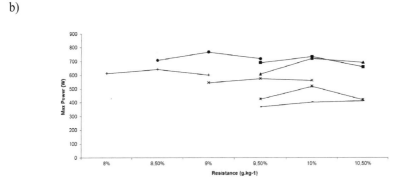

Figure 41.2. Pmax values attained by a) pubertal and b) postpubertal male swimmers in Wingate Test, when the optimal load was applied as it was determined in n x 10s test and added and subtracted 0.005 g·kg^{-1}.

Results of the n x 10 s pre-test found that the ideal resistance that should be applied in 30 s Wingate Tests performed by different maturational groups of swimmers is higher than the usual 0.075 g·kg^{-1}, proposed by Bar-Or (1996). The test seems to be accurate to determine optimal resistance load for pubertal and postpubertal male swimmers. When the optimal load was used in the Wingate Test as determined in the n x 10 s test and added and subtracted 0.005 g·kg^{-1}, an expected bell shape curve was found for Pmax plotted against the three tested loads. The same conclusion could not be applied to prepubertal swimmers, once, when optimal load was applied, a large number of swimmers (5 in 8) did not finish the 30s Wingate Test. This could probably be due to poor cycle ergometer ergonomic characteristics for children.

41.4 CONCLUSION

In conclusion, the proposed pre-test of n x 10 s maximal cycle ergometer test seems not to be accurate to determine the optimal resistance load to apply in the 30 s Wingate Test performed by prepubertal male swimmers, even though the same pre-test was shown to be accurate for pubertal and adult swimmers.

41.5 REFERENCES

Atkins, S.J., 2006, Performance of the Yo-Yo Intermittent Recovery Test by Elite Professional and Semiprofessional Rugby League Players. *Journal of Strength and Conditioning Research*, **20**, pp. 222-225.

Bampouras, T.M. and Marrin, K., 2009, Comparison of two anaerobic water polo-specific tests with the Wingate test. *Journal of Strength Conditioning Research*, **23**, pp. 336-340.

Bar-Or, O., 1987, The Wingate anaerobic test. An update on methodology, reliability and validity. *Sports Medicine*, **4**, pp. 381-394.

Bar-Or, O., 1996, Anaerobic performance. *Measurement in Pediatric Exercise Science*, edited by Docherty, D. (Windsor, Canada: Human Kinetics) pp. 161-182.

Bar-Or, O., Unnithan, V. and Illescas, C., 1994, Physiologic considerations in age-group swimming. *Medicine and Science in Aquatic Sports* edited by Myashita, M., Matoh, Y., Richardson, A.B.(Basel: Karger), pp.199-205.

Dore, E., Bedu, M., Franca, N.M. and Van Praagh, E., 2001, Anaerobic cycling performance characteristics in prepubescent, adolescent and young adult females. *European Journal of Applied Physiology*, **84**, pp. 476-481.

Dotan, R. and Bar-Or, O., 1983, Load optimization for the Wingate Anaerobic Test. *European Journal of Applied Physiology*, **51**, pp. 409-417.

Gastin, P.B., 2001, Energy system interaction and relative contribution during maximal exercise. *Sports Medicine*, **31**, pp. 725-741.

Guyton, A.C. and Hall, J.H., 2002, *Tratado de fisiologia médica*. (Rio de Janeiro: Editora Gunabara S.A.)

Inbar, O. and O. Bar-Or 1986, Anaerobic characteristics in male children and adolescents. *Medicine and Science in Sports and Exercise*, **18**, 264-269.

Salonia, M.A., Chu, D.A., Cheifetz, P.M. and Freidhoff, G.C., 2004, Upper-body power as measured by medicine-ball throw distance and its relationship to class level among 10- and 11-year-old female participants in club gymnastics. *Journal of Strength and Conditioning Research*, **18**, pp. 695-702.

Sands, W.A., McNeal, J. R., Ochi, M.T., Urbanek, T.L., Jemni, M. and Stone, M.H., 2004, Comparison of the Wingate and Bosco anaerobic tests. *Journal of Strength and Conditioning Research*, **18**, pp. 810-815.

Trappe, S.W., 1996, Metabolic demands for swimming. In *Biomechanics and Medicine in Swimming - Swimming Science VII*, edited by troup, J.P., Hollander, D., Strasse, S.W., Trappe, J.M., Cappaert, J.M., Trappe, T.A. (London: E and FN Spon), pp.127-134.

Troup, J.P., 1999, The physiology and biomechanics of competitive swimming. *Clinical Sports Medicine*, **18**, pp. 267-285.

Wilmore, J.H. and Costill, D.L., 1999, *Physiology of Sport and Exercise.* (Champaign, IL: Human Kinetics).

EXPLOSIVE LEG POWER AND BODY COMPOSITION IN 11–17-YEAR-OLD BOYS

A. Emeljanovas [1], R. Rutkauskaite[1], V. Volbekiene[1], R. Gruodyte[1,2]

[1]Lithuanian Academy of Physical Education, [2]University of Saskatchewan

42.1 INTRODUCTION

Explosive power and body composition are important components of health-related physical fitness, reflecting the health status of children and adolescents (Ortega *et al.*, 2008a,b; Hands *et al.*, 2009). Poor muscular and physical fitness in childhood has detrimental effects on a person's health in adulthood (Ruiz *et al.*, 2008). Numerous studies indicate that the physical fitness of children and adolescents is decreasing (Westerstahl *et al.*, 2003; Wedderkopp *et al.*, 2004; Volbekiene and Griciute, 2007). Physical fitness is not only a significant indicator of health (Ruiz *et al.*, 2006), but an essential factor, that must be taken into account when developing the policy of public health (Ortega *et al.*, 2008c).

Several studies have determined the interrelations between the components of body composition and physical fitness (including explosive power) in children and adolescents. Mak *et al.* (2010) have found significant relationships between body mass index (BMI) and some physical fitness components in 12-18-year-old boys from Hong Kong. Significant inverse relationships between fat mass and explosive power in adolescent Spanish boys were reported by Moliner-Urdiales *et al.* (2011). Furthermore, Houwen *et al.* (2010) ascertained significant inverse relationships between body mass, fat mass and explosive power in 6-12-year-old children from the Netherlands. However, these relationships were not investigated in regard to age, i.e. it is not clear whether the same relationships exist in different periods of age. According to Moliner-Urdiales *et al.* (2010), further studies are necessary to shed light on the relationships between muscular strength components and lean body mass in young people. We suggest that other components of body composition and their relationships with physical fitness in adolescents are also of interest to be investigated. The aim of this study was to examine the relationships between explosive power and body composition in 11-17-year-old boys.

42.2 METHODS

42.2.1 Experimental design and participants

In total, 430 schoolboys 11-17 years of age who fulfilled all requirements of the study (e.g. voluntarily agreed to take part in the tests; their parents or legal guardians gave written informed consent) provided all necessary data for performed vertical jump test and body components analysis were selected for the statistical analysis. Participants were randomly selected from secondary schools of Lithuania (11-year-old, n=64; 12-year-old, n=58; 13-year-old, n=67; 14-year-old, n=63; 15-year-old, n=68; 16-year-old, n=70; 17-year-old, n=40). The research was carried out under the bilateral agreements between the Lithuanian Academy of Physical Education and secondary schools.

Explosive leg power was measured by performing a maximal vertical jump (cm) on a Kistler forceplate. Body mass (kg), BMI ($kg \cdot m^{-2}$), body fat (%) and lean body mass (kg) were registered using bioelectrical impedance analysis (Tanita BC–418MA, Tanita Corporation, Tokyo, Japan). The tests were conducted by a specially trained team of qualified testers.

Statistical analysis was performed with *MS Excel* and *SPSS (16.0 version)* programmes. Means and standard deviations were determined. A one-way analysis of variance (ANOVA) and Tukey *post hoc* tests were used to compare the differences between age groups. Pearson's product moment correlation was used to examine relationships between explosive power results and body composition components. Stepwise multiple regression analysis was performed to determine the independent effect of the different anthropometric and body composition parameters to the explosive leg power. Statistical significance was set at $P < 0.05$.

42.3 RESULTS

The dynamics of vertical jump results of 11-17-year-old boys showed that with age the jumping height increases consistently from 28.2 ($\pm$ 5.1) cm in the group of 11 year-olds to 41 ($\pm$ 7.1) cm in the group of 17 year-olds ($P<0.05$) (Figure 42.1).

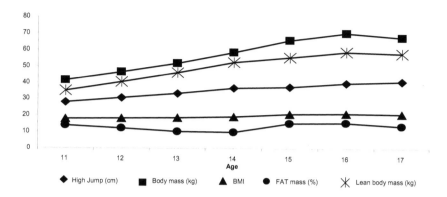

Figure 42.1. Explosive power and body composition of 11-17-year-old boys (n=430).

Body mass and BMI increased from 41.4 (± 12.4) kg to 70.4 (± 12.4) kg and 18.0 (± 3.6) kg·m^{-2} to 21.5 (± 3.1) kg·m^{-2} in 11 vs. 16-year-olds, respectively ($P<0.05$). Similar tendency was revealed in the lean body mass results, but the differences were not significant when comparing the different age groups ($P>0.05$). The dynamics of body fat increase were inconsistent. Significant inverse correlations of explosive leg power were found with: (a) body mass, BMI and body fat in 11 and 16-year-olds (r=-0.39–0.61; P<0.01); (b) BMI and body fat in 12-year-olds (r=-0.34–0.57; $P<0.01$); (c) body fat in 13 and 15-year-olds (r=-0.27–0.33; $P<0.05$). Lean body mass correlated with explosive leg power negatively in 11-year-old boys (r=-0.43; $P<0.01$) and positively in 14-year-olds (r=0.29; $P<0.05$). There were no significant correlations between explosive leg power and body composition components in the 17-year-old boys' group (Table 42.1).

Table 42.1. Relationships between explosive power and body composition components in 11-17-year-old boys (n=430).*$P<0.05$; **$P<0.01$.

Age (year)	N	Body mass (kg)	BMI (kg·m^{-2})	Body fat (%)	Lean body mass (kg)
11	64	−0.50**	−0.55**	−0.61**	−0.43**
12	58	−0.14	−0.34**	−0.57**	0.07
13	67	0.05	−0.18	−0.33**	0.14
14	63	0.11	0.01	−0.02	0.29*
15	68	−0.11	−0.15	−0.27*	0.01
16	70	−0.39**	−0.42**	−0.54**	−0.22
17	40	0.02	−0.05	−0.29	0.19
Total group	430	0.28**	0.38	−0.24**	0.42**

According to the correlational analysis, the relationships between explosive leg power and different components of body composition in boys were most pronounced at the ages of 11 and 16 years. The most frequent and strongest relationships of explosive leg power were with body fat (%). Stepwise multiple regression analysis indicated that age alone explained 31.9 % (r^2 x 100) of the total variance of jumping height (i.e. explosive leg power) in 11–17-year-old boys. Age and fat mass (%) together increased this influence to 42.7 % (r^2 x 100), while age, fat mass (%) and lean body mass together explained 44.4 % (r^2 x 100) of the total variance of jumping height in a studied population.

42.4 CONCLUSION

We suggest that 11 and 16 years of age are the periods when the relationships between explosive leg power and body composition in boys are most expressed. Age, fat mass (%) and lean body mass together explained 44.4 % (r^2 x 100) of the total variance of the explosive leg power in boys aged 11–17 years.

42.5 REFERENCES

Hands, B., Larkin, D., Parker, H., Straker, L. and Perry, M., 2009, The relationship among physical activity, motor competence and health-related fitness in 14-year-old adolescents. *Scandinavian Journal of Medicine and Science in Sports*, **19**, pp. 655–663.

Houwen, S., Hartman, E. and Visscher, C., 2010, The relationship among motor proficiency, physical fitness, and body composition in children with and without visual impairments. *Research Quarterly for Exercise and Sport*, **81**, pp. 290–299.

Mak, K.K., Ho, S.Y., Lo, W.S., Thomas, G.N., McManus, A.M., Day, J.R. and Lam, T.H., 2010, Health–related physical fitness and weight status in Hong Kong adolescents. *BMC Public Health*, **10**, pp. 88.

Moliner-Urdiales, D., Ortega F.B., Vincente-Rodriguez, G., Rey-Lopez, J.P, Gracia-Marco, L., Widhalm, K., Sjöström, M., Moreno, L.A., Castillo, M.J. and Ruiz, J.R., 2010, Association of physical activity with muscular strength and fat–free mass in adolescents: The HELENA Study. *European Journal of Applied Physiology*, **109**, pp. 1119–1127.

Moliner-Urdiales, D., Ruiz, J.R., Vicente-Rodriguez, G., Ortega, F.B., Rey-Lopez, J.P., España-Romero, V., Casajús, J.A., Molnar, D., Widhalm, K., Dallongeville, J., González-Gross, M., Castillo, M.J., Sjöström, M. and Moreno, L.A., 2011, Associations of muscular and cardiorespiratory fitness with total and central body fat in adolescents: The HELENA Study. *British Journal of Sports Medicine*, **45**, pp. 101–108.

Ortega, F.B., Artero, E.G., Ruiz, J.R., Vicente-Rodriguez, G., Bergman, P., Hagströmer, M., Ottevaere, C., Nagy, E., Konsta, O., Rey-López, J.P., Polito, A., Dietrich, S., Plada, M., Béghin, L., Manios, Y., Sjöström, M. and Castillo, M.J. 2008a, Reliability of health-related physical fitness tests in European adolescents. The HELENA Study. *International Journal of Obesity*, **32**, pp. 49–57.

Ortega, F.B., Ruiz, J.R., Castillo, M.J., Moreno, L.A. Urzanqui, A., González-Gross, M., Sjöström, M., Gutiérrez, A., 2008b, Health-related physical fitness according to chronological and biological age in adolescents. The AVENA Study. *Journal of Sports Medicine and Physical Fitness*, **48**, pp. 371–379.

Ortega, F.B., Ruiz, J.R., Castillo, M.J. and Sjöström, M., 2008c, Physical fitness in childhood and adolescence: A powerful marker of health. *International Journal of Obesity*, **32**, pp. 1–11.

Ruiz, J.R., Ortega, F.B. Gutierrez, A., Meusel, D., Sjöström, M. and Castillo, M.J., 2006, Health-related fitness assessment in childhood and adolescence: A European approach based on the AVENA, EYHS and HELENA studies. *Journal of Public Health*, **14**, pp. 269–277.

Ruiz, J.R., Sui, X., Lobelo, F., Morrow, J.R., Jackson, A.W., Sjostrom M. and Blair, S.N., 2008, Association between muscular strength and mortality in men: Prospective cohort study. *British Medical Journal*, **7661**, pp. 92–95.

Volbekiene, V. and Griciute, A., 2007, Health-related physical fitness among schoolchildren in Lithuania: A comparison from 1992 to 2002. *Scandinavian Journal of Public Health*, **35**, pp. 235–242.

Wedderkopp, N., Froberg, K., Hansen, H.S. and Andersen, L.B., 2004, Secular trends in physical fitness and obesity in Danish 9-year-old girls and boys: Odense School Child Study and Danish substudy of the European Youth Heart Study. *Scandinavian Journal of Medicine and Science in Sports*, **14**, pp. 150–155.

Westerstahl, M., Barnekow–Bergkvist, M., Hedberg, G. and Jansson, E., 2003, Secular trends in body dimensions and physical fitness among adolescents in Sweden from 1974 to 1995. *Scandinavian Journal of Medicine and Science in Sports*, **13**, pp. 128–137.

Part VII

Young Athlete and Sports Participation

TRAINING REDUCES CATABOLIC AND INFLAMMATORY RESPONSE TO A SINGLE PRACTICE BOUT IN FEMALE VOLLEYBALL PLAYERS

A. Eliakim[1], S. Portal[2], Z. Zadik[2], Y. Meckel[3],
and D. Nemet[1]

[1]Pediatric Department, Child Health and Sport Center, Meir Medical Center, Sackler School of Medicine, Tel-Aviv University, Tel-Aviv, Israel. [2]School of Nutritional Sciences, Hebrew University of Jerusalem, Jerusalem, Israel. [3]Zinman College of Physical Education and Sport Sciences at the Wingate Institute, Netanya, Israel

43.1 INTRODUCTION

In recent years, exercise-induced changes in the anabolic-catabolic hormonal balance and circulating inflammatory cytokines are used frequently by adolescent athletes and their coaches to optimize training (Eliakim and Nemet, 2010). One of the unique features of exercise is that it often leads to simultaneous increase of antagonistic mediators. On one hand, exercise stimulates anabolic components of the growth hormone (GH) → IGF-I (insulin-like growth factor-I) axis. On the other hand, exercise elevates catabolic pro-inflammatory cytokines such as Interlukin-6 (IL-6), IL-1 and tumor necrosis factor-α (Nemet and Eliakim, 2010). The very fine balance between the anabolic and inflammatory/catabolic response to exercise will dictate training effectiveness and the health implications of exercise. If the anabolic response dominates, exercise will probably lead ultimately to increased muscle mass and improved fitness. In contrast, if a greater catabolic response persists for a long duration and/or is combined with inadequate nutrition, this may lead to overtraining.

While the hormonal response to a single exercise bout has been previously determined, the effect of prolonged training on the response to a single exercise bout in adolescent athletes has not been studied. This is important because studies on the effect of fitness on hormonal responses to exercise yielded conflicting results (Eliakim and Nemet, 2008), and this has important implications for training of the young athlete. Moreover, these measurements are particularly important in adolescent athletes since puberty is characterized by rapid linear and muscle mass growth, and by spontaneous spurt of anabolic hormones. Therefore, the aim of the present study was to examine the effect of training on hormonal and inflammatory response to a single volleyball practice in elite female adolescent players.

43.2 METHODS

43.2.1 Participants

Thirteen healthy, female, elite, national team level, Israeli junior volleyball players (age 16.0 ± 1.4 y, Tanner stage for pubic hair 4-5) participated in the study. All participants were members of the Israeli national junior volleyball team.

43.2.2 Training regimen

The study was performed during the first 7 weeks of the volleyball season. Participants trained 18-22 hours per week. Training involved tactical and technical drills emphasizing volleyball skills and team strategies (~20 % of the time), power and speed drills with and without the ball (~25 % of the time), and interval sessions (~25 % of the time). About 15 % of the time consisted of endurance-type training (i.e. long-distance running). The additional 15 % of the time consisted of resistance training using mainly circuit training with free weights at 65-75 % of 1RM.

43.2.3 Anthropometric measurements and fitness assessment

Standard, calibrated scales and stadiometers were used to determine stature, body mass, and BMI. Fat percentage was calculated from skinfolds measurements. Fitness assessment, included anaerobic (vertical jump and the Wingate Anaerobic Test) and aerobic measures (VO_2 max predicted from the 20 m shuttle-run).

43.2.4 Exercise practice

The practice consisted of 20 minutes dynamic warm-up which included jogging, stretching and running drills at sub-maximal speed (up to 80 % of maximal speed), and additional 20 minutes of volleyball drills. The main part of the practice included seven repetitions of seven consecutive sprints from the back of the volleyball court to the net, maximal jump and a hit of the volleyball over the net in the end of each sprint. Each repetition lasted about 1.5 minutes with 1 minute rest to collect the balls between repetitions.

43.2.5 Blood sampling and analysis

Venous blood samples were collected, using an indwelling catheter, before and immediately after the 60 min volleyball practice, before and after 7 weeks of training. Measurements included the anabolic hormones GH, IGF-I, IGF binding protein-3 and testosterone, the catabolic hormone cortisol, the pro-inflammatory marker IL-6, and the anti-inflammatory marker IL-1 receptor antagonist, using commercially available kits.

43.2.6 Statistical analysis

A two-way repeated measure ANOVA (with Bonferroni post hoc test) was used to compare the effect of training on exercise practice associated changes. Statistical significance was set at $P<0.05$. Data are presented as mean (SD).

43.3 RESULTS

Training led to significant improvement of vertical jump, anaerobic properties and predicted VO_2max (Table 43.1). Volleyball practice, both before and after the training intervention, was associated with a significant increase of serum lactate, GH and IL-6 levels. The cortisol and the IL-6 response to the same relative intensity volleyball practice were significantly reduced at the end compared to before the training intervention (Table 43.2, Figure 43.1).

Table 43.1. Anthropometric and fitness characteristics of the participants.

	Pre training	Post training
Stature (cm)	175.6±6.3	175.9±6.1*
Body mass (kg)	64.1±6.5	65.7±6.3*
BMI (kg·m⁻²)	20.8±2.2	21.3±2.1*
Fat (%)	24.2±3.3	23.4±3.0*
VO₂ max (mL·kg⁻¹·min⁻¹)	38.2±3.2	40.1±3.7*
Anaerobic peak power (W·kg⁻¹)	11.4±0.7	12.4±0.7*
Anaerobic mean power (W·kg⁻¹)	7.9±0.6	8.6±0.8*
Vertical jump (m)	2.75±0.10	2.78±0.09*

(*$P<0.05$)

Table 43.2. Training effect on hormonal and inflammatory response to a single volleyball practice.

	Pre Training		Post Training	
	Pre practice	Post practice	Pre practice	Post practice
GH (ng·mL^{-1})	1.8±1.9	6.4±3.4*	1.5±2.1	4.8±2.7*
IGF-I (ng·mL^{-1})	519.8±89.1	537.8±63.9	493.7±81.2	507.5±65.6
IGFBP-3 (ng·mL^{-1})	6121.6±950.1	6268.8±772.5	5816.1±626.4	6015.4±844.0
Testosterone (ng·mL^{-1})	2.4±2.4	3.3±3.3	2.7±2.3	2.2±2.5
Cortisol (mcg·L^{-1})	28.4±9.8	32.6±17.5	30.9±9.8	26.5±15.0†
IL-6 (pg·mL^{-1})	1.2±0.5	2.5±1.1*	1.5±2.1	1.9±2.2*†
IL1ra (pg·mL^{-1})	360.8±112.5	381.0±146.2	310.6±93.2	328.5±119.2
Lactate (nmol·L^{-1})	3.0±0.9	5.7±1.7*	3.0±0.9	5.5±0.7*

* $P<0.05$ pre vs post practice; † $P<0.05$ pre vs post training

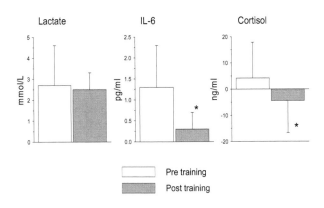

Figure 43.1. Effect of training on serum lactate, cortisol and IL-6 response to a single volleyball practice.

43.4 DISCUSSION

Training during the initial phases of the volleyball training season was associated with significant improvements in both anaerobic and aerobic properties. As previously described (Eliakim *et al.*, 2009), prior to the training intervention, a single, typical volleyball practice was associated with a significant increase of the anabolic hormone GH and the pro-inflammatory marker IL-6. Changes in GH may indicate exercise-related anabolic adaptations, and the IL-6 increase may indicate its important role in micro-traumatic muscle damage repair following volleyball training. The main contribution of the present study is that following 7 weeks of training during the initial phases of the volleyball season, we found a significantly reduced cortisol and IL-6 in response to the same relative intensity volleyball practice. Overall, this suggests that in addition to the training-related effect on improved anaerobic and aerobic properties, part of the training adaptation includes a reduced catabolic and inflammatory response to exercise. Changes in anabolic-catabolic balance and inflammatory cytokines can be used by athletes and coaches to determine training intensity in team sports like volleyball.

43.5 REFERENCES

Eliakim, A. and Nemet, D., 2008, Exercise provocation test for growth hormone secretion. *Pediatric Exercise Science*, **20**, pp. 370-378.

Eliakim, A. and Nemet, D., 2010, Exercise training, physical fitness and the growth hormone-insulin-like growth factor-I axis and cytokine balance. *Medicine and Sport Science*, **55**, pp. 128-140.

Eliakim, A., Portal, S., Zadik, Z., Rabinowitz, J., Adler-Portal, D., Cooper, D.M., Zaldivar, F. and Nemet, D., 2009, The effect of volleyball training on anabolic hormones and inflammatory markers in elite male and female adolescent players. *Journal of Strength and Conditioning Research*, **23**, pp. 1553-1559.

Nemet, D. and Eliakim, A., 2010, Growth hormone-insulin-like growth factor-I and inflammatory response to single exercise bout in children and adolescents. *Medicine and Sport Science*, **55**, pp. 141-155.

SHORT- AND LONG-TERM MAXIMAL PROTOCOLS AND THEIR CONTRIBUTION TO DIFFERENTIATE UNDER-17 HOCKEY PLAYERS BY COMPETITIVE LEVEL

J. Valente-dos-Santos[1], V. Vaz[1], A. Santos[1], A.J. Figueiredo[1],
M.T. Elferink-Gemser[2], R.M. Malina[3-4], and M.J. Coelho-e-Silva[1]

[1]University of Coimbra, Portugal, [2]University of Groningen, The Netherlands,
[3]University of Texas at Austin, TX, [4]Tarleton State University, Stephenville,
USA

44.1 INTODUCTION

Roller hockey was on the schedule of the 1992 Barcelona Olympic Games, but was not included in subsequent venues. Nevertheless, the popularity of the sport continues to grow in Europe in the form of U-20 and U-17 leagues. Research devoted to roller hockey in general and specifically among youth is scarce in the literature. Ice hockey and field hockey, in contrast, are reasonably well represented. For example, relationships among birth date, selection and competitive level were considered in adolescent ice hockey players (Sherar *et al.*, 2007). Other studies of youth ice hockey players tend to focus on functional parameters, e.g., validation of a skating protocol to predict aerobic power in players 9-25 years (Petrella *et al.*, 2007), validity and reliability of a maximal multistage shuttle run on-ice skate test (Leone *et al.*, 2007). Given the lack of information on youth roller hockey players, this study profiles the body size and performance characteristics of U-17 Portuguese male youth roller hockey players.

44.2 METHODS

44.2.1 Sample, training information and anthropometry

The sample comprised 73 adolescent hockey players, 14.5-16.5 years of age who were classified as juveniles (U-17) in the structure of Portuguese youth hockey. They were classified as club or elite based on whether or not they were selected for the national team. National team players (n=32) competed with their respective clubs during the season and were included in the group from which the Portuguese selection in 2007 and 2008 was chosen. The remainder (n=41) competed only at the club level with their respective teams and were labeled as local. All players participated in regular training sessions (2-5 sessions; ~180-510 min.week^{-1}) with their clubs and typically played one game per week. Stature was measured to the nearest 0.1 cm with a Harpenden stadiometer (model 98.603, Holtain Ltd, Crosswell, UK). Body mass was measured to the nearest 0.1 kg with a SECA balance (model 770, Hanover, MD, USA). Intra-observer technical errors of measurement for stature (0.27 cm) and mass (0.47 kg) were well within the range of intra- and inter-observer errors in several surveys in the United States and a variety of field surveys (Malina, 1995).

44.2.2 Field and laboratory tests

The 20 metre shuttle run (Leger *et al.*, 1988) was the measure of aerobic endurance. Based on a test-retest protocol (n=21, one week apart), technical errors of measurement (σ_e) and reliability coefficients (*r*) were determined: σ_e=6.3 runs, *r*=0.86. Laboratory testing was completed within one week and with at least 48 hours between sessions. Peak oxygen uptake was determined using an incremental running test on a motorized treadmill (Quasar, HP Cosmos, Germany). Participants started with 2 min at 8 km·h^{-1} with subsequent increments of 2 km·h^{-1} every minute until 16 km·h^{-1}. Exercise intensity was subsequently increased through increasing the treadmill grade by 2° every 2 min until exhaustion, that was reached in 8–12 min. Criteria for attainment of peak oxygen uptake were: RER $\geq$1.00 and heart rate within 5 % of the age predicted maximal HR (Armstrong and Welsman, 2001). Expiratory O_2 and CO_2 concentrations and flow were measured every 10 seconds using a mixing chamber system (MetaMax System, Cortex Biophysics, Leipzig, Germany). Before each test, flow and volume were calibrated using a 3 L capacity syringe (Hans Rudolph, Kansas City, USA). Gas analyzers were calibrated using gases of known concentrations. HR was measured throughout exercise with a commercially available HR-monitor (Polar Electro S-810, Finland). Athletes also completed the 30 s Wingate Test (WAnT) on a friction-loaded cycle ergometer (Monark 824E, Monark AB, Vargerg, Sweden) that was interfaced with a microcomputer and calibrated for pedal speed and applied resistance. Resistance was set at 0.075 kg (0.74 N) per unit of body mass. Test outputs concluded peak power (PP, highest generated mechanical power, watts), mean power (MP, average for the 30 s period, watts) and a fatigue index (FI), which corresponds to the peak power minus lowest power divided by peak power (Inbar *et al.,* 1996). Coefficients of variation based on replicate tests in 20 subjects were 2.8 %, 3.2 % and 8.7 % for PP, MP and FI, respectively

44.2.3 Statistical analysis

Analysis of variance was used to test differences by competitive level on anthropometry, field and laboratory tests. The alpha level was set at 0.05. Statistical analyses were performed using SPSS version 17.0 software (SPSS Inc., Chicago, IL).

44.3 RESULTS

Characteristics of players by competitive level are summarized in Table 44.1. Local and elite players did not differ in chronological age (CA). Elite players had fewer years of experience in competitive hockey, but had more practice sessions in the season and played more minutes. They also were 4.4 cm taller. Elite athletes attained better performances in aerobic endurance. In addition, the WAnT fatigue index was higher among local players (higher values correspond to poorer performance).

Table 44.1. Descriptive statistics for players by competitive level and results of ANOVAs

	Local (n=41)	Elite (n=32)	ANOVA F	p	η^2
CA (y)	15.43±0.75	15.43±0.42	0.01	0.93	0.00
Training experience (y)	8.9±1.3	8.3±0.9	4.20	0.04	0.06
Annual training sessions (n)	106.1±13.6	116.8±17.5	8.73	0.00	0.11
Annual playing time (min)	720±262	964±385	10.40	0.01	0.12
Body mass (kg)	62.1±12.7	66.4±9.0	2.64	0.11	0.04
Stature (cm)	168.0±7.7	172.4±4.7	8.12	0.01	0.10
20-m shuttle run (m)	1626±334	1880±290	11.69	0.00	0.14
Aerobic peak power (L·min^{-1})	3.90±0.69	3.87±0.52	0.04	0.84	0.00
WAnT: peak power (W)	583±152	612±91	0.99	0.32	0.01
WAnT: mean power (W)	489±116	530±67	2.96	0.09	0.04
WAnT: fatigue index	33.3±5.4	27.8±8.0	12.34	0.00	0.15

44.4 DISCUSSION

Players selected for the Portuguese national team were taller, had fewer years of experience in competitive hockey, but had more practice sessions in the season and played more minutes. Anthropometric characteristics differ between local and elite players only for height. Since reference data for Portuguese youth are not available, the height and weight of hockey players were compared to the United States reference (Kuczmarski *et al.,* 2000). Elite players had a mean height slightly above the median and a mean weight above the 75th percentile of the US reference. The elevated weight-for-height probably reflected the advanced maturity status of the players and perhaps the influence of training on fat-free mass and skinfold thickness.

Peak oxygen consumption of hockey players was comparable to those for young male athletes of similar age in several team sports but lower than participants in individual sports (Bunc, 2004). Hockey players had lower values in short-term power outputs compared to athletes of the same age and young adults in several team sports (Carvalho *et al.,* 2010). It is possible that laboratory-assessed peak oxygen uptake was less informative to selection in youth roller hockey in contrast to the 20 m shuttle run.

The two groups of hockey players did not significantly differ in WAnT peak and mean power. Elite players, however, were more resistant to short-term fatigue. Sport selection research has considered variables that discriminated local club and regional elite players (Coelho-e-Silva *et al.,* 2010).

In the current study of youth roller hockey players, two potential predictors of sport selection were derived: 20 m shuttle run and WAnT fatigue index. In addition, the study confirms the importance of playing time in the development of talent.

44.5 REFERENCES

Armstrong, N. and Welsman, J.R., 2001, Peak oxygen uptake in relation to growth and maturation in 11- to 17-year-old humans. *European Journal of Applied Physiology*, **85**, pp. 546–551.

Bunc, V., 2004, Physiological and functional characteristics of adolescent athletes in several sports: Implications for talent identification. In *Children and Youth in Organized Sports*, edited by Coelho-e-Silva M.J. and Malina R. (Coimbra: Coimbra University Press), pp. 247–257.

Carvalho, H.M., Coelho-e-Silva, M.J., Figueiredo, A.J., Goncalves, C.E., Philippaerts, R.M., Castagna, C. and Malina, R.M., 2010, Predictors of maximal short-term power outputs in basketball players 14-16 years. *European Journal of Applied Physiology*, **111**, pp.789-796

Coelho-e-Silva, M.J., Figueiredo, A.J., Simoes, F., Seabra, A., Natal, A., Vaeyens, R., Philippaerts, R.M., Cumming, S.P. and Malina, R.M., 2010, Discrimination of U-14 soccer players by level and position. *International Journal of Sports Medicine*, **231**, pp. 790–796.

Inbar, O., Bar-Or, O., and Skinner, J.S., 1996, *The Wingate Anaerobic Test*, (Champaign, IL: Human Kinetics).

Kuczmarski, R.J., Ogden, C.L., Grummer-Strawn, L.M., Felgal, K.M., Guo, S.S., Wei, R., Mei, Z., Curtin, L.R., Roche, A.F. and Johnson, C.L., 2000, CDC Growth Charts: United States, *Advance Data*, **313**, pp.1-27.

Leger, L.A., Mercier, D., Gadoury, C., and Lambert, J., 1988, The multistage 20 metre shuttle run test for aerobic fitness. *Journal of Sports Sciences*, **6**, pp. 93–101.

Leone, M., Leger, L.A., Lariviere, G., and Comtois, A.S., 2007, An on-ice aerobic maximal multistage shuttle skate test for elite adolescent hockey players. *International Journal of Sports Medicine*, **28**, pp. 823–828.

Malina, R.M., 1995, Anthropometry. In *Physiological Assessment of Human Fitness*, edited by Maud P.J. and Foster C. (Champaign, IL: Human Kinetics), pp. 205–220.

Petrella, N.J., Montelpare, W.J., Nystrom, M., Plyley, M., and Faught, B.E., 2007, Validation of the FAST skating protocol to predict aerobic power in ice hockey players. *Applied Physiology, Nutrition, and Metabolism*, **32**, pp. 693–700.

Sherar, L.B., Baxter-Jones, A.D., Faulkner, R.A., and Russell, K.W., 2007, Do physical maturity and birth date predict talent in male youth ice hockey players? *Journal of Sports Sciences*, **25**, pp. 879–886.

THE EVALUATION OF SMALL-SIDED GAMES AS A TALENT IDENTIFICATION MECHANISM IN ELITE YOUTH FOOTBALL

V.B. Unnithan[1], A. Georgiou[1], J. Iga[2], and B. Drust[3]

[1]Staffordshire University, UK, [2]Wolverhampton Wanderers Football Club, UK
[3]Liverpool John Moores University, UK

45.1 INTRODUCTION

Until recently, talent identification programmes have not been based on rigorous scientific criteria and this could be important in supporting the subjective decision made by the coaches (Williams and Reilly, 2000). It is well documented that performance in football is a consequence of an individual's tactical and technical ability, their psychological skills and their physiological attributes (Reilly and Gilbourne, 2003). There is a vast amount of data on the technical aspects of the sport, the activity profiles of the players and the physiological loads imposed (Reinzi *et al.,* 2001). The combination, however, of these characteristics as an overall performance indicator within real match-play situations has received relatively little attention.

Small-sided games (SSG) are being used as a useful way of training because of the multiple benefits achieved. These types of games combine technical, tactical and physiological training (Drust *et al.,* 2000). The broader benefit for the player is that they acquire skills (technical/tactical) of real match-play situations in a small-sided game situation. Jones and Drust (2007) have shown that the work rate profiles observed in a 4 vs. 4 small-sided games seem to be similar in pattern to those observed in elite 11-a-side match-play.

Heart rate measurements have been used in many football research projects to compare physiological loads among different types of exercises, playing ages and field dimensions (Rampinini *et al.,* 2007). Recent football studies have also used the movement characteristics of the players as another physiological variable which may help to quantify the physiological load of different football training sessions and games (Harley *et al.,* 2010).

Consequently, the aims of the study were to: i) Evaluate the physiological loading of players during multiple small-sided games and, ii) to determine whether multiple SSG could act as a talent identification tool in elite youth football.

45.2 METHODS

45.2.1 Experimental design

Sixteen, male, elite young footballers from an English Premier League club volunteered to participate in the study (age: 15.2 ± 0.6 y, stature: 175.7 ± 6.7 cm and mass: 66.0 ± 9.1 kg). Participants were randomly allocated into two groups of eight players. Each group played six (4 vs. 4) matches, each of 5 min duration, on a pitch 25 x 35 m in dimension. A 3 min rest period was given between matches, at which time, the players were re-organised into different 4 vs. 4 combinations. Each combination was different, therefore no player played with the same 3 team-mates on two occasions. Telemetric (Activio Monitoring System, Stockholm, Sweden) heart rate (HR) data were obtained from all players. The movement characteristics of the players were also obtained using Global Positioning Systems data (Minimax S4, Catapult Innovations, Victoria, Australia). Each player was awarded 2 points for a win, 1 point for a draw and 0 points for a loss during each match (TP).

The football coaches completed a game technical scoring chart (GTSC) based on the performance of each player, during each 4 vs. 4 game and a comprehensive technical football scoring chart (CFS) that evaluated the players' performances during all matches and training. All players were evaluated with regard to their performance on 10 football elements: cover/support, communication/team work, decision making, receiving/first touch, control, running with the ball, 1 vs. 1, shooting, assists, marking. Each element had a range of points between 0-5. Each point described a player's performance on a certain skill as follows: 1-poor, 2-below average, 3-average, 4-very good, 5-excellent. Technical and tactical characteristics of each player were covered through this skill evaluation.

45.2.2 Statistical analyses

Mann Whitney tests were used to test for differences in the HRs and GPS data between the two teams during each 4 vs. 4 match. Pearson correlation coefficients were used to examine the relationship between: TP and GTSC, TP and CFS and GTSC and CAS. An unpaired t-test was used to compare GTSC and CAS for those players that scored less than 7 points across the 6 matches vs. those players that scored 7 or more points. The alpha level was set at 0.05. SPSS Version 17 (Chicago, IL, USA) was used to analyse the data.

45.3 RESULTS

There were no significant differences in peak HR between the winning and losing teams across the 12 matches that were played. Game 1: (winning team: 196 ± 10 b·min^{-1} vs. losing team: 189 ± 3 b·min^{-1}) and Game 12: (winning team: 186 ± 8 b·min^{-1} vs. losing team: 184 ± 6 b·min^{-1}). Similarly, there were no significant differences with respect to any of the GPS data when comparing the winning and losing teams from Games 1 to 12. Game 1 (Total distance covered): (winning team: 555 ± 60 m vs. losing team: 506 ± 27 m) and Game 12: (winning team: 549 ± 73 m vs. losing team: 581 ± 18 m). Game 1 (Number of high speed runs above 15 km·h^{-1}): (winning team: 54 ± 11 vs. losing team: 42 ± 16) and Game 12: (winning team: 51 ± 34 vs. losing team: 61 ± 25). The relationship between TP and GTSC approached significance ($r=0.39$, $P=0.07$) and between GTSC and CFS was ($r=0.55$, <0.05). There was no significant relationship between TP and CFS ($r=0.199$). There were no significant differences for both GTSC (TP of 7 or above: 31.6 ± 2.6 points vs. TP of less than 7: 31.6 ± 2.8 points) and CFS (TP of 7 or above: 32.1 ± 3.9 points vs. TP of less than 7: 31.6 ± 4.1 points), when the players were divided based on their total points scored in the matches.

45.4 CONCLUSION

Physiological responses during the 4 vs. 4 small-sided games were similar to previous studies (Jones and Drust, 2007; Hill-Haas et al., 2009). The physiological and movement characteristics of the winning teams were not significantly different to the losing teams during any of the SSG. These findings suggest that the structure of the multiple SSG generated a physiological load similar to that seen in 11-a-side football for all participants. There did appear to be a meaningful association between the players who were more successful in SSG and the coaches' technical evaluation of their skills during the SSG. It is possible to speculate that the predictive power of SSG in the present study could have been enhanced further by increasing participant numbers. Furthermore, the elite status of the footballers may have led to a relative homogeneity of their technical skills, thereby reducing the predictive power of SSG. Consequently, the real utility of SSG as a talent identification tool may be for those individuals who are aspiring to reach the elite level.

Acknowledgement

We would like to thank Mr. Steve Barrett and Perform Better Ltd. for their technical support in the collection of the GPS data.

45.5 REFERENCES

Drust, B., Reilly, T. and Cable, N.T., 2000, Physiological responses to laboratory-based soccer-specific intermittent and continuous exercise. *Journal of Sport Sciences*, **18**, pp. 885-892.

Harley, J.A., Barnes, C.A., Portas, M., Lovell, R., Barrett, S., Paul, D. and Weston, M., 2010, Motion analysis of match-play in elite U12 to U16 age-group soccer players. *Journal of Sports Sciences*, **28**, pp. 1391-1397.

Hill-Haas, S.V., Dawson, B.T., Coutts, A.J. and Rowsell, G.J. 2009, Physiological responses and time-motion characteristics of various small-sided soccer games in youth players. *Journal of Sports Sciences*, **27**, pp. 1-8.

Jones, S. and Drust, B., 2007, Physiological and technical demands of 4v4 and 8v8 games in elite youth soccer players. *Kinesiology*, **39**, pp. 150-156.

Rampinini, E., Impellizzeri, F., Castagna, C., Abt, G., Chamari, K., Sassi, A. and Marcora, S.M., 2007, Factors influencing physiological responses to small-sided soccer games. *Journal of Sports Sciences*, **25**, pp. 659-666.

Reilly, T. and Gilbourne, D., 2003. Science and football: A review of applied research in the football codes. *Journal of Sports Sciences*, **21**, pp. 693-705.

Reinzi, E., Drust, B., Reilly, T., Carter, J. and Martin, A., 2001. Investigation of anthropometric and work-rate profiles of elite South American international soccer players. *Journal of Sports Medicine and Physical Fitness*, **40**, pp. 162-169.

Williams, A.M. and Reilly, T., 2000. Talent identification and development in soccer. *Journal of Sports Sciences*, **18**, pp. 657-667.

ARE THERE ANY DETECTABLE SECULAR GROWTH CHANGES IN YOUNG MALE ATHLETES?

A. Farkas, G. Ag, and M. Szmodis

Semmelweis University, Budapest, Hungary

46.1 INTRODUCTION

When speaking about secular trends we mean the changes in the population ruled by a biological phenomenon which manifests itself in mostly positive changes in body dimensions such as stature, body mass, in body proportions and also in maturation, in earlier occurrence of menarche and spermarche (Van Wieringen, 1978; Wolanski, 1978). Secular trend is usually characterized by changes over decades but the velocity of differences in body parameters can alter within short(er) periods of time, as well. In Hungary several studies on the secular changes in Hungarian youth were carried out (Mohácsi and Mészáros, 1987; Eiben, 1989; Bodzsár and Pápai, 1994; Mohácsi et al., 1994; Tóth and Eiben 2004).

Our question was whether, in a selected group of male basketball players, could any of the secular growth changes be registered now?

46.2 SUBJECTS AND METHODS

In our present sample male basketball players aged between 11 and 14 years were studied (n=257). Anthropometric measurements were taken according to the methods of the International Biological Programme (Weiner and Lourie, 1969), metric and plastic indices of Conrad's growth type (1963). Metric index describes body proportions or linearity of the body by the roundness of the trunk related to stature, while the plastic index characterises the musculo-skeletal developmental level. Body fat % was assessed by Pařížková's (1961) method. A complex body composition four component analysis was performed by the Drinkwater and Ross technique (1980). BMI was calculated as well. For somatotyping the Heath and Carter method was used (1967). Data were analyzed and compared by Statistica Statsoft Version 9 computer program, basic statistics, interrelationships and Student t-test were ($P<0.05$) used.

Table 46.1. The number of the boys in the age-groups

Age (y)	1988	2004	2009	Σ
11	14	37	21	72
12	20	32	15	67
13	34	29	7	70
14	26	22	-	48
ΣΣ	94	120	43	257

46.3 RESULTS

We found a constant but not significant age-dependent increase between the subsequent years in stature. In the first period – between 1998 and 2004 – this increase seemed more marked but it levelled off between 2004 and 2009. Also the increasing standard deviations showed the more heterogeneity of the sample.

Table 46.2. The means (SD) of stature

Age	1998		2004		2009	
(y)	mean (cm)	SD	mean (cm)	SD	mean (cm)	SD
11	152.78	6.88	154.34	6.70	154.20	7.55
12	157.18	7.44	156.78	7.46	155.66	3.44
13	163.75	8.97	167.41	9.29	166.63	9.33
14	173.19	9.46	172.93	12.70	-	-

The largest difference was found between the stature values of the 13 and 14 year-old-boys in 1998 and a year earlier between that of the 12 and 13 year-olds in 2004. Similar tendencies occurred in the change of the boys' body mass values.

Table 46.3. Mean (SD) of body mass

Age	1998		2004		2009	
(y)	(kg)	SD	(kg)	SD	(kg)	SD
11	40.95	7.21	43.88	8.67	41.59	8.92
12	44.16	10.73	44.10	7.79	43.43	6.55
13	49.01	9.84	53.01	9.80	53.97	6.95
14	56.26	9.83	56.64	12.05	-	-

No significant changes were found in the subsequent groups mostly because of the limited subject numbers. When considering the body fat % a tendencious and slight constant decrease can be seen in the 1998 and 2004 sample while the opposite tendency occurred in the latest year. In BMI we found a regular age-dependent mild increase. We observed the same high values in the 1st component, in relative fatness of the Heath-Carter somatotyping (1967). By these two phenomena we can state that there is a disadvantageous tendency even in the sample of athletic, basketball player boys, i.e. the increasing tendency of their body mass could not be explained because of the higher muscle content but fat mass.

It seems that at least two to three sessions of regular training per week could not "override" the bad civilizational effects such as high energy intake, sedentary lifestyle even in athletic boys. We can also suppose that hormonal changes in boys did not reach yet the level that can elicit marked, clear tendencies in body composition changes.

Table 46.4. Means (SD) of body fat % and BMI

Age	1998		2004		2009	
(y)	mean	SD	mean	SD	mean	SD
11	20.14	4.99	18.93	6.61	19.37	4.97
% BMI	17.44	2.00	18.30	2.78	17.32	2.49
12	19.22	5.17	18.85	6.32	19.73	5.27
% BMI	17.71	3.18	17.88	2.56	17.89	2.39
13	18.33	4.66	18.07	4.58	20.69	4.81
% BMI	18.16	2.48	18.77	2.09	19.46	2.27
14	16.77	3.15	16.03	4.54	-	-
% BMI	18.64	2.04	18.77	2.48	-	-

46.4 CONCLUSION

In summarising the interrelationships between all the studied variables we can state that most of the body composition parameters were closely related to the characteristics of the physique, such as metric and plastic indices of Conrad's growth type (1963) in the 1998 sample. In metric index – which is highly genetically determined – the more picnomorphic physique was related to higher body fat content as reported previously (Mészáros and Mohácsi, 1987) but in our samples in 2004 and 2009 there were no further constant significant relationships between fat % and the characteristics of the physique and other body composition parameters.

In the results, the lack of proportional growth and the changes in body composition focus our attention on disadvantageous environmental effects.

Some questions arise from these facts: Does it mean that no further secular trend changes could be proved among the youngest generations? Has it happened because of the changes in environmental factors such as economic recession or is there an unknown biological explanation? In the future, we have to confirm our present results in other larger athletic as well as in non-athletic samples.

46.5 REFERENCES

Bodzsár, É.B. and Pápai, J., 1994, Secular trend in body proportions and composition. In Eiben, O.G. (Ed.) Auxology '94. Children and youth at the end of the 20th century. *Humanbiologia Budapestinensis*, **25**, pp. 245-254.

Conrad, K., 1963, *Der Konstitutionstypus* (2. Aufl.), Springer, Berlin.

Drinkwater, D.T. and Ross, W.D., 1980, Anthropometric fractionation of body mass. In *Kinanthropometry II*. Edited by Ostyn, M., Beunen, G. and Ross, W.D. (Baltimore: University Park Press), pp. 178-189.

Eiben, O.G., 1989, Secular trend in Hungary. *Humanbiologia Budapestinensis*, **19**, pp. 161-168.

Heath, B.H. and Carter, J.E.L., 1967, A modified somatotype method. *American Journal of Physical Anthropology*, **1**, pp. 57-74.

Mészáros, J. and Mohácsi, J., 1987, The growth type of 7 to 18 years old schoolchildren in Hungary. *Eighth International Anthropological Poster Conference*, Zagreb, pp. 17-19.

Mohácsi, J. and Meszáros, J., 1987, Stature and body mass in Hungarian schoolchildren between 7 to 18. *13th School of Biological Anthropology, Abstracts*, Zagreb, p. 23.

Mohácsi, J., Mészáros, J., and Farkas, A., 1994, Secular growth trend in height, body weight and growth type indices of boys aged between 14 to 8. In Eiben, O.G. (Ed.) Auxology '94. Children and youth at the end of the 20th century. *Humanbiologia Budapestinensis*, **25**. pp. 369-372.

Pařižková, J., 1961, Total body fat and skinfold thickness in children. *Metabolism*, **10,** pp. 794-807.

Tóth G.A. and Eiben O.G., 2004, Secular changes of body measurements in Hungary. *Humanbiologia Budapestinensis*, **28**, pp. 7-72.

Van Wieringen, J.C., 1978. Secular growth changes. In *Human Growth 2, Postnatal Growth*. Edited by Faulkner, F. and Tanner, J.M. (New York: Plenum Press). pp. 445-473.

Weiner, J.E.S. and Lourie, J.A., 1969, (Eds.) *Human Biology*. A Guide to Field Methods. IBP Handbook, No. 9, (Oxford: Blackwell).

Wolanski, N., 1978, Secular trend in man: Evidence and factors. *Collegium Antropologicum*, **2**, pp. 69-86.

ISOKINETIC STRENGTH AND RISK OF MUSCLE IMBALANCE IN U-17 HOCKEY PLAYERS BY COMPETITIVE LEVEL

M.J.Coelho-e-Silva, H.M. Carvalho, V. Vaz, J. Valente-dos-Santos, A.J. Figueiredo, M.T. Elferink-Gemser, and R.M. Malina
University of Coimbra, Portugal

47.1 INTRODUCTION

Research focusing on sport selection and talent development is often considered to enhance world-class performance as a result of several factors (Reilly *et al.*, 2000). Multidisciplinary approaches have distinguished adolescent players classified as local and elite players (Elferink-Gemser *et al.*, 2004; Vaeyens *et al.*, 2008; Mohamed *et al.*, 2009). Testing batteries are mainly based on field assessments and not surprisingly the literature using dynamometer assessment of muscle strength in young athletes by competitive level is still lacking. In addition, isokinetic testing can provide useful information regarding muscle balance which is very relevant for injury prevention and understanding the effects of intensive training. Research devoted to youth roller hockey is scarce. Hence, this study profiles the body size and isokinetic assessment of U-17 Portuguese male youth roller hockey players by competitive level.

47.2 METHODS

The sample comprised 73 adolescent hockey players, 14.5-16.4 years of age. They were classified as club or elite based on whether or not they were selected for the national team. National team players (n=32) competed with their respective clubs during the season and were included in the group from which the Portuguese selection in 2007 and 2008 was chosen. The remainder (n=41) competed only at the club level with their respective teams and were categorized as club players. Information about sessions and minutes of training and competition was collected on a weekly basis.

A single trained observer measured body mass, to the nearest 0.1 kg with a SECA balance (model 770, Hanover, MD, USA) and stature, measured to the nearest 0.1 cm with a Harpenden stadiometer (model 98.603, Holtain Ltd, Crosswell, UK). Intra-observer technical errors of measurement for stature (0.27 cm) and body mass (0.47 kg) were well within the range of intra- and inter-observer errors in several surveys in the United States and a variety of field surveys (Malina et al., 2004). Isokinetic concentric (CON) and eccentric (ECC) modes of knee extension (KE) and flexion (KF) were assessed using a calibrated dynamometer (Biodex System 3, Shirley, NY, USA) at angular velocities of $60°·s^{-1}$ after a 10 min warm-up on a Monark cycle ergometer (Monark 814E, Varberg, Sweden) with minimal resistance (basket supported) at 60 $rev·min^{-1}$ and 2 min of static stretching of the hamstring and quadriceps muscles. Athletes were placed in a seated position in a standardized 85° hip flexion from the anatomical position. Range of motion was set using voluntary maximal full KE (0°) to 90° KF. Visual feedback of moment versus time was provided during the test, but no verbal feedback was given (Baltzopoulos et al., 1991). Each subject performed five continuous and reciprocal maximal repetitions on each mode and leg. Maximal KF and KE peak torque from the best repetition in both CON and ECC muscular actions were retained and expressed as N·m. Thigh muscle function was assessed by calculating the functional hamstring-quadriceps ratios (Aagaard et al., 1998). Reliability estimates of the observer for the used protocol (repeated measurements in 13 university students, age 21.1 ± 3.1 y), were: $KE_{(CON)}$, coefficient of variation (CV) = 4.1 % and intra-class correlation (ICC) = 0.98; $KF_{(CON)}$, CV = 4.1 % and ICC = 0.98; $KE_{(ECC)}$, CV = 5.2 % and ICC = 0.97; $KF_{(ECC)}$, CV = 4.8 % and ICC = 0.97.

The differences by competitive level (club and elite) were tested using t-tests. The effect size correlations (ES-r) were estimated using the square root of the ratio of t-value squared and the difference between t-value squared and degrees of freedom (total amount of variance in the sample) (Rosnow et al., 1996). Significance level was always set at 5 %. Statistical analyses were performed using SPSS version 17.0 software (SPSS, Chicago, IL).

47.3 RESULTS

Descriptive statistics and comparisons between groups are summarized in Table 47.1. Elite players showed more annual training exposure (t=2.74, P<0.01), competed more minutes (t=2.92, P<0.01), were taller (t=3.02, P<0.01) and evidenced higher thigh strength in concentric actions than their club level peers (KE: t=2.57, P<0.01; KF: t=1.95, t<0.05). Interestingly, the values of functional hamstring-quadriceps ratios for the elite group were further away from muscle balance in both extension and flexion.

47.4 DISCUSSION

Coaches are interested in the recruitment of players who suggest potential to attain higher performance-levels but also are ready for intensive training loads and international competition without risk of injuries. The present study confirms the importance of training volume and playing time in talent development, but simultaneously noted a risk of imbalances developing in lower limb strength which may correspond to an excessive specialization in particular aspects of roller hockey. Note that elite players accumulated less years of sport training.

The maximal isokinetic strength outputs in youth roller hockey players were similar to those for young male athletes of the same age in other team sports, in particular young soccer and basketball players (Gerodimos et al., 2003; Buchanan and Vardaxis, 2009; Forbes et al., 2009; Iga et al., 2009). Given the consistency of results, lower-body dynamic strength is likely essential for participation in roller hockey. During fast KE and towards full extension, the eccentrically acting hamstrings have been shown to produce a braking joint flexor moment that is equal to or greater than the extensor moment exerted by the quadriceps (Aagaard et al., 1998), thus an $ECC_{(KE)}/CON_{(KE)}$ ratio of 1.0 indicates that the eccentrically acting hamstrings have the ability to fully brake the action of the concentrically contracting quadriceps (Coombs and Garbutt, 2002). The lower values of $ECC_{(KF)}/CON_{(KF)}$ ratio indicate that the specific length tension and force-velocity properties were impaired for the hamstring muscles and enhanced for the quadriceps muscles during fast forceful knee flexion (Coombs and Garbutt, 2002). The functional ratios of the present study indicated an effect of competitive level in youth roller hockey. Elite athletes presented lower values of $ECC_{(KE)}/CON_{(KE)}$ and higher values of $ECC_{(KF)}/CON_{(KF)}$ suggesting that specific training in the sport may produce thigh muscles imbalances. For the knee joint, co-activation of hamstrings and quadriceps may be critical to prevent or to reduce knee motion and loads that increase the risk of ACL injury (Alentorn-Geli et al., 2009). Compensatory strategies to prevent injuries should be considered.

Table 47.1 Comparison of young roller hockey players by competitive level

	Club (n=41)	Elite (n=32)	t	p	ES-r
Chronological age (y)	15.43±0.75	15.43±0.42	0.02	0.98	0.00
Training experience (y)	8.9±1.3	8.3±0.9	-2.15	0.03	0.25
Annual training sessions (n)	106.1±13.6	116.8±17.5	2.74	0.01	0.44
Annual playing time (min)	720±262	964±385	2.92	0.01	0.44
Body mass (kg)	62.1±12.7	66.4±9.0	1.69	0.09	0.20
Stature (cm)	168.0±7.7	172.4±4.7	3.02	0.00	0.34
Peak Torque CON $_{(KE)}$ (N·m)	168.1±40.7	188.1±25.5	2.57	0.01	0.30
Peak Torque ECC $_{(KF)}$ (N·m)	240.4±62.0	251.8±78.6	-0.69	0.49	0.08
Peak Torque CON $_{(KF)}$ (N·m)	98.4±23.2	108.0±17.7	1.95	0.05	0.22
Peak Torque ECC $_{(KE)}$ (N·m)	155. 6±35.8	148.7±32.9	-0.85	0.40	0.10
Ratio: ECC $_{(KE)}$ /CON $_{(KE)}$	0.94±0.15	0.79±0.16	-4.10	0.00	0.44
Ratio: CON $_{(KF)}$ /ECC $_{(KF)}$	0.42±0.07	0.46±0.13	1.82	0.08	0.27

Acknowledgement

Supported by *Portuguese Foundation for Science and Technology* FCT [PTDC/DES/121772/2010, SFRH/BD/41647/2007, SFRH/BD/64648/2009].

47.5 REFERENCES

Aagaard, P., Simonsen, E.B., Magnusson, S.P., Larsson, B., and Dyhre-Poulsen, P., 1998, A new concept for isokinetic hamstring: Quadriceps muscle strength ratio, *American Journal of Sports Medicine*, **26**, pp.231-237.

Alentorn-Geli, E., Myer, G.D., Silvers, H.J., Samitier, G., Romero, D., Lazaro-Haro, C., and Cugat, R., 2009, Prevention of non-contact anterior cruciate ligament injuries in soccer players. Part 1: Mechanisms of injury and underlying risk factors, *Knee Surgery, Sports Traumatology, Arthroscopy*, **17**, pp.705-729.

Baltzopoulos, V., Williams, J.G., and Brodie, D.A., 1991, Sources of error in isokinetic dynamometry: Effects of visual feedback on maximum torque, *Journal of Orthopaedic and Sports Physical Therapy*, **13**, pp.138-142.

Buchanan, P.A., and Vardaxis, V.G., 2009, Lower-extremity strength profiles and gender-based classification of basketball players ages 9-22 years, *Journal of Strength and Conditioning Research*, **23**, pp.406-419.

Coombs, C., and Garbutt, G., 2002, Developments in the use of the hamstring/quadriceps ratio for the assessment of muscle balance, *Journal of Sports Science and Medicine*, **1**, pp.56-62.

Elferink-Gemser, M.T., Visscher, C., Lemmink, K.A., and Mulder, T.W., 2004, Relation between multidimensional performance characteristics and level of performance in talented youth field hockey players, *Journal of Sports Sciences*, **22**, pp.1053-1063.

Forbes, H., Bullers, A., Lovell, A., McNaughton, L.R., Polman, R.C., and Siegler, J.C., 2009, Relative torque profiles of elite male youth footballers: Effects of age and pubertal development, *International Journal of Sports Medicine*, **30**, pp.592-597.

Gerodimos, V., Mandou, V., Zafeiridis, A., Ioakimidis, P., Stavropoulos, N., and Kellis, S., 2003, Isokinetic peak torque and hamstring/quadriceps ratios in young basketball players. Effects of age, velocity, and contraction mode, *Journal of Sports Medicine and Physical Fitness*, **43**, pp.444-452.

Iga, J., George, K., Lees, A., and Reilly, T., 2009, Cross-sectional investigation of indices of isokinetic leg strength in youth soccer players and untrained individuals, *Scandinavian Journal of Medicine and Science in Sports*, **19**, pp.714-719.

Malina, R.M., Bouchard, C., and Bar-Or, O., 2004. *Growth, Maturation, and Physical Activity*, 2nd ed., (Champaign, IL: Human Kinetics).

Mohamed, H., Vaeyens, R., Matthys, S., Multael, M., Lefevre, J., Lenoir, M., and Philppaerts, R., 2009, Anthropometric and performance measures for the development of a talent detection and identification model in youth handball, *Journal of Sports Sciences,* **27**, pp.257-266.

Reilly, T., Williams, A.M., Nevill, A., and Franks, A., 2000, A multidisciplinary approach to talent identification in soccer, *Journal of Sports Sciences*, **18**, pp.695-702.

Rosnow, R.L., and Rosenthal, R., 1996, Computing contrasts, effect sizes, and counternulls on other people's published data: General procedures for research consumers, *Psychological Methods*, **1**, pp.331-340.

Vaeyens, R., Lenoir, M., Williams, A.M., and Philippaerts, R.M., 2008, Talent identification and development programmes in sport: Current models and future directions, *Sports Medicine*, **38**, pp.703-714.

Part VIII

Methodology in Longitudinal Research

CHAPTER NUMBER 48

THE ADVANTAGES AND DISADVANTAGES OF LONGITUDINAL RESEARCH IN GROWTH AND HEALTH OF KIDS

H.C.G. Kemper
VU University Medical Center, EMGO+ Institute,
Amsterdam, The Netherlands

48.1 INTRODUCTION

Individual changes in growth, development and health can only be studied if the same individuals are measured repeatedly over a period of time. This is called a longitudinal study. However, longitudinal designs also have their constraints: No matter which design has been used, always confounding effects will occur. Three classical research designs can be discerned: (1) a cross-sectional design, (2) a time-lag design and (3) a longitudinal design (see Figure 48.1).

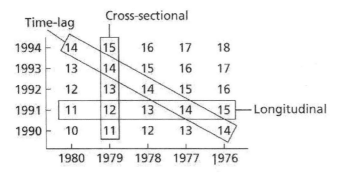

Figure 48.1. Graphical representation of the three classical research designs: vertical bar, cross-sectional design; diagonal bar, time lag design; and horizontal bar, longitudinal design

Each measurement taken on a subject at a particular point of time is influenced by three factors: (1) The chronological age of the subject, defined as the period that elapses between the date of birth and the time of measurement. The age effects produce the mean growth curve. (2) The birth cohort to which the subject belongs. This is defined as the group of individuals born in the same year.

Cohort effects can be used to study secular trends. (3) The time of measurement is the moment at which the measurement in the subject is taken. Time of measurement effects are related to changes in environmental conditions that can occur over a period of time.

The three classical designs are characterized in the following ways. In a cross-sectional design, the time of measurement is kept constant (and cohort and age varied), and different groups are measured at the same point in time. Conversely, in a time-lag design, different groups of the same age are measured at different points in time, thus age is kept constant (cohort and time of measurement are varied. In a longitudinal study, information is gathered from the same cohort at different points in time, thus at different ages. Because the cohort is kept constant (age and time of measurement are varied), the same group is measured repeatedly. None of the three designs allows all three effects to be isolated (Schaie, 1965).

Descriptions can be found in the literature of several longitudinal designs to overcome confounding effects (Tanner, 1962; Rao and Rao, 1966; Kowalski and Prahl-Andersen, 1979). The multiple longitudinal design, with repeated measurements on more than one cohort and overlapping ages, has the advantage of isolating the main age effect from interfering effects such as time of measurement and cohort effects (Kemper and van't Hof , 1978).

48.2 METHODS

In the Amsterdam Growth and Health Longitudinal Study (AGAHLS) a multiple longitudinal design is used in 600 boys and girls to isolate confounding effects of cohort- and time of measurement effects from the main age effect of interest. The AGAHLS research design used at the start four yearly repeated measurements (chronological age between 12 and 17 years) and continued later with repeated measurements with about 5 years in between (age 21-23; age 26-28; age 31-33: age 36-38 and age 41-43 y). It concerned three birth cohorts (1962, 1963 and 1964) resulting in overlapping age groups.

Another problem with repeated measurements in longitudinal studies is a testing or learning effect. Many variables, physical as well as psychological, require a certain motivation or habituation of the subject while being measured. This can introduce differences between periods of measurement that are solely caused by changes in attitudes towards the measurement procedure itself. Such testing effects may be positive (i.e. when habituation or learning of the subject is important) or negative (i.e. when motivation in the subject decreases). Systematic testing effects can be estimated if the design also includes a comparable control group of boys and girls, in which repeated measurements are not made. Therefore, apart from this longitudinal group of boys and girls, during the first 4 years a cross-sectional group of boys and girls was created with the same birth cohorts. But these boys and girls were only measured once during the four annual measurement years, using only one (different) quarter of the total population.

48.3 RESULTS

Using the multiple longitudinal design with repeated measurements in three cohorts with overlapping calendar ages, has the advantage of isolating the main age effects from interfering effects such as time of measurement and cohort effects.

In Figure 48.2 the data of maximal oxygen uptake (VO_2max), directly measured with a running test on a treadmill (Kemper, 1991) are given in the three cohorts repeatedly measured between the calendar age of 12 and 23 years. Because of the overlap in age groups at the age 13, 14, 15 and 16 years, the mean values of the three cohorts can be combined if there are no significant cohort effects. Because this was the case, the mean values of the cohorts can be combined to construct the true and mean age curve for this parameter.

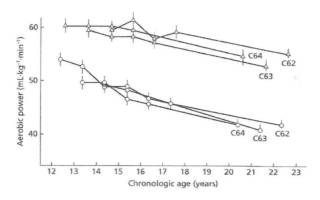

Figure 48.2. Mean and standard error of maximal aerobic power, measured in the in the Amsterdam Growth and Health Study in boys (open triangles) and girls (open circles) of the three cohorts (C64, C63 and C62).

48.3.1 Cohort effects

A cohort effect however was indicated in the measurement of the Netherlands Personality test (NPV-j; Luteijn *et al*, 1981): One of the five subscales is called Rigidity: it is a personality trait characterized by the need for regularity, having fixed habits and principles, a great responsibility and a positive conception of duty. In Figure 48.3 the mean rigidity scores of both boys and girls are given against calendar age. There is a strong decrease in both sexes from the age of 12 years. The age curves are based on measurements in three cohorts. In the boys the decreasing trend is visible till the age of 17 years, but in girls the rigidity score is increasing from 16 to 17 years of age. This increase is however the result of an effect caused by the birth cohort from 1962. This 1962 birth cohort of the girls shows on all ages a higher rigidity score compared with the other two birth cohorts. Because the mean score at age 17 is built up by only the mean scores of the 1962 cohort this confounds the age trend of the girls.

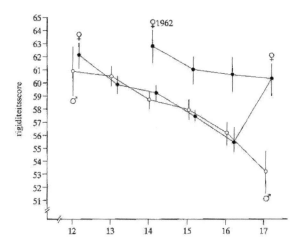

Figure 48.3. Mean rigidity scores of boys (open circles) and girls (closed) between the age of 12-17 years. The sudden increase of the score in 17 year old girls is caused by the separate depicted scores of the 1962 birth cohort.

48.3.2 Time of measurement effects

A time of measurement effect was discovered in the measurement of daily physical activity.

One of the methods used to measure daily physical activity was the pedometer week score (Montoye *et al.*, 1996). The pedometer is an instrument, that when attached to the waist of a child, counts the number of vertical movements of the body's centre of gravity. These pedometers were used during 1 week on school and weekend days, resulting in a pedometer week score.

In Figure 48.4 are the mean scores given of the three birth cohorts of boys measured longitudinally over the 4 years. Although the mean scores with increasing age seem to diminish, this decrease is not always the case. In the first year of measurement in each birth cohort the mean pedometer week score is lower than in the second year. In the third and fourth year of measurement the decreasing trend is visible in all three birth cohorts. A plausible explanation of the high activity scores in the second year of measurement are the climatic circumstances in that particular year: in the winter of 1978 it was relatively cold with unusual snow and ice for a long period. These exceptional circumstances resulted in a massive participation of the Dutch youth in ice skating (figure and speed skating), ice hockey and snow ball games. Therefore the higher mean scores are traceable at three different ages from the same year of measurement.

The same phenomenon is also seen in the 13/14 year old boys from the control group, measured in 1978 (see interrupted line).

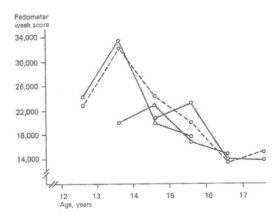

Figure 48.4. Age trend of the mean week score of the pedometers in boys from 12-17 years. The three full lines are longitudinal data and the interrupted line from cross-sectional data.

48.3.3 Test and learning effects

Comparing the longitudinal cohorts with the cross-sectional cohorts enabled us to trace possible test and learning effects. This could be demonstrated in different measurements: the test effects were positive and significant in two physical fitness tests, the arm pull and the flexed arm hang test, and negative in the 12-min endurance run in both boys and girls. The positive effects can be explained by habituation and learning and the negative effects by decrease of motivation.

Also the measurement of daily energy intake by a cross-check dietary history interview (Post, 1989) showed a significant and positive test effect in the girls but not in boys (see Fig 48.5).

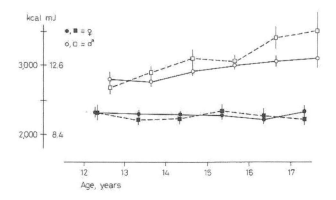

Figure 48.5. The mean (SE) of the energy intake (in kcal and MJ) from 12-17 years of age from the longitudinal measured boys and girls (full lines) compared with the cross-sectional measured boys and girls (interrupted lines).

The mean energy intake per week is higher in boys than in girls all through the teenage periods. The mean energy intake is increasing with age in boys but not in girls. However comparing the mean energy intake in the longitudinal groups (full lines) with the cross-sectional groups (interrupted lines) the data in the girls are identical, but the longitudinally measured boys show a systematic faster increase in the mean energy intake than the boys in the cross-sectional group. This testing effect in boys can be explained by an increasing under reporting of their food intake caused by repeated measurement with the dietary interview. This effect is the greatest at age 16 and 17 years: after 4 years of repeated measurement it seems that boys are less interested in to report their food intake than girls at this age.

48.4 CONCLUSIONS

With the research design applied to the Amsterdam Growth and Health Longitudinal Study it could be shown that age related trends could be confounded by birth cohort effects, time of measurement effects and test effects. If control measurements are carefully collected with a multiple longitudinal design and combined with cross sectional measured control groups, confounding can be quantified and the study results corrected accordingly.

48.5 REFERENCES

Kemper, H.C.G. and Van't Hof, M.A., 1978, Design of a multiple longitudinal study of growth and health of teenagers. *European Journal of Pediatrics*, **129**, pp. 147-155.

Kemper, H.C.G., 1991, Sources of variation in longitudinal assessment of maximal aerobic power in teenage boys and girls: The Amsterdam Growth and Health Study. *Human Biology*, **63**, pp. 533-546.

Kowalski, C.J. and Prahl-Andersen, B., 1979, General considerations in the design of studies of growth and development. In: A mixed longitudinal interdisciplinary study of growth and development, edited by Kowalski C.J., Prahl-Andersen, B., Heyendael, P. (New York: Academic Press), pp. 3-13.

Luteijn, F., Dijk, H. and van Ploeg, A.E.A van der., 1981, *Dutch Personality Inventory. Youth Version.* (Swets and Zeitlinger: Lisse, The Netherlands)

Montoye, H.J., Kemper, H.C.G., Saris, W.H.M. and Washburn, R.A., 1996, *Measuring Physical Activity and Energy Expenditure.* (Champaign, IL: Human Kinetics,).

Post, G.B., 1989, Nutrition in adolescence: A longitudinal study in dietary patterns from teenager to adult. Thesis (PhD), Wageningen University. Haarlem, NL.

Rao, M.N. and Rao, C.R., 1962, Linked cross-sectional study for determining norms and growth rates: A pilot survey of Indian school-going boys, *Saykgya*, **68**, pp. 237-258.

Schaie, K.W., 1965, A general model for the study of developmental problems. *Psychological Bulletin*, **64,** pp. 92-107.

Tanner, J.M., 1962, *Growth at Adolescence* (Blackwell Scientific Publications: Oxford, UK).

Author Index

A

B

C

D

General Index

H

HRV	72, 202
Hydration	101
Hypertension	29, 51

I

IGF-1	289
IL-1	291
Injury	22, 24, 309
Interval training	269
Intervention	23, 239
Intima-media thickness	30

L

Lipids	110, 115, 122, 240
Lung function	211, 260

M

Maturation	5, 65, 78, 116, 217
Metabolism	7, 43, 68, 74, 124, 224, 262,
Muscle fibre type	9, 39
Motor function	42, 91, 228, 245
Muscle function	40, 216, 218, 310

N

NIRS	83
Nitric oxide	30, 233

O

Obesity	19, 97, 139, 167
Osteoporosis	155, 161, 187, 195, 215

P

Peak VO_2	9, 85, 109, 129, 141, 202, 210, 234, 259
Physioflow	234
^{31}PMRS	8, 12, 14
Power output	43, 210, 276
Psychosocial	167, 171

R

Reliability	74, 134, 246

Printed and bound by CPI Group (UK) Ltd, Croydon, CR0 4YY

05/11/2024

01784077-0001